Knowledge Translation in Health Care: Moving from Evidence to Practice

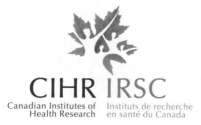

CIHR IRSC

Canadian Institutes of   Instituts de recherche
Health Research   en santé du Canada

Knowledge Translation in Health Care: Moving from Evidence to Practice

Edited by

Sharon E. Straus

Li ka Shing Knowledge Institute
St. Michael's Hospital
and
Department of Medicine
University of Toronto
Toronto, Ontario, Canada

Jacqueline Tetroe

Knowledge Translation Portfolio
Canadian Institutes of Health Research
Ottawa, Ontario, Canada

Ian D. Graham

Knowledge Translation Portfolio
Canadian Institutes of Health Research
Ottawa, Ontario, Canada

WILEY-BLACKWELL

A John Wiley & Sons, Ltd., Publication

BMJ|Books

Library of Congress Cataloging-in-Publication Data
Knowledge translation in health care : moving from evidence to practice / edited by Sharon Straus, Jacqueline Tetroe, Ian Graham.
        p. : cm.
    Includes bibliographical references.
    ISBN 978-1-4051-8106-8
    1. Evidence-based medicine. 2. Knowledge, Theory of. I. Straus, Sharon E. II. Tetroe, Jacqueline. III. Graham, Ian D.
    [DNLM: 1. Evidence-Based Medicine 2. Health Services Research–standards. 3. Quality of Health Care–standards. WB 102.5 K73 2009]
    R723.7.K663   2009
610–dc22
ISBN: 978-14051-8106-8

2008045643

A catalogue record for this book is available from the British Library.

Set in 9.5/12 pt Minion by Aptara® Inc., New Delhi, India
Printed and bound in Singapore by Fabulous Printers Pte Ltd

4   2010

Contents

Contributors, viii

Foreword, xii

Preface, xvii

Section 1 Introduction

1.1 Knowledge to action: what it is and what it isn't, 3
Sharon E. Straus, Jacqueline Tetroe, Ian D. Graham

Section 2 Knowledge Creation

2.1 The K in KT: knowledge creation, 13
Sharon E. Straus

2.2 Knowledge synthesis, 15
Jennifer Tetzlaff, Andrea C. Tricco, David Moher

2.3 Knowledge translation tools, 35
Melissa C. Brouwers, Dawn Stacey, Annette M. O'Connor

2.4 Searching for research findings and KT literature, 46
K. Ann McKibbon, Cynthia Lokker

Section 3 The Knowledge-to-Action Cycle

3.1 The action cycle, 59
Sharon E. Straus

3.2 Identifying the knowledge-to-action gaps, 60
Alison Kitson, Sharon E. Straus

3.3 Adapting knowledge to a local context, 73
Margaret B. Harrison, Ian D. Graham, Beatrice Fervers

3.4 Assessing barriers and facilitators to knowledge use, 83
France Légaré

3.5 Selecting KT interventions, 94

    3.5.1 Selecting, tailoring, and implementing knowledge translation interventions, 94
    Michel Wensing, Marije Bosch, Richard Grol

    3.5.2 Educational interventions, 113
    Dave Davis, Nancy Davis

    3.5.3 Linkage and exchange interventions, 123
    Martin P. Eccles, Robbie Foy

    3.5.4 Audit and feedback interventions, 126
    Robbie Foy, Martin P. Eccles

    3.5.5 Informatics interventions, 131
    Samir Gupta, K. Ann McKibbon

    3.5.6 Patient-mediated interventions, 137
    Annette M. O'Connor

    3.5.7 Organizational interventions, 144
    Ewan Ferlie

3.6 Monitoring and evaluating knowledge, 151

    3.6.1 Monitoring knowledge use and evaluating outcomes of knowledge use, 151
    Sharon E. Straus, Jacqueline Tetroe, Ian D. Graham, Merrick Zwarenstein, Onil Bhattacharyya

    3.6.2 Framework for evaluating complex interventions, 159
    Sasha Shepperd

3.7 Sustaining knowledge use, 165
    Barbara Davies, Nancy Edwards

3.8 Case examples, 174
    Sumit R. Majumdar

Section 4 Theories and Models of Knowledge to Action

4.1 Planned action theories, 185
    Ian D. Graham, Jacqueline Tetroe, KT Theories Group

4.2 Cognitive psychology theories of change, 196
    Alison Hutchinson, Carole A. Estabrooks

4.3 Educational theories, 206
    Alison Hutchinson, Carole A. Estabrooks

4.4 Organizational theory, 215
    Jean-Louis Denis, Pascale Lehoux

4.5 Quality improvement, 226
Anne Sales

Section 5 Knowledge Exchange

5.1 Knowledge dissemination and exchange of knowledge, 235
Michelle Gagnon

Section 6 Evaluation of Knowledge to Action

6.1 Methodologies to evaluate effectiveness of knowledge translation
interventions, 249
Onil Bhattacharyya, Merrick Zwarenstein

6.2 Economic evaluation of knowledge-to-action interventions, 261
Deborah J. Kenny, Evelyn Cornelissen, Craig Mitton

Appendixes

1 Approaches to measurement, 269
Robert Parent

2 Knowledge management and commercialization, 280
Réjean Landry

3 Ethics in knowledge translation, 291
Burleigh Trevor-Deutsch, Kristiann Allen, Vardit Ravitsky

Index, 301

Contributors

Kristiann Allen MA
Ethics Office
Canadian Institutes of Health Research
Ottawa, ON, Canada

Onil Bhattacharryya MD
Li Ka Shing Knowledge Institute
St. Michael's Hospital
and
Department of Family and Community
   Medicine, University of Toronto
Ontario, Canada

Marije Bosch MSc
Scientific Institute for Quality of Healthcare
Radboud University Nijmegen Medical
   Centre
Nijmegen, The Netherlands

Melissa C. Brouwers PhD
Department of Clinical Epidemiology and
   Biostatistics, McMaster University
and
Canadian Partnership Against Cancer
   Corporation
Hamilton, ON, Canada

Evelyn Cornelisson
Faculty of Health and Social Development
University of British Columbia—Okanagan
Kelowna, BC, Canada

Barbara Davies RN, PhD
University of Ottawa School of Nursing
Ottawa, ON, Canada

Dave Davis MD
Association of American Medical Colleges
Washington DC, USA

Nancy Davis PhD
National Institute for Quality and
   Education
Pittsburgh, PA, USA

Jean-Louis Denis PhD
Department of Health Administration
University of Montréal
Montréal, QC, Canada

Martin P. Eccles MD
Institute of Health and Society
Newcastle University
Newcastle upon Tyne, UK

Nancy Edwards MSc, PhD
University of Ottawa School of Nursing
Ottawa, ON, Canada

Carole A. Estabrooks RN, PhD
Faculty of Nursing
University of Alberta
Edmonton, AL, Canada

Ewan Ferlie PhD
School of Management
Royal Holloway University of London
Egham, Surrey, UK

Béatrice Fervers MD, MSc
Oncology Guideline Programme
French Federation of Cancer Centers
   (FNCLCC), Centre Léon Bérard
and
Université Lyon
Lyon, France

Robbie Foy MBChB, MSc, PhD
Institute of Health and Society
Newcastle University
Newcastle upon Tyne, UK

Michelle Gagnon MBA, PhD
Knowledge Synthesis and Exchange Branch
Canadian Institutes of Health Research
   (CIHR)
Ottawa, ON, Canada

Ian D. Graham PhD
Knowledge Translation Portfolio
Canadian Institutes of Health Research
and
School of Nursing
University of Ottawa
Ottawa, ON, Canada

Richard Grol PhD
Scientific Institute for Quality of Healthcare
Radboud University Nijmegen Medical
   Centre
Nijmegen, The Netherlands

Samir Gupta MSc, MD
Li Ka Shing Knowledge Institute
St. Michael's Hospital
Toronto, ON, Canada

Margaret B. Harrison
RN, PhD
Practice and Research in Nursing (PRN)
   Group, Queen's University
Kingston, ON, Canada

Alison Hutchinson Mbioeth,
PhD
Knowledge Utilization Studies Program
Faculty of Nursing
University of Alberta
Edmonton, AB, Canada

Deborah J. Kenny
TriService Nursing Program, Uniformed
   Services
University of Health Sciences
Bethesda, MD, USA

Alison Kitson BSc(Hons) PhD,
RN, FRCN
Templeton College
University of Oxford
Oxford, UK

Réjean Landry PhD
Department of Management
Faculty of Business
Laval University
Quebec City, QC, Canada

France Légaré PhD
Centre de Recherche
Hospital St. François-d'Assise
and
Department of Family Medicine
Laval University
Quebec, Canada

Pascale Lehoux
Department of Health Administration
University of Montreal
Montreal, QC, Canada

Cynthia Lokker PhD
Department of Clinical Epidemiology and
  Biostatistics
McMaster University
Hamilton, ON, Canada

Sumit R. Majumdar MD, MPH
Department of Medicine
University of Alberta
Edmonton, AB, Canada

K. Ann McKibbon MLS, PhD
Department of Clinical Epidemiology and
  Biostatistics
McMaster University
Hamilton, ON, Canada

Craig Mitton PhD
Health Services Priority Setting
University of British Columbia
  —Okanagan,
Kelowna, BC, Canada

David Moher PhD
Ottawa Health Research Institute
Ottawa, ON, Canada

Annette M. O'Connor RN,
PhD, FCAHS
Department of Epidemiology
University of Ottawa School of Nursing
and
Ottawa Health Research Institute
Ottawa, ON, Canada

Robert Parent
University of Sherbrooke
Quebec, Canada

Vardit Ravitsky PhD
Ethics Office
Canadian Institutes of Health Research
Ottawa, ON, Canada

Anne Sales RN, PhD
Faculty of Nursing
University of Alberta
Edmonton, AB, Canada

Sasha Shepperd MSc, DPhil
Department of Public Health
University of Oxford
Headington, Oxford, UK

Dawn Stacey RN, PhD
University of Ottawa School of Nursing
Ottawa, ON, Canada

Sharon E. Straus MD, FRCPC,
MSc
Li Ka Shing Knowledge Institute
St. Michael's Hospital
and
Department of Medicine
University of Toronto,
Toronto, ON, Canada

Jacqueline Tetroe MA
Knowledge Translation Portfolio
Canadian Institutes of Health Research
Ottawa, ON, Canada

Jennifer Tetzlaff BSc
Clinical Epidemiology Program
Ottawa Health Research Institute
Ottawa, ON, Canada

**Burleigh Trevor-
  Deutsch** PhD, LLB
Ethics Office
Canadian Institutes of Health Research
Ottawa, ON, Canada

Andrea C. Tricco
Institute of Population Health
University of Ottawa
Ottawa, ON, Canada

Michel Wensing PhD
Scientific Institute for Quality of Healthcare
Radboud University Nijmegen Medical
    Centre
Nijmegen, The Netherlands

Merrick Zwarenstein MB,
BCh(Med), MSc(CHDC)
Sunnybrook Research Institute
University of Toronto
and
Institute for Clinical Evaluative Sciences
Toronto, ON, Canada

Foreword

Improving research dissemination and uptake in the health sector: beyond the sound of one hand clapping

Jonathan Lomas

Introduction

Science is both a collection of ideological beliefs and an agency for liberation, it substitutes democracy for political and religious authority. Demanding evidence for statements of fact and providing criteria to test the evidence, it gives us a way to distinguish between what is true and what powerful people might wish to convince us is true [1].

The above quote provides a justification for concern about improving the link between research and decision making—good information is a tool in the maintenance of democracy and a bulwark against domination of the diffuse broad interests of the many by the concentrated narrow interests of the powerful few. Current concern with evidence-based decision making (EBDM) is about improving the quantity, quality, and breadth of evidence used by all participants in the health care system: legislators, administrators, practitioners, industry, and, increasingly, the public. Better dissemination and uptake of health research is integral to EBDM. Current failings in this area have more to do with unrealistic expectations between the various decision-maker audiences and researchers than they are with unavailability of research or an absent need for it in decision making. Understanding the roots of unrealistic expectations on both sides helps to point the way to improved dissemination and uptake of health research.

Understanding the roots of unrealistic expectations

There appear to be at least four areas of misunderstanding between researchers and decision makers:

1. *Research and decision making as processes not products*

There is a tendency for decision makers to treat the research community as a retail store. They interact only when they wish to acquire the product of many years of conceptualization and effort emerging from the research team's process of investigation. Thus, the research is often of limited relevance because the constraints, priorities, and concerns of the decision maker were neither communicated nor sought out early enough and often enough to be incorporated into the conduct of the research. Similarly, researchers tend to treat decision making as an event rather than a process. Thus, they often arrive too late with their findings and try to insert them into the decision-making process after the problem has been formulated, feasible options delineated, and causal models incompatible with their approach adopted. The multiple stages of the decision-making and research processes argue for far more ongoing communication of priorities, approaches, choice points, and constraints between the two communities.

2. *The political and institutional context of decision making*

Trained as rational scientists, most researchers confuse their desire for *rational* decision making with the reality of politically and institutionally constrained *sensible* decision making. Researchers therefore underestimate the importance of values in decision making and overestimate the role of their "facts." These facts are contestable in the decision-making environment, and vie with other sources of information and become transformed in the hands of various interested (stakeholders) and disinterested (media) purveyors of information for decision making. Receptivity to "facts" from research is based on system values as expressed through the preconceived notions of the participants, predilictions of those with the decision-making power, and the precedents of the institutions responsible for the decision process. Failure of researchers to understand this political and institutional environment leads to naive expectations regarding the adoption of their findings; over-commitment to *rational* decision making may even lead to wilful disregard of these political and institutional realities.

3. *Decision makers' views and expectations of research communities*

Researchers, especially those based in universities, organize around disciplines rather than issues. Integrated knowledge addressing a specific problem is therefore a rare commodity. The desire of decision makers for one-stop-shopping to acquire "trans-disciplinary" relevant knowledge is often frustrated by these disciplinary divisions. Furthermore, the historical incentive in universities is to engage in discovery research (designed to serve future, often as yet unspecified, needs) more than applied research (designed to address current perceived needs). To the extent that most decision makers confront current problems, there is a mismatch between where researchers spend their time and where decision makers would wish them to spend their time.

Although some rebalancing of university effort is needed toward more applied research, there is a danger that decision makers, in their haste to acquire research for their decision making, may divert excessive resources away from discovery research. Not all research is (or should) be dedicated to serving today's decision makers. At least some capacity has to be dedicated to discovery research that produces the feedstock of methods, new approaches, and innovations for future applied research.

4. *Researchers' views and expectations of decision-making communities*

Researchers tend to treat decision makers as a homogeneous community. Many fail to discriminate between (and do not tailor dissemination of findings to) at least four audiences consisting of different types of individuals with different needs from research, different preferred formats for its dissemination, and different degrees of skill and motivation in extracting findings from the research community.

Legislative decision makers—politicians, bureaucrats, and various interest groups—are more likely to use research and analysis to form policy agendas (e.g., should health consequences be an integral part of debates on unemployment?) or to justify already chosen courses of action (e.g., how many deaths per year can we claim to have averted with gun controls?) than they are to engage in open-ended searches for the most scientifically valid solution to a problem. Health policy analysis is of most use to them. Decision making at this level is more about policy ideas, about ways of framing issues and defining manageable problems than it is about selecting solutions. Research information communicated via dense and jargon-laden publications is less appropriate for this busy audience than are person-to-person or brief memo formats.

Administrative decision makers—program managers, hospital executives, regional administrators, insurers, and board members—may use the more applied health services research and sometimes clinical research to make decisions, such as facility location, program design, human resource mix, budget allocations, and quality improvement strategies. Often specialists in some aspect of health care, they wish to make more instrumental use of health research and may establish ongoing contacts with particular researchers to reduce search time and assure reliability of information. Synthesized knowledge around a concrete issue, provided within the time frame of the decision process, is of most use to them, either in written form or via workshops and seminars or their personal contacts.

Clinical decision makers—individual practitioners, specialty and professional society officials, and expert panel members—are concerned with specific questions of patient selection criteria, schedules for preventive regimens, safely delegable acts, effective monitoring, and disciplinary procedures. Clinical research is of most interest to them. With perhaps the most circumscribed needs of any audience, their clinical information needs are increasingly served by mediating organizations, such as the Cochrane Collaboration or by journals dedicated to the synthesis of clinically relevant knowledge. Nevertheless, the time constraints and informal communication channels of this audience still require attention to the use of innovations in dissemination, such as local opinion leaders and peer bench-marking.

Industrial decision makers—pharmaceutical companies, software and device manufacturers, and venture capitalists—are interested in potentially profitable products and can be distinguished from the other audiences by their high degree of motivation to "pull" marketable findings from researchers. Consequently, this audience most obviously raises the ethical and allocational question of proprietary-oriented versus publicly oriented (or profit-oriented versus need-oriented) objectives for health research. Although clinical and biomedical research has historically been of most interest to them, health services research with software or other system implications is of increasing importance to this audience. Because of their high degree of motivation in finding marketable products, the formats for dissemination can be closer to "raw" research findings than for other audiences.

The failure of many researchers to distinguish between the needs and preferred dissemination formats of these audiences has led them to an inappropriate "one-size-fits-all" journal publication approach to dissemination of research findings.

Conclusion

Achieving improved dissemination and uptake of health research will depend on interested applied researchers, committed decision makers, and both research sponsors and universities willing to consider new ways of doing business. This discussion document identifies four elements in a campaign to achieve this improvement:

1. An umbrella message from a national level that communicates a cultural change toward more conduct of relevant, good quality research and

greater attention to the application of findings from such research to decision making.

2. New structures to improve the opportunities for ongoing fruitful communication between researchers and decision makers, and to concentrate both applied research production and research receptor skills as a critical mass in universities and decision-making organizations, respectively.

3. New activities and processes:

   i. By researchers to synthesize and disseminate their work in a way that is more sensitive to the needs of their target audiences,

   ii. By decision makers to both receive and apply research findings, as well as to communicate audience-specific priorities,

   iii. By universities to reward instead of penalize employees interested in applied research, and

   iv. By research sponsors to both encourage greater relevance in funded research and to recognize issue-specific bodies of knowledge as an important unit of research production and transfer.

4. New human resource approaches to give both decision makers and researchers a better understanding of each others' environments and to produce new categories of personnel (e.g., knowledge brokers) skilled in bridging the not insignificant cultural gap between the two communities.

August, 1997

Reference

1 Tesh SN. *Hidden Arguments: Political Ideology and Disease Prevention Policy*. London: Rutgers University Press; 1989, p. 167.

Preface

In 1997, Jonathan Lomas wrote a commentary describing the gap between research and decision making and postulated why this may occur. He described areas of misunderstanding between researchers and decision makers that may contribute to this gap and suggested that improved communication across these groups was necessary to enhance knowledge uptake. We reproduced part of his analysis as Foreword to outline challenges in knowledge implementation that were identified at that time. He went on to implement many of the ideas emerging from his work during his 1998–2007 tenure as the inaugural Chief Executive Officer of the Canadian Health Services Research Foundation.

This book attempts to demonstrate the progress that has been made in implementing knowledge in health care and describes strategies to bridge the gap between knowledge and action. We believe that both the science and practice of knowledge implementation have advanced in the last decade, and efforts in these areas are growing exponentially. This book highlights some of these efforts, provides a framework for implementation activities, and demonstrates future areas of research, where gaps still exist.

Section 1
Introduction

Section
introduction

1.1 Knowledge to action: what it is and what it isn't

Sharon E. Straus[1,2], Jacqueline Tetroe[3], and Ian D. Graham[3,4]

[1]Department of Medicine, University of Toronto, Toronto, ON, Canada
[2]Li Ka Shing Knowledge Institute, St. Michael's Hospital, Toronto, ON, Canada
[3]Knowledge Translation Portfolio, Canadian Institutes of Health Research, Ottawa, ON, Canada
[4]School of Nursing, University of Ottawa, Ottawa, ON, Canada

---

KEY LEARNING POINTS

- Gaps between evidence and decision making occur across decision makers including patients, health care professionals, and policy makers.
- Knowledge translation (KT) is the synthesis, dissemination, exchange, and ethically sound application of knowledge to improve health, provide more effective health services and products, and strengthen the health care system.

Health care systems are faced with the challenge of improving the quality of care and decreasing the risk of adverse events [1]. Globally, health systems fail to optimally use evidence, resulting in inefficiencies and reduced quantity and quality of life [2,3]. The science and practice of knowledge translation (KT) can answer these challenges. The finding that providing evidence from clinical research is necessary but not sufficient for providing optimal care delivery has created interest in KT, which we define as the methods for closing the knowledge-to-action gaps.

What is knowledge translation?

Many terms are used to describe the process of putting knowledge into action [4]. In the United Kingdom and Europe, the terms *implementation science* and *research utilization* are commonly used in this context. In the United States, the terms *dissemination* and *diffusion, research use, knowledge transfer,* and *uptake* are often used. Canada commonly uses the terms *knowledge transfer* and *exchange.* In this book, we use the terms *knowledge translation* (KT) and *knowledge to action* interchangeably. For those who want a formal definition of KT, the Canadian Institutes of Health Research (CIHR) defines

---

Knowledge Translation in Health Care: Moving from Evidence to Practice. Edited by S. Straus, J. Tetroe, and I. Graham. © 2009 Blackwell Publishing, ISBN: 978-1-4051-8106-8.

KT as "a dynamic and iterative process that includes the synthesis, dissemination, exchange and ethically sound application of knowledge to improve health, provide more effective health services and products and strengthen the healthcare system." This definition has been adapted by the U.S. National Center for Dissemination of Disability Research and the World Health Organization (WHO). The move beyond simple dissemination of knowledge to actual use of knowledge is the common element to these different terms. It is clear that knowledge creation, distillation, and dissemination are not sufficient on their own to ensure implementation in decision making.

Some organizations may use the term *knowledge translation* synonymously with *commercialization* or *technology transfer*. However, this narrow view does not consider the various stakeholders involved or the actual process of using knowledge in decision making. Similarly, some confusion arises around continuing education versus KT. Certainly, educational interventions are a strategy for knowledge implementation, but it must be kept in mind that the KT audience is larger than the number of health care professionals who are the target for continuing medical education or continuing professional development. KT strategies may vary according to the targeted user audience (e.g., researchers, clinicians, policy makers, public) and the type of knowledge being translated (e.g., clinical, biomedical, policy) [2].

Why is KT important?

Failure to use research evidence to inform decision making is apparent across all key decision-maker groups, including health care providers, patients, informal carers, managers, and policy makers, in developed and developing countries, in primary and specialty care, and in care provided by all disciplines. Practice audits performed in a variety of settings have revealed that high-quality evidence is not consistently applied in practice [5]. For example, although several randomized trials have shown that statins can decrease the risk of mortality and morbidity in poststroke patients, statins are considerably underprescribed [6]. In contrast, antibiotics are overprescribed in children with upper respiratory tract symptoms [7]. A synthesis of 14 studies showed that many patients (26–95%) were dissatisfied with information given to them [8]. Lavis and colleagues [9] studied eight health policy-making processes in Canada. Citable health services research was used in at least one stage of the policy-making process for only four policies; only one of these four policies had citable research used in all stages of the policy-making process. Similarly, evidence from systematic reviews was not frequently used by WHO policy makers [10]. And, Dobbins and colleagues observed that although systematic reviews were used in making public health guidelines in Ontario, Canada, policy-level recommendations were not adopted [11].

Increasing recognition of these issues has led to attempts to effect behavior, practice, or policy change. Changing behavior is a complex process that requires the evaluation of the entire health care organization, including systematic barriers to change (e.g., lack of integrated health information systems) and targeting of those involved in decision making, including clinicians, policymakers, and patients [2]. Effort must be made to close knowledge-to-practice gaps with effective KT interventions, thereby improving health outcomes. These initiatives must include all aspects of care, including access to and implementation of valid evidence, patient safety strategies, and organizational and systems issues.

What are the KT determinants?

Multiple factors determine the use of research by different stakeholder groups [12–16]. A common challenge that all decision makers face relates to the lack of knowledge-management skills and infrastructure (the sheer volume of research evidence currently produced, access to research evidence, time to read, and skills to appraise, understand, and apply research evidence). Better knowledge management is necessary, but is insufficient to ensure effective KT, given other challenges that may operate at different levels [16], including the health care system (e.g., financial disincentives), health care organization (e.g., lack of equipment), health care teams (e.g., local standards of care not in line with recommended practice), individual health care professionals (e.g., knowledge, attitudes, and skills), and patients (e.g., low adherence to recommendations). Frequently, multiple challenges operating at different levels of the health care system are present. KT interventions and activities need to keep abreast with these challenges and changes in health care.

The knowledge-to-action framework: a model for KT

There are many proposed theories and frameworks for achieving knowledge translation that can be confusing to those responsible for KT [17–21]. A conceptual framework developed by Graham and colleagues, termed the knowledge-to-action cycle, provides an approach that builds on the commonalities found in an assessment of planned-action theories [4]. This framework was developed after a review of more than 30 planned-action theories that identified their common elements. They added a knowledge creation process to the planned-action model and labeled the combined models the

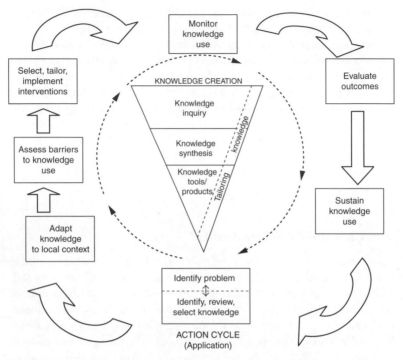

Figure 1.1.1 The knowledge-to-action framework.

knowledge-to-action cycle. The CIHR, Canada's federal health research funding agency, has adopted the cycle as the accepted model for promoting the application of research and as a framework for the KT process.

In this model, the knowledge-to-action process is iterative, dynamic, and complex, concerning both knowledge creation and application (action cycle) with fluid boundaries between creation and action components. Figure 1.1.1 illustrates the knowledge creation funnel and the major action steps or stages comprising the knowledge-to-action model.

Knowledge creation

Knowledge creation, or the production of knowledge, consists of three phases: knowledge inquiry, knowledge synthesis, and knowledge tools and/or product creation. As knowledge is filtered or distilled through each stage of the knowledge creation process, the resulting knowledge becomes more refined and potentially more useful to end users. For example, the synthesis stage brings together disparate research findings that may exist globally on a topic and attempts to identify common patterns. At the tools/products development stage, the best quality knowledge and research is further synthesized and distilled into a decision-making tool, such as practice guidelines or algorithms.

The action cycle

Seven action phases can occur sequentially or simultaneously, and the knowledge phases can influence the action phases at several points in the cycle. At each phase, multiple theories from different disciplines can be brought to bear. Action parts of the cycle are based on planned-action theories that focus on deliberately engineering change in health care systems and groups [17,18]. Included are the processes needed to implement knowledge in health care settings, namely, identification of the problem; identifying, reviewing, and selecting the knowledge to implement; adapting or customizing knowledge to local context; assessing knowledge use determinants; selecting, tailoring, implementing, and monitoring KT interventions; evaluating outcomes or impact of using the knowledge; and determining strategies for ensuring sustained knowledge use. Integral to the framework is the need to consider various stakeholders who are the end users of the knowledge that is being implemented.

In this book, we attempt to provide an approach to the science and practice of KT. We will describe the roles of synthesis and knowledge tools in the knowledge creation process, as well as present key elements of the action cycle and outline successful KT strategies targeted to relevant stakeholders including the public, clinicians, and policy makers. Each chapter was created following a systematic search of literature and appraisal of individual studies for validity. Gaps in the literature will be identified; the science of KT is a relatively new field, and we will attempt to reflect this by highlighting future areas of research.

References

1 Kohn LT, Corrigan JM, Donaldson MS (eds). *To Err Is Human: Building a Safer Health System*. Washington, DC: National Academy Press, 1999.
2 Davis D, Evans M, Jadad A, Perrier L, Rath D, Ryan D, et al. The case for KT: shortening the journey from evidence to effect. *BMJ* 2003 Jul 5;327[7405]: 33–5.
3 Madon T, Hofman KJ, Kupfer L, Glass RI. Public health. Implementation science. *Science* 2007 Dec 14;318[5857]:1728–9.

4 Graham ID, Logan J, Harrison MB, Straus SE, Tetroe J, Caswell W, et al. Lost in knowledge translation: time for a map? *J Contin Ed Health Prof* 2006 Winter;26[1]:13–24.

5 Majumdar SR, McAlister FA, Furberg CD. From knowledge to practice in chronic cardiovascular disease—a long and winding Road. *J Am Coll Cardiol* 2004;43[10]:1738–42.

6 LaRosa JC, He J, Vupputuri S. Effect of statins on the risk of coronary disease: a meta-analysis of randomised controlled trials. *JAMA* 1999;282[24]:2340–6.

7 Arnold S, Straus SE. Interventions to improve antibiotic prescribing practices in ambulatory care. *Cochrane Database Syst Rev* 2005 Oct 19;[4]:CD003539.

8 Kiesler DJ, Auerbach SM. Optimal matches of patient preferences for information, decision-making and interpersonal behavior: evidence, models and interventions. *Patient Educ Couns* 2006 Jun;61[3]:319–41.

9 Lavis J, Ross SE, Hurley JE, Hohenadel JM, Stoddart GL, Woodward CA, et al. Examining the role of health services research in public policy making. *Milbank Q* 2002;80[1]:125–54.

10 Oxman A, Lavis JN, Fretheim A. Use of evidence in WHO recommendations. *Lancet* 2007 Jun 2;369[9576]:1883–9.

11 Dobbins M, Thomas H, O-Brien MA, Duggan M. Use of systematic reviews in the development of new provincial public health policies in Ontario. *Int J Technol Assess Health Care* 2004 Fall;20[4]:399–404.

12 Cabana MD, Rand CS, Powe NR, Wu AW, Wilson MH, Abboud PA, et al. Why don't physicians follow clinical practice guidelines? A framework for improvement. *JAMA* 1999;282[15]:1458–65.

13 Gravel K, Legare F, Graham ID. Barriers and facilitators to implementing shared decision-making in clinical practice: a systematic review of health professionals' perceptions. *Implement Sci* 2006 Aug 9;1:16.

14 Legare F, O'Connor AM, Graham ID, Saucier D, Cote L, Blais J, et al. Primary health care professionals' views on barriers and facilitators to the implementation of the Ottawa Decision Support Framework in practice. *Patient Educ Couns* 2006;63[3]:380–90.

15 Milner M, Estabrooks CA, Myrick F. Research utilisation and clinical nurse educators: a systematic review. *J Eval Clin Pract* 2006;12[6]:639–55.

16 Grimshaw JM, Eccles MP, Walker AE, Thomas RE. Changing physician's behaviour: what works and thoughts on getting more things to work. *J Contin Educ Health Prof* 2002 Fall;22[4]:237–43.

17 Graham ID, Harrison MB, Logan J, and the KT Theories Research Group. *A review of planned change (knowledge translation) models, frameworks and theories.* Presented at the JBI International Convention, Adelaide, Australia, Nov 2005.

18 Graham ID, Tetroe J, KT Theories Research Group. Some theoretical underpinnings of knowledge translation. *Acad Emerg Med* 2007 Nov;14[11]:936–41.

19 Estabrooks CA, Thompson DS, Lovely JJ, Hofmeyer A. A guide to knowledge translation theory. *J Contin Educ Health Prof* 2006 Winter;26[1]:25–36.

20 McDonald KM, Graham ID, Grimshaw J. Toward a theoretic basis for quality improvement interventions. In: KG Shojania, KM McDonald, RM Wachter, & DK Owens (eds), *Closing the quality gap: a critical analysis of quality improvement strategies, volume 1 – series overview and methodology.* Technical Review 9. 2004 (Contract No. 290-02-0017 to the Stanford University-UCSF Evidence-Based Practices Center). AHRQ Publication No. 04-0051-1. Rockville, MD: Agency for Healthcare Research and Quality. Aug 2004. URL http://www.ncbi.nlm.nih.gov/books/bv.fcgi?rid=hstat2.chapter.26505.

21 Wensing M, Bosch M, Foy R, van der Weijden T, Eccles M, Grol R. *Factors in theories on behaviour change to guide implementation and quality improvement in healthcare.* Nijmegen, the Netherlands: Centres for Quality of Care Research (WOK), 2005.

Section 2
Knowledge Creation

2.1 The K in KT: knowledge creation

Sharon E. Straus

Li Ka Shing Knowledge Institute, St. Michael's Hospital, and Department of Medicine, University of Toronto, Toronto, ON, Canada

In the center of the knowledge-to-action cycle is the knowledge funnel, which represents knowledge creation [1]. As knowledge moves through the funnel, it is refined and, ideally, becomes more useful to end users of the knowledge, which can include researchers, health care professionals, policy makers, and the public. During each phase of knowledge creation, knowledge producers tailor their activities to the needs of the end users. First-generation knowledge is derived from primary studies such as randomized trials and interrupted time series. Knowledge synthesis is second-generation knowledge. Systematic reviews are examples of this knowledge product and are described in Chapter 2.2. Third-generation knowledge includes tools and products such as decision aids and educational modules. Their purpose is to present knowledge in user-friendly, implementable formats, and they are outlined in Chapter 2.3. Each format can be tailored to the needs of the end users of the knowledge.

Chapter 2.4 reviews strategies for identifying research findings, specifically knowledge syntheses and practice guidelines. For people interested in the science and practice of KT, understanding how to search the literature for articles about KT is helpful. Although searching the literature around any topic can be challenging, searching for KT literature has several distinct challenges, including the varying terminology that is used to describe KT. Tetroe and colleagues have found 33 different terms to describe KT, including *implementation science, research utilization,* and *knowledge exchange and uptake* [2]. Cognizant of these challenges, we provide an approach to searching for KT literature in this chapter.

Knowledge Translation in Health Care: Moving from Evidence to Practice. Edited by S. Straus, J. Tetroe, and I. Graham. © 2009 Blackwell Publishing, ISBN: 978-1-4051-8106-8.

References

1 Graham ID, Logan J, Harrison MB, Straus SE, Tetroe J, Caswell W, et al. Lost in knowledge translation: time for a map? *J Contin Ed Health Prof* 2006;26:13–24.
2 Tetroe J, Graham I, Foy R, Robinson N, Eccles MP, Wensing M, et al. Health research funding agencies' support and promotion of knowledge translation: an international study. *Milbank Quarterly* 2008;86[1].

2.2 Knowledge synthesis

Jennifer Tetzlaff[1,2], Andrea C. Tricco[1,3], and David Moher[1,2]

[1] Chalmers Research Group, Children's Hospital of Eastern Ontario Research Institute, Ottawa, ON, Canada

[2] Faculty of Medicine, Department of Epidemiology & Community Medicine, University of Ottawa, Ottawa, ON, Canada

[3] Institute of Population Health, University of Ottawa, Ottawa, ON, Canada

---

KEY LEARNING POINTS

- Knowledge synthesis interprets the results of individual studies within the context of global evidence and bridges the gap between research and decision making.

- Many groups worldwide conduct knowledge syntheses, and some general methods apply to most reviews. However, variations of these methods are apparent for different types of reviews, such as realist reviews and mixed models reviews.

- Review validity is dependent on the validity of the included primary studies and the review process itself. Steps should be taken to avoid bias in knowledge synthesis conduct. Transparency in reporting will help readers assess review validity and applicability, thus increasing its utility.

- Given the magnitude of existing literature, increasing demands on systematic review teams, and the diversity of approaches, continuing methodological efforts will be important to increase the efficiency, validity, and applicability of systematic reviews.

- Research should focus on increasing the uptake of knowledge synthesis, how best to update reviews, comparing different types of reviews (e.g., rapid versus comprehensive reviews), and prioritizing knowledge synthesis topics.

"Knowledge synthesis" is not a new concept. Examples date to the early 1900s [1]. In the 1960s, research syntheses were common in social science, education, and psychology [1]. Along with recognizing the importance of evidence-based decision making in health care came an understanding of the need for making decisions based on the best available evidence and a demand for this evidence [2]. Since then, knowledge syntheses have become increasingly important in health care. Knowledge translation that focuses on the results of individual studies may be misleading due to bias in conduct or random variations in findings [3]. This suggests that knowledge syntheses that interpret the results of individual studies within the context of

---

Knowledge Translation in Health Care: Moving from Evidence to Practice. Edited by S. Straus, J. Tetroe, and I. Graham. © 2009 Blackwell Publishing, ISBN: 978-1-4051-8106-8.

global evidence should be considered the basic unit of knowledge translation (KT) [4]. Syntheses provide evidence for other KT tools, such as policy briefs, patient decision aids, and clinical practice guidelines [4], which are discussed in Chapter 2.3. Additionally, granting agencies, such as the Canadian Institutes of Health Research, require knowledge syntheses to justify the need to fund and conduct randomized controlled trials [5]. Knowledge synthesis is central to KT, bridging the gap between research and decision making [6].

The terms used to describe specific approaches to synthesis have evolved over time. There is no consistent use of these terms, but we will adopt definitions used by The Cochrane Collaboration. Systematic reviews consist of a clearly formulated question and use systematic and explicit methods to identify, select, critically appraise, and extract and analyze data from relevant research. A meta-analysis consists of statistical techniques to quantitatively integrate the results of included studies. A knowledge synthesis may not necessarily include a meta-analysis.

Many groups worldwide conduct systematic reviews (see Chapter 2.4). The Cochrane Collaboration often answers questions about efficacy and effectiveness of interventions [7]. As such, it places strong reliance on synthesizing evidence from randomized controlled trials (RCTs). Other organizations include study designs in their systematic reviews. Examples include the Campbell Collaboration [8], which addresses questions related to crime and justice, education, and social welfare; the Evidence-Based Practice Centre (EPC) program [9], which completes knowledge syntheses in health care and policy areas; and the Joanna Briggs Institute, which conducts knowledge syntheses on health issues of interest to nursing [10]. These groups may use different templates for conducting systematic reviews. Explicit methods will depend, in part, on the question being considered. Nevertheless, some general methods apply to most reviews (Table 2.2.1), and we focus on these in the following sections.

The review team

Prior to a review, a systematic review team should be identified. The type of question being addressed determines the optimal team, and the team generally consists of clinical or content experts with extensive knowledge of the review topic, methodologists with expertise in systematic reviews, a librarian to search the literature comprehensively [11], and epidemiologists or other researchers with experience in conducting primary research on the topic. The funder or commissioning agency may help inform the context of the question, and a statistician may be consulted if statistical pooling (i.e., meta-analysis) is being considered. Some review teams also involve end users of the review, such as policy makers, health care professionals, or patients, in the initial stages of the review process.

Table 2.2.1 Conducting a systematic review

- Develop the review question
- Develop a review protocol
  - Outline the background
  - Define/clarify objectives and eligibility criteria
  - Develop search strategies
  - Identify methods to assess bias risk
  - Describe data to be abstracted
  - Prespecify outcomes and analysis methods
- Locate studies
  - Search electronic databases
  - Use other methods, if applicable (e.g., trial registers, hand searching, contacting experts)
- Select studies
  - Broad screen of citations
  - Strict screen of full-text articles
- Assess bias risk in included studies
  - Use bias risk instrument outlined in protocol
- Extract data
  - Develop and pilot test forms
  - Extract data for primary and secondary outcomes outlined in protocol
- Analyze results
  - Include a narrative synthesis of main findings and bias risk results
  - Synthesize results quantitatively (e.g., meta-analysis) or qualitatively, if appropriate
  - Consider bias risk across studies (e.g., publication bias)
- Present results
  - Present screening results (e.g., flow diagram)
  - Present characteristics of included studies and results of bias risk assessment (e.g., table)
  - Present quantitative data (e.g., forest plot) and/or qualitative data (e.g., thematic matrix)
- Interpret and discuss results
  - Consider quality, strength, and applicability of results
  - Discuss relevance of findings to key stakeholders
  - Describe study-level and review-level limitations
  - Carefully derive conclusions
- Disseminate results
  - For example, through peer-reviewed journals, media, reports

How do we formulate the question, eligibility criteria, and protocol?

Developing a clear and concise question is the first and one of the most important steps in conducting a systematic review. This will guide the review process. Formulating relevant questions can be complex, and the Popula-tion, Intervention, Comparators, Outcome, and (Study design) (PICO[S]) acronym is proposed as a structured way to facilitate this process [12]. With this approach, the question addresses the population, participants, or problem (P); the interventions, independent variables or index test (for diagnostic reviews) (I); the comparators (C) (e.g., placebo, standard of care, or context, in the case of qualitative studies); and dependent variables, endpoints, or outcomes of interest (O). Sometimes an additional component, the study design (S), limits the systematic review to certain study types, such as RCTs or cohort studies. This paradigm will not fit all questions but may be a useful guideline. For example, systematic reviews of epidemiological studies may substitute *intervention* with *exposure*.

Once the review team has been assembled and the objectives defined, a protocol prespecifying the systematic review methods should be developed to guide the process for the review team. Protocol use may decrease the likelihood of biased *posthoc* changes to methods and selective outcome reporting. Important elements of the review protocol are provided elsewhere but include details on the methods used for the search, retrieval, and appraisal of literature and data abstraction [13]. The systematic review process may be iterative. As such, the protocol may change over time; this is especially the case for qualitative reviews [14]. Changes to the review protocol may be acceptable; however, these should be transparently described in the final report.

The eligibility criteria of studies to be included in the synthesis should extend from the components of the review question and may be based on study or report characteristics. Study characteristics may include the PICO(S) criteria, as well as others, such as length of follow-up. Report characteristics may include publication language and status (e.g., published material). Evidence suggests that selectively including studies based on report characteristics (e.g., publication status or publication language) may bias the effect estimate in meta-analyses [15–20]. Conversely, caution may be needed in all-inclusive approaches to study selection due to potential differences in the risk of bias from some sources, such as selective reporting in abstracts versus full-text reports [21–25]. Regardless of the choices, eligibility should be thoroughly considered, properly defined, and transparently reported to avoid ambiguity in the review process and to inform the validity of the review.

How do we find relevant studies?

The review question or PICO(S) components guide the location of relevant studies, usually entailing bibliographic database searches and other methods. Commonly searched electronic databases for health-related research are MEDLINE [26], EMBASE [27], and The Cochrane Central Register of Controlled Trials [28]. Reviewers may also search subject-specific databases, such as the Cumulative Index of Nursing and Allied Health (CINAHL), or geographical databases, such as the Latin American Caribbean Health Sciences Literature (LILACS). The scope of the database and the review should be considered to select the most relevant databases for the review, and searching more than one database is highly recommended to overcome potential indexing biases [29]. Consulting a librarian ensures that the search strategies are comprehensive.

Systematic reviewers often use other methods to supplement their searches, such as hand-searching journals, searching reference lists of included studies, or searching trial registries. Searching grey literature[1] should be considered, including Web sites from funding agencies, health policy groups, and ministries of health. More detailed searching information can be found elsewhere [13].

How do we select studies?

Systematic reviewers generally separate the study selection process into two stages: (1) a broad screen of titles and citation abstracts retrieved from the literature search, and (2) a strict screen of full-text articles passing the broad screen to select the final included studies. This selection is usually facilitated through the use of eligibility criteria. Having two or more reviewers screen the material independently is helpful. Results are then compared and conflicts may be resolved by discussion or with the involvement of a third reviewer. Recording and reporting agreement across reviewers is useful.

The process of identifying and selecting studies requires detailed record-keeping because it must be reported in sufficient detail for the end user to determine validity. The ratio of reports to studies is not always 1:1; some reports will describe multiple studies and some studies are described in more than one report. Duplicate publications are not always obvious [31–34], and authors should attempt to identify duplicate data.

How do we assess risk of bias of included studies?

The validity of the results of a systematic review will depend on the risk of bias in the individual studies. Risk of bias assessment can be completed using scales, checklists, or components, and many tools are available for different

---

[1] Information produced on all levels of government, academics, business, and industry in electronic and print formats not controlled by commercial publishing—that is, where publishing is not the primary activity of the producing body [30].

study designs [35,36]. Assessing the risk of bias in qualitative research is widely debated, although numerous tools have been developed [14]. Regardless of the instrument used, individual components should be reported for each study. Simply reporting a score from an assessment scale is not as helpful to the end user because there is insufficient detail to understand where sources of bias arise. Excluding studies from a review based on their risk of bias is generally not advisable. Rather, the impact of this potential bias can be addressed through sensitivity analyses, which explore whether results of the review are robust to differences in the trials, such as methodology (e.g., examining studies with and without concealed allocation separately) and populations examined.

How do we extract data from individual studies?

At the time of protocol development, information sought from the included studies should be considered. The outcome(s) of primary importance (e.g., clinical, patient, or policy relevant) should be differentiated from "secondary" outcomes. Recent surveys have found that authors of randomized trials modified primary outcomes between the protocol and the final report in approximately 50% of trials [37] and that the outcomes selectively reported in final reports were significantly more likely to be statistically significant than those omitted [38,39]. Therefore, if a review is limited only to variables reported in the included studies rather than those considered important at the outset, the review risks being subject to bias.

It is advisable to develop a data extraction form *a priori,* including the variables to be collected and clear definitions for them. The form can be pilot-tested by review team members to increase the reliability of the data extraction process. Having two or more people independently extract study data may also decrease the potential for error. Reviewers should consider contacting authors to verify assumptions for missing or unclear information.

How do we analyze the data?

The analysis method will depend on the question(s) being asked and the type of data collected; however, all systematic reviews should at least include a narrative synthesis describing the results and risk of bias in included studies. For a typical intervention review that includes quantitative data, standard effect measures will need to be chosen, if possible, to compare studies (e.g., odds ratio, standardized mean difference, hazard ratio). The next step usually involves determining whether statistical synthesis (i.e., meta-analysis) is possible and appropriate. For example, if outcome assessment across the included studies is inconsistent or evidence of substantial clinical, methodological, or statistical heterogeneity of included studies exists, quantitative synthesis may not be suitable [13]. Guidance on effect measures, approaches to detect heterogeneity, and meta-analysis techniques are available elsewhere [13,40,41].

Qualitative analytical approaches differ from quantitative methods. For example, qualitative data may be input into matrices or tables to allow comparison across studies [42]. Some knowledge syntheses will include qualitative and quantitative data for which a variety of methods are available [42]. Examples include a quantitative case survey, in which qualitative data are converted into quantitative form and analyzed statistically (e.g., through meta-analysis) [42], and Bayesian meta-analysis, which allows the incorporation of qualitative research into a quantitative synthesis to provide policy makers with decision support [43,44].

How do we present the results of the review?

Results of knowledge syntheses may be presented in numerous ways. The screening process may be described in the text and/or presented as a flowchart (Figure 2.2.1) [45]. Many journals require this information to be presented as a flowchart to facilitate process transparency. Characteristics of included studies, such as descriptions of study designs, participant populations, and interventions, are generally presented in tabular form and/or synthesized textually. Results of risk-of-bias assessments may also be presented in a table or text, and sufficient detail should be presented to allow the end user to determine potential validity threats.

Quantitative data should be presented as summary data (e.g., 2×2 tables of counts, means, and standard deviations) and effect estimates (e.g., odds ratio, difference in means) with confidence intervals for each study, where possible. This data may be presented for each outcome in a table or in a forest plot, with the combined effect estimate of the meta-analysis, if relevant (Figure 2.2.2; [e.g., 46]). Qualitative data may also be presented visually, for example, through a conceptual framework. Results of all other analyses, such as assessment of publication bias, should also be reported.

How can we interpret the results?

Reviewers should discuss quality, strength, and applicability of the evidence for each main outcome when summarizing results. Formal assessment approaches do exist [47], although no standard method is universally recommended. Relevance of the results should also be considered for key

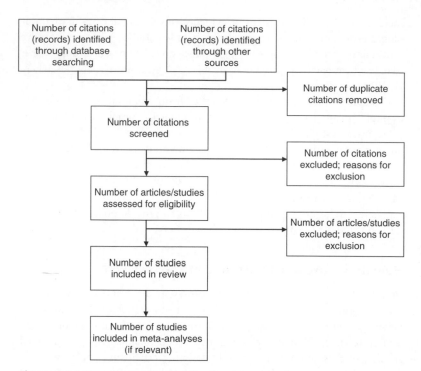

Figure 2.2.1 Flow diagram documenting literature retrieval.

stakeholders (e.g., policy makers, patients, health care providers) because this will help increase applicability of the results for these groups. As mentioned earlier, involving these groups at the review's outset (e.g., defining the research question, choosing eligibility criteria and outcomes) will increase applicability of results.

Reviewers should consider both study and review-level limitations. If the conduct or reporting of included studies is poor, review conclusions may be biased, and this should be stated explicitly. Furthermore, knowledge syntheses themselves can be susceptible to bias. A recent systematic review summarized evidence of possible bias and confounding in systematic reviews [29]. Reviewers should be aware of and take steps to avoid bias potential in review conduct by comprehensively searching for relevant literature and enlisting content and methodological support for the review team. Despite these efforts, some review limitations will exist and should be noted.

Finally, reviewers should draw conclusions based on the available evidence. Conclusions may include specific recommendations for decision making or

Description	Tetracycline-rifampicin n/N	Tetracycline-streptomycin n/N	Relative risk (fixed) (95% CI)	Relative risk (fixed) (95% CI)
Acocella 1989[w72]	3/63	2/53		1.26 (0.22 to 7.27)
Ariza 1985[w73]	7/18	2/28		5.44 (1.27 to 23.34)
Ariza 1992[w74]	5/44	3/51		1.93 (0.49 to 7.63)
Baylndir 2003[w75]	5/20	6/41		1.71 (0.59 to 4.93)
Colmenero 1989[w76]	7/52	5/59		1.59 (0.54 to 4.70)
Colmenero 1994[w77]	2/10	0/9		4.55 (0.25 to 83.70)
Dorado 1988[w78]	8/27	4/24		1.78 (0.61 to 5.17)
Ersoy 2005[w79]	7/45	4/32		1.24 (0.40 to 3.90)
Kosmidis 1982[w80]	1/10	2/10		0.50 (0.05 to 4.67)
Montejo 1993[w81]	6/46	4/84		2.74 (0.81 to 9.21)
Rodriguez Zapata 1987[w82]	3/32	1/36		3.38 (0.37 to 30.84)
Solera 1991[w83]	12/34	3/36		4.24 (1.31 to 13.72)
Solera 1995[w84]	28/100	9/94		2.92 (1.46 to 5.87)
Total (95% CI)	501	557		2.30 (1.65 to 3.21)

Total events: 94 (tetracycline-rifampicin),
45 (tetracycline-streptomycin)

0.1 0.2   0.5   1   2   5   10

Favours tetracycline-rifampicin   Favours tetracycline-streptomycin

Test for heterogeneity: $\chi^2 = 7.64$, df = 12, P = 0.81, $I^2 = 0\%$

Test for overall effect: z = 4.94, P < 0.001

Figure 2.2.2 Example of forest plot. This forest plot depicts the meta-analysis of overall failure (defined as failure of assigned regimen or relapse) with tetracycline-rifampicin (T-R) versus tetracycline-streptomycin (T-S) (42). In the forest plot, the relative risk is depicted by a square, the size of which is relative to the size or weight of each study, and a line depicting the 95% confidence interval (CI). The diamond at the bottom of the figure depicts the combined effect estimate and 95% CI across studies and shows that T-S is more effctive than T-R (more failures for the latter) with a relative risk of 2.30 (95% CI: 1.65-3.21). In other words, the odds of treatment failure or relapse when treated with T-R are over twice those for treatment with T-S and this difference is significant. The figure also includes, from left to right, the references of the included studies, the event rates, and number of subjects in the intervention and control arms, the numerical values of the effect sizes, and 95% confidence intervals for each study and the combined effect estimate. The bottom of the figure includes statistical output for tests for heterogeneity.

for research [48]. If no conclusions can be drawn because of insufficient evidence, this point should be stated as it may indicate a need for further research.

How do we disseminate the results of our review?

The final step in the review process is making the results accessible. The most common form of dissemination is publication in peer-reviewed journals, with recent estimates suggesting that over 2500 English language systematic reviews are indexed annually in MEDLINE [49]. Other forms may include targeted dissemination via media for the public [50] and brief reports for health care providers, policy makers, and consumers [51]. Many factors may impede the uptake of the results of systematic reviews; however, one factor that is in the author's control is the quality of the review report. Transparent descriptions of the review methods and results allow readers to assess the methods, risk bias of included studies and the review, and inform them of the applicability of the review.

Recent evidence suggests that systematic review reporting is suboptimal [49]. The QUOROM Statement (Quality Of Reporting Of Meta-analyses) was developed to improve the reporting of systematic reviews and meta-analysis [45]. This reporting guideline has been recently updated and expanded (PRISMA, Preferred Reporting Items for Systematic reviews and Meta-Analyses) to address advances in systematic review methodology and changes in terminology. Similar initiatives are also available for reviews of observational studies [52].

How do we increase the uptake of our review results?

There is limited evidence to support how systematic reviews should be presented to enhance uptake in decision making. Despite advances in the conduct and reporting of systematic reviews (and recognition of their importance in KT), current evidence suggests that they may be used infrequently by clinicians, patients, and others to make decisions. A systematic review of physicians' information-seeking behavior found that textbooks (many of which do not rely on evidence from systematic reviews) are still the most frequent source of information, followed by advice from colleagues [53].

Given that systematic reviews of randomized trials are less susceptible to bias than expert opinions and observational data, why are they used so infrequently? There are many answers to this question, and answers can be broadly categorized according to the relevance of the questions being addressed, the lack of contextualization, and the format of presentation. Whereas much attention is paid to enhancing the quality of systematic reviews, relatively little attention is given to the format for presentation of the review. Because systematic reviews tend to focus on methodological rigor more than clinical context, they often do not provide crucial information for clinicians. In one study, researchers found that of systematic reviews published in *ACP JC* and *EBM Journal* (journals of secondary publication), less than 15% had sufficient information about the intervention to allow clinicians or policy makers to implement it [54].

Table 2.2.2 Variations in questions and methods for different types of systematic reviews

Type of review	Type of question	Example of question	Variation of review methods
TRADITIONAL SYSTEMATIC REVIEWS*			
Intervention review [13]	Does the intervention of interest work for a particular outcome?	What is the effectiveness of vitamin E for the treatment of cardiovascular disease? [64]	• Studies: often limited to data from experimental studies • Bias risk assessment: often focused on experimental studies • Analysis: may be qualitative or quantitative (meta-analysis)
Network meta-analysis [65]	Does the intervention of interest work for a particular outcome?	What are the odds of developing diabetes during long-term treatment with an initial class of antihypertensive drug? [66]	• Studies: often limited to data from experimental studies • Bias risk assessment: often focused on experimental studies • Analysis: often allows both direct and indirect comparisons (i.e., when the strategies have not been directly compared)
Diagnostic test review [67]	How well does the diagnostic test work for a particular group of patients?	What is the diagnostic accuracy of sentinel node biopsy, positron emission tomography, magnetic resonance imaging, and computed tomography in determining lymph node status in patients with cervical cancer? [68]	• Studies: focused on studies of test accuracy, for example • Bias risk: focused on issues pertinent to diagnostic studies • Analysis: combined results will be based on the summary statistic and sources of heterogeneity, especially variation in diagnostic thresholds

(Continued)

Table 2.2.2 (*Continued*)

Type of review	Type of question	Example of question	Variation of review methods

Human genome epidemiology reviews [69]	Which genes are associated with particular outcomes?	What is the susceptibility of 160A allele carriers to seven types of cancers? [70]	• Studies: often limited to data from observational studies
			• Bias risk: focuses on issues pertinent to genome association studies
			• Analysis:
			  ○ Quantitative test of bias and confounding usually performed (i.e., Hardy-Weinberg Equilibrium)
			  ○ Statistical methods used to combine results will be strongly based on heterogeneity

Prognostic review [71]	How can you predict a disease outcome more accurately or efficiently?	Does B-type natriuretic peptide (BNP) predict mortality or other cardiac endpoints in persons diagnosed with coronary artery disease? [72]	• Studies: often limited to data from observational studies
			• Bias risk: often focused on issues pertinent to prognostic studies
			• Analysis:
			  ○ Compares the outcome for groups with different prognostic variables
			  ○ Must adjust for many confounding variables
			  ○ May involve survival analysis if reported outcome is time-to-event

OTHER TYPES OF REVIEWS

Metanarrative review [58]	How best can one explain complex bodies of evidence?	How best to explain the diffusion of innovation in evidence-based medicine? [58]	• Questions: framed in broad, open-ended format • Literature search: involves browsing relevant perspectives and approaches, finding seminal conceptual papers by tracking references of references • Analysis: involves mapping and comparing storylines
Realist review [73]	How do complex programs work (or why do they fail) in certain contexts and settings?	Which aspects of school feeding programs in disadvantaged children determine success and failure in various situations? [74]	• Question: scope of the review involves additional steps, such as identifying key theories to be explored • Literature search: involves searching for theories explaining why the program works • Data abstraction: includes contextual data, such as theory, process detail, and historical aspects of the study • Analysis: often involves an iterative process

(Continued)

Table 2.2.2 (Continued)

Type of review	Type of question	Example of question	Variation of review methods
Metaethnography review [57]	How can qualitative evidence explain why certain interventions work and others do not?	What are the types of factors that could influence adherence to tuberculosis treatment from the patient's experience? [57]	• Question: question must be answerable with qualitative research • Literature search: involves searching electronic databases beyond the medical domain as well as books and theses • Data abstraction: involves abstracting metaphors, quotations, and common themes • Analysis: focuses on narrative summary of the evidence, data may be arranged in a matrix to show the commonalities of themes across studies

*Note: There are many ways to categorize this table. One possibility is to categorize it by the four pillars from the CIHR perspective. For example, intervention reviews may be best suited for biomedical and clinical research, whereas realist reviews may be more relevant to health services and population health.

Although most systematic review publications use structured abstracts, there is little data on the impact of their use on the clinician's ability to apply evidence [55]. There is even less data on the impact of the presentation of a complete systematic review on clinicians' understanding of evidence or their ability to apply it to individual patients. A study by McDonald and colleagues concluded that a focused systematic review was perceived to be more useful than a traditional narrative review [56]. This area represents a gap in KT research that should be addressed.

Variations of review methods

Knowledge synthesis is increasingly being accepted as a science, and it consists of a family of methodologies for synthesizing data [13]. There is an ever-increasing number of different types of knowledge synthesis, ranging from the general approach described earlier to reviews that use only some of these elements (Table 2.2.2). The development of these various approaches to conducting reviews likely reflects the fact that only a minority of health care publications is on randomized trials that adequately address the question of "what works." However, there is a need to develop reviews that incorporate the rich information from other types of health research that address broader questions.

Realistic reviews use a more flexible and adaptive approach to some of the steps in a "what works" systematic review; however, the steps are applied differently, and new and different steps are introduced into the review process, such as "articulating key theories to be investigated" as part of addressing a policy-oriented question. Meta-ethnography reviews may only sample some identified studies [57]. Similarly, there is no consensus on whether quality assessment of included studies should be part of such reviews. Metanarrative reviews focus on interpretations of how stories are told within individual studies when answering a review question [58]. Finally, there are efforts to combine elements of the quantitative and qualitative review processes into a mixed-model approach [59]. Variations in how systematic reviews are conducted demonstrate the creative component (or the "art") of knowledge synthesis. Although these variations are exciting, there are limited examples of their use and even less methodological research validating them.

Future research

Research to assess various aspects of systematic review methodology and to help guide review prioritization and updating is needed. For example, is there sufficient evidence for duplicate screening in reviews given resource implications, or are sampling methods to check validity sufficient? Although new research is emerging on the importance of updating systematic reviews [60,61], suggested frequency, and methods of updating [62,63], more research is required on these topics. Additionally, the comparability of different systematic review approaches to answer the same question is unknown. For example, as rapid reviews emerge as a method to address timely but pressing topics, is there any evidence that different methods provide consistent results compared to more comprehensive reviews? Finally, methods to prioritize systematic review topics (e.g., scoping exercises) are becoming of interest and may warrant future research.

References

1 Chalmers I, Hedges LV, Cooper H. A brief history of research synthesis. *Eval Health Prof* 2002;25[1]:12–37.

2 Naylor CD. Clinical decisions: from art to science and back again. *Lancet* 2001;358[9281]:523–4.

3 Grimshaw JM, Santesso N, Cumpston M, Mayhew A, McGowan J. Knowledge for knowledge translation: the role of the Cochrane Collaboration. *J Contin Educ Health Prof* 2006;26[1]:55–62.

4 Graham ID, Logan J, Harrison MB, Straus SE, Tetroe J, Caswell W, et al. Lost in knowledge translation: time for a map? *J Contin Educ Health Prof* 2006;26[1]: 13–24.

5 Canadian Institutes of Health Research. Randomized controlled trials registration/application checklist. [document on the Internet]. 2006. URL http://www.cihr-irsc.gc.ca/e/documents/rct_reg_e.pdf [accessed July 30, 2008].

6 Graham ID, Tetroe J. Some theoretical underpinnings of knowledge translation. *Acad Emerg Med* 2007;14[11]:936–41.

7 The Cochrane Collaboration. [homepage on the Internet]. 2008. URL http://www.cochrane.org/ [accessed July 30, 2008].

8 Campbell Collaboration. [homepage on the Internet]. 2008. URL http://www.campbellcollaboration.org [accessed July 29, 2008].

9 Atkins D, Fink K, Slutsky J. Better information for better health care: the Evidence-based Practice Center program and the Agency for Healthcare Research and Quality. *Ann Intern Med* 2005;142[12 Pt 2]:1035–41.

10 Joanna Briggs Institute. [homepage on the Internet]. 2008. URL http://www.joannabriggs.edu.au/about/home.php [accessed July 29, 2008].

11 Petticrew M. Systematic reviews from astronomy to zoology: myths and misconceptions. *BMJ* 2001;322[7278]:98–101.

12 Stone PW. Popping the (PICO) question in research and evidence-based practice. *Appl Nurs Res* 2002;15[3]:197–8.

13 Higgins JPT, Green S (eds.). Cochrane handbook for systematic reviews of interventions. Version 5.0.0. [document on the Internet]. 2008. URL http://www.cochrane-handbook.org [accessed July 30, 2008].

14 Dixon-Woods M, Bonas S, Booth A, Jones DR, Miller T, Sutton AJ, et al. How can systematic reviews incorporate qualitative research? A critical perspective. *Qual Res* 2006;6[1]:27–44.

15 Gregoire G, Derderian F, Le LJ. Selecting the language of the publications included in a meta-analysis: is there a Tower of Babel bias? *J Clin Epidemiol* 1995;48[1]: 159–63.

16 Egger M, Zellweger-Zahner T, Schneider M, Junker C, Lengeler C, Antes G. Language bias in randomised controlled trials published in English and German. *Lancet* 1997;350[9074]:326–9.

17 Moher D, Pham B, Klassen TP, Schulz KF, Berlin JA, Jadad AR, et al. What contributions do languages other than English make on the results of meta-analyses? *J Clin Epidemiol* 2000;53[9]:964–72.

18 Juni P, Holenstein F, Sterne J, Bartlett C, Egger M. Direction and impact of language bias in meta-analyses of controlled trials: empirical study. *Int J Epidemiol* 2002;31[1]:115–23.

19 Pan Z, Trikalinos TA, Kavvoura FK, Lau J, Ioannidis JP. Local literature bias in genetic epidemiology: an empirical evaluation of the Chinese literature. *PLoS Med* 2005;2[12]:e334.

20 Hopewell S, McDonald S, Clarke M, Egger M. Grey literature in meta-analyses of randomized trials of health care interventions. *Cochrane Database Syst Rev* 2007; Issue 2. Art. No.: MR000010. DOI: 10.1002/14651858.MR000010. pub3.

21 Bhandari M, Devereaux PJ, Guyatt GH, Cook DJ, Swiontkowski MF, Sprague S, et al. An observational study of orthopaedic abstracts and subsequent full-text publications. *J Bone Joint Surg Am* 2002;84-A[4]:615–21.

22 Rosmarakis ES, Soteriades ES, Vergidis PI, Kasiakou SK, Falagas ME. From conference abstract to full paper: differences between data presented in conferences and journals. *FASEB J* 2005;19[7]:673–80.

23 Toma M, McAlister FA, Bialy L, Adams D, Vandermeer B, Armstrong PW. Transition from meeting abstract to full-length journal article for randomized controlled trials. *JAMA* 2006;295[11]:1281–7.

24 Scherer RW, Langenberg P, vonElm E. Full publication of results initially presented in abstracts. *Cochrane Database Syst Rev* 2007; Issue 2. Art. No.: MR000005. DOI: 10.1002/14651858.MR000005.pub3.

25 von Elm E, Costanza MC, Walder B, Tramer MR. More insight into the fate of biomedical meeting abstracts: a systematic review. *BMC Med Res Methodol* 2003;3:12.

26 U.S. National Library of Medicine. Medical literature analysis and retrieval system online - PubMed. [homepage on the Internet]. 2008. URL http://www.ncbi.nlm .nih.gov/PubMed [accessed March 19, 2008].

27 Excerpta Medica Database. [homepage on the Internet]. 2008. URL http://www .embase.com/ [accessed March 19, 2008].

28 Cochrane Central Register of Controlled Trials. The Cochrane Library. [homepage on the Internet]. 2008. URL http://www3.interscience.wiley.com/cgi-bin/ mrwhome/106568753/HOME [accessed March 18, 2008].

29 Tricco AC, Tetzlaff J, Sampson M, Fergusson D, Cogo E, Horsley T, et al. Few systematic reviews exist documenting the extent of bias: a systematic review. *J Clin Epidemiol*. In press 2008.

30 Luxembourg Convention Definition of Grey Literature: 3rd International Conference on Grey Literature: Luxembourg, 1997; updated in New York, 2004.

31 Gotzsche PC. Multiple publication of reports of drug trials. *Eur J Clin Pharmacol* 1989;36[5]:429–32.

32 Tramer MR, Reynolds DJ, Moore RA, McQuay HJ. Impact of covert duplicate publication on meta-analysis: a case study. *BMJ* 1997;315[7109]:635–40.

33 Bailey BJ. Duplicate publication in the field of otolaryngology-head and neck surgery. *Otolaryngol Head Neck Surg* 2002;126[3]:211–6.

34 Barden J, Edwards JE, McQuay HJ, Moore RA. Oral valdecoxib and injected parecoxib for acute postoperative pain: a quantitative systematic review. *BMC Anesthesiol* 2003;3[1]:1.

35 Moher D, Soeken K, Sampson M, Ben-Porat L, Berman B. Assessing the quality of reports of systematic reviews in pediatric complementary and alternative medicine. *BMC Pediatr* 2002;2:3.

36 Sanderson S, Tatt ID, Higgins JP. Tools for assessing quality and susceptibility to bias in observational studies in epidemiology: a systematic review and annotated bibliography. *Int J Epidemiol* 2007;36[3]:666–76.

37 Chan AW, Hrobjartsson A, Haahr MT, Gotzsche PC, Altman DG. Empirical evidence for selective reporting of outcomes in randomized trials: comparison of protocols to published articles. *JAMA* 2004;291[20]:2457–65.

38 Chan AW, Krleza-Jeric K, Schmid I, Altman DG. Outcome reporting bias in randomized trials funded by the Canadian Institutes of Health Research. *CMAJ* 2004;171[7]:735–40.

39 Chan AW, Altman DG. Identifying outcome reporting bias in randomised trials on PubMed: review of publications and survey of authors. *BMJ* 2005; 330[7494]:753.

40 Fleiss JL. The statistical basis of meta-analysis. *Stat Methods Med Res* 1993;2[2]: 121–45.

41 Egger M, Davey SG, Altman D. (eds.). *Systematic Reviews in Health Care: Meta-Analysis in Context*. 2nd ed. London: British Medical Journal Publishing Group; 2001.

42 Mays N, Pope C, Popay J. Systematically reviewing qualitative and quantitative evidence to inform management and policy-making in the health field. *J Health Serv Res Policy* 2005;10[Suppl 1]:6–20.

43 Sutton AJ, Abrams KR. Bayesian methods in meta-analysis and evidence synthesis. *Stat Methods Med Res* 2001;10[4]:277–303.

44 Spiegelhalter DJ, Myles JP, Jones DR, Abrams KR. Bayesian methods in health technology assessment: a review. *Health Technol Assess* 2000;4[38]:1–130.

45 Moher D, Cook DJ, Eastwood S, Olkin I, Rennie D, Stroup DF. Improving the quality of reports of meta-analyses of randomised controlled trials: the QUOROM statement. *Onkologie* 2000;23[6]:597–602.

46 Skalsky K, Yahav D, Bishara J, Pitlik S, Leibovici L, Paul M. Treatment of human brucellosis: systematic review and meta-analysis of randomised controlled trials. *BMJ* 2008;336[7646]:701–4.

47 Guyatt GH, Oxman AD, Vist GE, Kunz R, Falck-Ytter Y, onso-Coello P, et al. GRADE: an emerging consensus on rating quality of evidence and strength of recommendations. *BMJ* 2008;336[7650]:924–6.

48 Clarke L, Clarke M, Clarke T. How useful are Cochrane reviews in identifying research needs? *J Health Serv Res Policy* 2007;12[2]:101–3.

49 Moher D, Tetzlaff J, Tricco AC, Sampson M, Altman DG. Epidemiology and reporting characteristics of systematic reviews. *PLoS Med* 2007;4[3]:e78.

50 Atallah AN, de Silva EM, Paiva EV. Disseminating results of systematic reviews through a tv show in Brazil. *Syst Rev Evid Action Int Cochrane Colloq 6th 1998*, Baltimore; 2008, p. 77.

51 Oermann MH, Floyd JA, Galvin EA, Roop JC. Brief reports for disseminating systematic reviews to nurses. *Clin Nurse Spec* 2006;20[5]:233–8.

52 Stroup DF, Berlin JA, Morton SC, Olkin I, Williamson GD, Rennie D, et al. Meta-analysis of observational studies in epidemiology: a proposal for reporting. Meta-analysis of Observational Studies in Epidemiology (MOOSE) group. *JAMA* 2000;283[15]:2008–12.

53 Dawes M, Sampson U. Knowledge management in clinical practice: a systematic review of information seeking behavior in physicians. *Int J Med Inform* 2003;71[1]:9–15.

54 Glasziou P, Shepperd S. Ability to apply evidence from systematic reviews. *Society for Academic Primary Care* 2007;Jul 5.

55 Hartley J. Clarifying the abstracts of systematic literature reviews. *Bull Med Libr Assoc* 2000;88[4]:332–7.

56 McDonald JW, Mahon J, Zarnke K, Feagan B, Simms L, Tucker W. A randomized survey of the preference of gastroenterologists for a Cochrane review versus a traditional narrative review. *Can J Gastroenterol* 2002;16[1]:17–21.

57 Atkins S, Lewin S, Smith H, Engel M, Fretheim A, Volmink J. Conducting a meta-ethnography of qualitative literature: lessons learnt. *BMC Med Res Methodol* 2008;8:21.

58 Greenhalgh T, Robert G, Macfarlane F, Bate P, Kyriakidou O, Peacock R. Storylines of research in diffusion of innovation: a meta-narrative approach to systematic review. *Soc Sci Med* 2005;61[2]:417–30.

59 Harden A, Thomas J. Methodological issues in combining diverse study types in systematic reviews. *Int J Social Research Methodology* 2005;8: 257–71.

60 Shojania KG, Sampson M, Ansari MT, Ji J, Doucette S, Moher D. How quickly do systematic reviews go out of date? A survival analysis. *Ann Intern Med* 2007;147[4]:224–33.

61 Sampson M, Shojania KG, Garritty C, Horsley T, Ocampo M, Moher D. Systematic reviews can be produced and published faster. *J Clin Epidemiol* 2008;61[6]: 531–6.

62 Moher D, Tsertsvadze A, Tricco AC, Eccles M, Grimshaw J, Sampson M, et al. A systematic review identified few methods and strategies describing when and how to update systematic reviews. *J Clin Epidemiol* 2007;60[11]:1095–104.

63 Moher D, Tsertsvadze A, Tricco AC, Eccles M, Grimshaw J, Sampson M, et al. When and how to update systematic reviews. *Cochrane Database Syst Rev* 2008;[1]:MR000023.

64 Shekelle PG, Morton SC, Jungvig LK, Udani J, Spar M, Tu W, et al. Effect of supplemental vitamin E for the prevention and treatment of cardiovascular disease. *J Gen Intern Med* 2004;19[4]:380–9.

65 Lumley T. Network meta-analysis for indirect treatment comparisons. *Stat Med* 2002;21[16]:2313–24.

66 Elliott WJ, Meyer PM. Incident diabetes in clinical trials of antihypertensive drugs: a network meta-analysis. *Lancet* 2007;369[9557]:201–7.

67 Deeks J, Glanville J, Sheldon TA. *Undertaking Systematic Reviews of Research on Effectiveness: CRD Guidelines for Those Carrying Out or Commissioning Reviews.* Chichester, UK: John Wiley & Sons, Ltd; 1996.

68 Selman TJ, Mann C, Zamora J, Appleyard TL, Khan K. Diagnostic accuracy of tests for lymph node status in primary cervical cancer: a systematic review and meta-analysis. *CMAJ* 2008;178[7]:855–62.

69 Little J, Higgins JPT. (eds.). The HuGENet™ HuGE review handbook, version 1.0. [document on the Internet]. 2008. URL http://www.hugenet.ca [accessed July 30, 2008].

70 Wang GY, Lu CQ, Zhang RM, Hu XH, Luo ZW. The E-cadherin gene polymorphism 160C->A and cancer risk: a HuGE review and meta-analysis of 26 case-control studies. *Am J Epidemiol* 2008;167[1]:7–14.

71 Altman DG. Systematic reviews of evaluations of prognostic variables. *BMJ* 2001;323[7306]:224–8.

72 Oremus M, Raina PS, Santaguida P, Balion CM, McQueen MJ, McKelvie R, et al. A systematic review of BNP as a predictor of prognosis in persons with coronary artery disease. *Clin Biochem* 2007.

73 Pawson R, Greenhalgh T, Harvey G, Walshe K. Realist review–a new method of systematic review designed for complex policy interventions. *J Health Serv Res Policy* 2005;10[Suppl 1]:21–34.

74 Greenhalgh T, Kristjansson E, Robinson V. Realist review to understand the efficacy of school feeding programmes. *BMJ* 2007;335[7625]:858–61.

2.3 **Knowledge translation tools**

Melissa C. Brouwers[1], Dawn Stacey[2], and Annette M. O'Connor[3]

[1] Department of Clinical Epidemiology and Biostatistics, McMaster University, and
Canadian Partnership against Cancer Corporation, Hamilton, ON, Canada
[2] University of Ottawa School of Nursing, Ottawa, ON, Canada
[3] Department of Epidemiology, University of Ottawa School of Nursing, and Ottawa
Health Research Institute, Ottawa, ON, Canada

KEY LEARNING POINTS

Clinical practice guidelines:
- Translate evidence into clinical practice recommendations to assist in decisions by
  patients and providers
- Have the capacity to impact quality of care and systems performance
- Can be quality appraised using the Appraisal of Guideline Research and Evaluation
  (AGREE) tool

Patient decision aids:
- Translate evidence to inform patients about their options, help patients clarify the
  value they place on the benefits and harms of these options, and subsequently guide
  them in the process of decision making
- Improve patient participation in decision making, knowledge of options, and
  agreement between patient values and subsequent care decisions
- Can be quality appraised using International Patient Decision Aid Standards (IPDAS)

In Chapter 2.2, we outlined how knowledge syntheses can form the base unit
of KT tools, such as clinical practice guidelines and patient decision aids, that
are discussed in this chapter. When scientific evidence is available for decision making, outcomes can be classified as "black" (i.e., harmful: harms far
outweigh benefits) or "white" (i.e., beneficial: benefits far outweigh harms)
[1,2]. The goal in evidence based health care is to reduce overuse of black zone
treatments and improve underuse of white zone treatments. Clinical practice
guidelines represent an explicit approach to the outlining of black and white
zones within a defined clinical area. However, a review of 2500 treatments
found that only 17% had adequate scientific evidence to be classified as black
or white; the majority were "grey" either because of insufficient evidence or
because the balance between benefits and harms was close [2]. For grey zone

---

Knowledge Translation in Health Care: Moving from Evidence to Practice. Edited by S. Straus,
J. Tetroe, and I. Graham. © 2009 Blackwell Publishing, ISBN: 978-1-4051-8106-8.

decisions, patient decision aids have the potential to reduce practice variations and improve decision quality [1,3]. Together, clinical practice guidelines and patient decision aids represent vital elements of the knowledge creation component of the knowledge-to-action cycle [4].

Knowledge translation using clinical practice guidelines

What are clinical practice guidelines?

Evidence-based clinical practice guidelines are knowledge tools defined as systematically developed statements that help clinicians and patients make decisions about appropriate health care for specific clinical circumstances [5]. In addition, practice guidelines may inform decisions made by health care policy makers and clinical managers [6]. This definition is important because it articulates and defines what clinical practice guidelines are and what they are not. They are tools that, in addition to many other factors (e.g., values and preferences of patients, providers, and society; costs) aim to assist in decision making, not supplant it. They are not dictum or formulaic tactics to drive patient care. Indeed, clinical practice guidelines should facilitate high-quality practice informed by evidence, enable appropriate resource allocation, and advance research by identifying research gaps and areas in which additional research will not advance knowledge further.

How are clinical practice guidelines developed?

Well-articulated systematic and rigorous methodologies exist to ensure the creation of high-quality clinical practice guidelines. Guideline development requires a combination of methodological rigor and social engagement (Table 2.3.1). Ensuring that the appropriate stakeholders are involved is a key strategy to facilitate successful guideline development and implementation. Methodologically, clinical practice guidelines begin with a clinical question informed by a clinical or health care problem. As mentioned in Chapter 2.2, the PICO format can be used to formulate the question. Starting with a good question is key because it then informs the specific inclusion and exclusion of criteria used to design and execute a systematic review of research evidence. The evidentiary base is the foundation on which to make clinical recommendations. Recommendations should explicitly state the level of evidence that supports them. This process can be done with grading systems (e.g., GRADE [7]) or with language that explicitly describes the evidentiary base and study designs they are based on. There are pros and cons to both strategies [8,9].

The next step is an external review of draft clinical practice guidelines by key stakeholders and intended users of the recommendations. This review can improve the quality of clinical practice guidelines by identifying evidence that was missed and enabling stakeholders to endorse the interpretation of the

Table 2.3.1 Clinical practice guidelines: essential elements

- Establish multidisciplinary guideline team
- Identify clinical question that explicitly defines the patients, intervention/exposure, comparisons (if relevant), outcomes of interest and setting
- Conduct a systematic review of evidence
- Appraise and interpret evidence and come to consensus on its meaning
- Draft guideline recommendations that align with evidentiary base
- Complete an external review of draft report among intended users and key stakeholders
- Revise the guidelines in response to external review
- Read the final guideline report for distribution and dissemination
- Prepare implementation strategy

evidence by the developers, or by offering alternative interpretations. Furthermore, the review provides an opportunity to explore the "implementability" of recommendations, including an analysis of barriers and enablers, by their intended users and administrative and system leaders involved in the organization of health care services [10].

From a social engagement perspective, clinical practice guidelines can facilitate a culture of stakeholders who are receptive to, understand, and can apply evidence. To this end, the highest-quality and most effective clinical practice guidelines involve a development group consisting of a multidisciplinary team of stakeholders, including clinical and content experts, methodologists, and other users, such as patient representatives, researchers, policy makers, and funders. External review is also a form of social engagement. It creates a system of accountability between developers and the intended users of the clinical practice guidelines. It also provides a forum from which to engage stakeholders' endorsement of and intentions to use the recommendations. Only with the engagement of relevant stakeholders can a viable strategy for implementing the guidelines be developed.

There are several resources available to help in the development of clinical practice guidelines [10–13]. In addition, recent efforts by a group of international researchers, ADAPTE, have resulted in a rigorous methodology to enable clinical practice guidelines from one jurisdiction or context to be adapted for use in another [14], and this is discussed in Chapter 3.1. Within the guidelines enterprise, adaptation is identified as an important step toward reducing duplication in *de novo* guideline development, which can result in a tremendous financial and human resource cost.

Do clinical practice guidelines work?
The impact of clinical practice guidelines on practice and outcomes is complex. Systematic reviews by Grimshaw and others suggest that interventions to

implement clinical practice guidelines, or similar statements, do, on average, influence both the processes and the outcomes of care, although the effect sizes tend to be modest [15,16]. Interventions for implementation ranged from mass media interventions to use of local opinion leaders and include interventions that target the public, health care professionals, and managers, among others. However, the potential benefits of clinical practice guidelines are only as good as the quality of clinical practice guidelines. Interestingly, Grimshaw and colleagues [15] found in their review of 235 studies that the majority of studies used process outcomes for primary endpoints despite only three guidelines being explicitly based on evidence!

Although faithfulness to evidence-based principles is important, other factors believed to influence guideline uptake include adopters' perceptions of guideline characteristics and messages, perceptions of the development process, and factors related to norms and context [10,15–19]. An implementation strategy that includes analysis of enablers and barriers (Chapter 3.2), selection of appropriate and feasible KT interventions (Chapter 3.5.1), and indicators to measure impact (Chapter 3.6.1) increases the likelihood of success [4,10,15–19].

How do we determine the quality of clinical practice guidelines?

In reality, the quality of clinical practice guidelines can be variable and often falls short of basic standards. For example, Graham and colleagues appraised the quality of 217 Canadian drug therapy clinical practice guidelines produced between 1994 and 1999 and found that less than 15% of those reviewed met half or more of the 20 criteria for assessing the rigor of development; the overall mean score was 30% [20].

In response to this challenge, the Appraisal of Guidelines Research and Evaluation (AGREE) Collaboration was established to develop a valid and reliable instrument for assessing the quality of clinical practice guidelines (Table 2.3.2). AGREE defines guideline quality as the confidence that the biases linked to the rigor of development, presentation, and applicability of a clinical practice guideline have been minimized and that each step of the development process is clearly reported [21,22]. The AGREE instrument consists of 23 items targeting six quality domains (i.e., scope and purpose, stakeholder involvement, rigor of development, clarity of presentation, applicability, and editorial independence) and one global rating scale. The AGREE Next Steps initiative continues to build on this original work to improve the reliability and firmly establish validity of the instrument.

Although the AGREE instrument provides important criteria on which to evaluate clinical practice guidelines, the clinical validity, appropriateness of recommendations, and thorough analysis of the capacity to implement

Table 2.3.2 AGREE instrument domains

- Scope and purpose
- Stakeholder involvement
- Rigor of development
- Clarity and presentation
- Applicability
- Editorial independence

recommendations are not within its scope. Indeed, although there are currently no gold standards for these measures of quality, some advances have been made. For example, the Guideline Implementability Assessment (GLIA) tool provides a unique perspective by assessing the extent to which recommendations are computable in an information system [23,24]. The ADAPTE tool (Chapter 3.3) also provides criteria to evaluate the clinical fidelity of recommendations and their link to evidence [14].

Knowledge translating for patients using decision aids

What are patient decision aids?

Patient decision aids translate evidence into patient-friendly tools to inform patients about their options, help them clarify the value they place on benefits versus harms, and guide them in the process of decision making [25]. Evidence included in patient decision aids is defined as up-to-date scientific information on options, benefits and risks of options, and associated probabilities [26]. Formats for these tools include paper-based booklets, video/DVDs, decision boards, and internet-based materials. Patient decision aids are used as adjuncts to practitioner counselling for grey zone decisions in which the best choice depends on how patients weigh the benefits, risks, and scientific uncertainty (e.g., birth control, genetic testing, breast and prostate cancer treatment, options for menopause symptoms, back pain, osteoarthritis, level of end-of-life care). They differ from educational materials by not only providing option information but also by tailoring it to the patient's clinical risk profile and guiding patients to express their personal values. Figure 2.3.1 provides a sample page from a patient decision aid. Others are available on the website http://www.ohri.ca/DecisionAid/ (accessed May 8, 2008).

How are patient decision aids developed?

High-quality patient decision aids are developed using a systematic process and explicit guidelines and are available elsewhere [26]. The first step is to

1.0 Patient Decision Aid presentation of outcome probabilities

Blocks of 100 faces show a "best estimate" of what happens to **100 people** who choose different options [**specify time period**]. Each face [☺] stands for one person. The shaded areas show the number of people affected. There is no way of knowing in advance if you will be the one who is affected.

	OPTION A	OPTION B

Benefits

* [Fewer/More] people get a if they [insert option] .... →

15 get this   4 get this

Describe what it is like to experience this

85 avoid this   96 avoid this

Risks and Side Effects

* More people who [insert option] have **risk/side effect a** .... →

25 get this   52 get this

Describe what it is like to experience this

75 avoid this   48 avoid this

✳ or ✱ symbols mean stronger study results; ★ or ✚ mean weaker results.

2.0 Patient Decision Aid exercise to clarify patients' values for outcomes

Common reasons to choose each option are listed below.
Check ✓ how much each reason matters *to you* on a scale of 0 to 5.
"**0**" means it is **not** important to you. "**5**" means it is **very** important to you.

Reasons to choose OPTION A	Not Important	Very Important
How important is it to you to [get the benefit of option A]?	⓪ ① ② ③ ④ ⑤	
How important is it to you to [avoid a risk/side effect/inconvenience] of the option B]?............................	⓪ ① ② ③ ④ ⑤	
Reasons to choose OPTION B	Not Important	Very Important
How important is it to you to [get the benefit of option B]?	⓪ ① ② ③ ④ ⑤	
How important is it to you to [avoid a risk/side effect/inconvenience] of the option A]?	⓪ ① ② ③ ④ ⑤	

Figure 2.3.1 Example of selected components of a patient decision aid.

determine the decision-making needs of potential users (e.g., patients and practitioners). Needs assessments focus on the users' perceptions of the decision (i.e., options, outcomes, values), perceptions of others involved in the decision (e.g., decisional roles, opinions, pressures), and resources needed to make and/or implement the decision [27]. Second, the patient decision aid is based on a synthesis of the evidence and includes essential elements outlined in Table 2.3.3. To minimize bias and improve patient ability to understand the chances of outcomes, there are evidence-based criteria for

Table 2.3.3 Patient decision aids: essential elements

- Evidence-based information on the condition, options, and outcomes relevant to the patient's clinical situation
- Risk communication on the chances of outcomes and the level of scientific uncertainty
- Values clarification to ascertain which benefits, harms, and scientific uncertainties are most important to the patient
- Structured guidance in the steps of deliberating and communicating with practitioners and significant others

Table 2.3.4 IPDAS criteria for presenting probabilities of option outcomes

- Use event rates specifying the population and time period
- Compare outcome probabilities using the same denominator, time period, and scale
- Describe uncertainty around probabilities
- Use multiple methods to view probabilities [words, numbers, diagrams]
- Allow patient to view probabilities based on their own situation
- Place probabilities in context of other events
- Use both positive and negative frames

From [25,26].

displaying probabilities within patient decision aids (Table 2.3.4). Third, the decision aid is reviewed by a panel of experts, external to the development process. The panel may include clinicians, researchers, and patients among others. Finally, the patient decision aid is evaluated by end users. Defining a "good decision" is a challenge when there is no single "best" therapeutic action and choices depend on how patients value benefits versus harms. The International Patient Decision Aids Standards Collaboration (IPDAS) has reached a consensus on the criteria for judging decision quality (informed, preference-based) and processes leading to decision quality: recognize that a decision needs to be made; know options and their features; understand that values affect the decision; be clear about the option features that matter most; discuss values with their practitioner; and become involved in preferred ways. These standards are available at http://www.ipdas.ohri.ca.

Do patient decision aids work?

A recent review of 10 systematic reviews of patient decision aids showed that knowledge tools improve patients' participation in decision making, knowledge of options, and agreement between patients' values and the subsequent treatment or screening decisions [29]. However, impact on clinical outcomes is less clear [29]. When probabilities of outcomes are presented, patients have more realistic expectations of the chances of benefits, harms, and side effects. The use of elective surgery (e.g., hysterectomy, prostatectomy, mastectomy, coronary bypass surgery, back surgery) decreased in favor of more conservative options, without apparent adverse effects on health outcomes or anxiety. One trial evaluated the cost effectiveness of patient decision aids for women experiencing benign abnormal uterine bleeding [30]. Although there was no consistent effect on health status, those women who received information plus coaching to help them express their preferences had reduced hysterectomy rates compared to those in the control group (odds ratio 0.60 [95% confidence interval 0.38 to 0.96]) and to those who received information but no coaching (odds ratio 0.52 [95% confidence interval 0.33 to 0.82]). Health system costs were lower for those who received education and coaching around preferences.

A systematic review of 28 studies found that barriers to implementing patient decision aids in clinical practice include practitioner perception of patients' readiness to use them, forgetting to offer them to patients, practitioner belief that content was too complex or too simple, time required to make them available, outdated evidence, costs, and limited accessibility [31]. This review also found that patient decision aids are more likely to be used when there are positive effects on patient outcomes and/or the clinical process, when patients prefer to actively participate in decision making, and when health professionals are motivated to use them.

How do we determine the quality of patient decision aids?

Although many patient decision aids are available, like clinical practice guidelines, they are of varying quality [32]. As a result, the IPDAS Collaboration was established to reach agreement on criteria for developing and appraising their quality [26]. The IPDAS checklist has domains that include (1) essential content (providing information, presenting probabilities, clarifying values, guiding deliberation and communication); (2) development (systematic development process, balance, evidence base, plain language, disclosure); and (3) evaluation (decision quality) [26,33]. The IPDAS checklist is used to appraise available patient decision aids in the Cochrane Inventory at a publicly available website (www.ohri.ca/decisionaid). Validity and reliability of an IPDAS instrument is underway.

Future research

Research that is focused on developing strategies to enhance implementation of guidelines will be useful. And, more work is needed to show the impact of patient decision aids on clinical outcomes.

Summary

In view of findings from systematic reviews, clinical practice guidelines may improve patient outcomes and patient decision aids, therefore improving decision quality. Both knowledge translation tools show promise in decreasing practice variations and preventing overuse or underuse of health care options. Important in the development of high-quality clinical practice guidelines and patient decision aids is the systematic synthesis of the evidence to be used within these tools and the systematic iterative process of obtaining feedback from potential users. Ideally, systematic reviewers of clinical interventions should consider using these knowledge translation tools for communicating their findings in clinical practice.

References

1 Wennberg JE. Unwarranted variations in healthcare delivery: implications for academic medical centres. *BMJ* 2002;325[7370]:961–4.

2 Clinical Evidence. A guide to the text: Summary page. 2005. URL http://www .clinicalevidence.bmj.com/ceweb/about/knowledge.jsp [accessed May 27, 2008].

3 O'Connor AM, Bennett C, Stacey D, Barry MJ, Col NF, Eden KB, et al. Do patient decision aids meet effectiveness criteria of the International Patient Decision Aid Standards Collaboration? *Med Decis Making* 2007;27[5]:554–74.

4 Graham ID, Logan J, Harrison MB, Straus SE, Tetroe J, Caswell W, et al. Lost in knowledge translation: time for a map? *J Contin Educ Health Prof* 2006;26[1]:13–24.

5 Committee to Advise the Public Health Service on Clinical Practice Guidelines. Clinical Practice Guidelines: Directions for a New Program. Washington, DC: National Academy Press, 1990.

6 Browman GP, Snider A, Ellis P. Negotiating for change. The healthcare manager as catalyst for evidence-based practice: changing the healthcare environment and sharing experience. *Health Pap* 2003;3[3]:10–22.

7 Atkins D, Briss PA, Eccles M. Systems for grading the quality of evidence and the strength of recommendations. 2: Pilot study of a new system. *BMC Health Serv Res* 2005;5:25.

8 Guyatt G, Oxman A, Vist G, Kunz R, Falck-Ytter Y, Alonso-Coello P, et al. GRADE working group. An emerging consensus on rating quality of evidence and strength of recommendations. *BMJ* 2008;336:924–26.

9 Brouwers MC, Somerfield MR, Browman GP. A for effort: learning from the application of the GRADE approach to cancer guideline development. *JCO* 2008;26[7]:1025–26.

10 Palda VA, Davis D, Goldman J. A guide to the Canadian Medical Association Handbook on Clinical Practice Guidelines. *CMAJ* 2007;177[10]:1221–6.

11 Program in Evidence-Based Care Guidelines Manual [Web site of Cancer Care Ontario]. 2008. URL http://www.cancercare.on.ca.

12 Clinical guideline development methods [Web site of the National Institute for Health and Clinical Excellence]. 2007. URL http://www.nice.org.uk/aboutnice/howwework/developingniceclinicalguidelines/clinicalguidelinedevelopment methods/theguidelinesmanual2007/the_guidelines_manual_2007.jsp [accessed May 27, 2008].

13 SIGN 50a. A guideline developer's handbook. [Web site of the Scottish Intercollegiate Guidelines Network]. 2008. URL http://www.sign.ac.uk/guidelines/fulltext/50/index.html [accessed May 27, 2008].

14 ADAPTE Group. Adapte manual for guideline adaptation. 2007. URL http://www.adapte.org [accessed May 27, 2008].

15 Grimshaw J, Eccles M, Thomas R, MacLennan G, Ramsay C, Fraser C, et al. Toward evidence-based quality improvement. Evidence [and its limitations] of the effectiveness of guideline dissemination and implementation strategies 1966–1998. *J Gen Intern Med* 2006;21 Suppl 2:S14–S20.

16 Grimshaw JM, Thomas RE, MacLennan G, Fraser C, Ramsay CR, Vale L, et al. Effectiveness and efficiency of guideline dissemination and implementation strategies. *Health Technol Assess* 2004;8[6]:iii–iv,1–72.

17 Grol R. Successes and failures in the implementation of evidence-based guidelines for clinical practice. *Med Care* 2001;39[8 Suppl 2]:II46–54.

18 Grol R, Dalhuijsen J, Thomas S, Veld C, Rutten G, Mokkink H. Attributes of clinical guidelines that influence use of guidelines in general practice: observational study. *BMJ* 1998;317[7162]:858–61.

19 Grol R, Buchan H. Clinical guidelines: what can we do to increase their use? *Med J Aust* 2006;185[6]:301–2.

20 Graham ID, Beardall S, Carter AO, Glennie J, Hebert PC, Tetroe JM, et al. What is the quality of drug therapy clinical practice guidelines in Canada? *CMAJ* 2001;165[2]:157–63.

21 AGREE Collaboration Writing Group. Development and validation of an international appraisal instrucment for assessing the quality of clinical practice guidelines: the AGREE project. *Qual Saf Health Care* 2003[12]:18–21.

22 AGREE Research Trust. 2008. URL http://www.agreetrust.org [accessed May 27, 2008].

23 Schiffman R, Dixon J, Brandt C, Essaihi A, Hsiao A, Michel G, et al. The GuideLine Implementability Appraisal [GLIA]: development of an instrument to identify obstacles to guideline implementation. *BMC Medical Informatics and Decision Making* 2005;5:23.

24 Guideline Implementability Appraisal. 2008. URL http://www.nutmeg.med.yale .edu/glia/login.htm:jsessionid=CD3941C2E319D1A4D8B40718019A3B96 [accessed May 27, 2008].

25 O'Connor AM, Rostom A, Fiset V, Tetroe J, Entwistle V, Llewellyn-Thomas H, et al. Decision aids for patients facing health treatment or screening decisions: A Cochrane systematic review. *BMJ* 1999;319[7212]:731–4.

26 Elwyn G, O'Connor A, Stacey D, Volk R, Edwards A, Coulter A, et al. Developing a quality criteria framework for patient decision aids: online international Delphi consensus process. *BMJ* 2006;333[7565]:417.

27 Jacobsen MJ, O'Connor A. Population needs assessment: a workbook for assessing patients' and practitioners' decision making needs. 2006. URL http://decisionaid .ohri.ca/docs/implement/Population [accessed May 27, 2008].

28 Trevena LJ, Davey HM, Barratt A, Butow P, Caldwell P. A systematic review on communicating with patients about evidence. *J Eval Clin Pract* 2006[1]:13–23.

29 Coulter A, Ellins J. Effectiveness of strategies for informing, educating, and involving patients. *BMJ* 2007;335[7609]:24–7.

30 Kennedy AD, Sculpher MJ, Coulter A, Dwyer N, Rees M, Abrams KR, et al. Effects of decision aids for menorrhagia on treatment choices, health outcomes, and costs. A randomized controlled trial. *JAMA* 2002;288[21]:2701–8.

31 O'Connor AM, Stacey D, Entwistle V, Llewellyn-Thomas H, Rovner D, Holmes-Rovner M, et al. Decision aids for people facing health treatment or screening decisions. *Cochrane Database Syst Rev* 2003;[2]:CD001431.

32 Sepucha KR, Fowler FJ, Jr., Mulley AG, Jr. Policy support for patient-centered care: the need for measurable improvements in decision quality. *Health Aff* [Millwood] 2004;Suppl Web Exclusives:VAR54-62.

33 Gravel K, Legare F, Graham ID. Barriers and facilitators to implementing shared decision-making in clinical practice: a systematic review of health professionals' perceptions. *Implement Sci* 2006;1:16.

2.4 Searching for research findings and KT literature

K. Ann McKibbon and Cynthia Lokker

Department of Clinical Epidemiology and Biostatistics, McMaster University, Hamilton, ON, Canada

---

KEY LEARNING POINTS

- KT practitioners need to identify published and unpublished material related to elements of the KT action cycle. This material can be summaries of existing knowledge, demonstration projects, and summaries of successful and unsuccessful KT interventions, and material related to KT theory (e.g., models and frameworks).
- Many resources must be used to identify this material. Bzdel and colleagues have produced a document that helps those who want material important to KT practice.
- Many Internet sites include resources and tools useful for general and more focused KT areas. The abundance of sites makes finding material both easier and harder because the documents and resources one needs may be found in multiple places.
- The varied terminology across disciplines and geographic areas complicates retrieval. Standardization of definitions and acknowledgment of equivalent terms will make finding material easier.

Searching for evidence in health literature is difficult for almost any topic. The major problems involved in searching center around the time it takes, knowing the most promising resources to use, and how best to use the resource once it is selected [1]. The knowledge-to-action cycle prescribes the need to identify studies, research, synthesis, and knowledge tools comprising the knowledge creation funnel, as well as the need to identify literature on the KT process (e.g., KT theories, KT interventions).

People involved in KT research and practice benefit from using information from several categories. We need to identify evidence and evidence summaries (e.g., systematic reviews, clinical practice guidelines, health technology assessments [HTAs]). We also may need to identify evidence to develop knowledge syntheses that form the basis of guidelines, as discussed in Chapters 2.2 and 2.3. We need to identify successful KT interventions—evidence showcasing

---

Knowledge Translation in Health Care: Moving from Evidence to Practice. Edited by S. Straus, J. Tetroe, and I. Graham. © 2009 Blackwell Publishing, ISBN: 978-1-4051-8106-8.

KT applications that we can use to model projects. Also, information describing the theoretical basis (e.g., KT models or frameworks) is important for designing and evaluating KT [2].

This chapter has two purposes. First, we want to provide a description of where information we refer to above can be found. Second, we want to provide the vocabulary to use when searching in resources that may be encountered. We incorporate information from Bzdel and colleagues' useful Web resource [3] and encourage people to consult this guide as a starting point for almost any KT project or proposal.

Getting started: how do we find knowledge syntheses?

Evidence summaries or syntheses should provide the foundation of KT interventions. Busy practitioners do not have time to summarize the total evidence on important questions; researchers starting studies can also benefit from existing summaries. It is more efficient to use or build on existing well-done summaries of evidence than to produce new summaries. These summaries are even more useful if they are published in specific, multiple formats for such audiences as the public, patients, physicians, nurses, and policy staff. Several categories of summaries exist, and their identification varies by category. The largest category is systematic reviews, including meta-analyses. These are often published and indexed in large bibliographic databases, such as Medline and CINAHL (Cumulative Index to Nursing and Allied Health Literature) or in smaller databases. The health-evidence.ca site (http://www.health-evidence.ca/) provides systematic reviews in public health that are useful to decisionmakers. The Cochrane and Campbell Collaborations produce high-quality clinically important systematic reviews on all areas of health care (http://www3.interscience.wiley.com/cgi-bin/mrwhome/106568753/HOME?CRETRY=1&SRETRY=0) and social science (http://www.campbellcollaboration.org/frontend.aspx). The Joanna Briggs Institute in Australia produces systematic reviews in nursing and other health disciplines and provides access to many health discipline-specific resources (http://www.joannabriggs.edu.au/about/home.php). Reviews are also available from the UK Centre for Reviews and Dissemination at York University (http://www.york.ac.uk/inst/crd/crddatabases.htm). Their databases include reviews (Database of Reviews of Effects or DARE), economics studies (National Health Service Economic Evaluation Database), and health technology assessments (HTA Database). A searching guide for health technology assessments and similar material can be found at http://www.ahfmr.ab.ca/publications/?search=Internet+sources+of+information&type=1.

As mentioned in Chapter 2.3, clinical practice guidelines can be seen as evidence summaries that provide directions or recommendations for patient care. The largest site for guidelines is produced by the U.S. Agency for Healthcare Research and Quality (National Guidelines Clearinghouse at http://www.guideline.gov/). Although its title indicates national coverage, it includes many guidelines from other countries. The Canadian Medical Association provides links to Canadian guidelines (CMA infobase http://mdm.ca/cpgsnew/cpgs/index.asp). NICE (UK National Institute for Health and Clinical Evidence) produces UK guidelines [http://www.nice.org.uk/ and Chapter 2.3]). GIN or the Guidelines International Network brings together individuals and organizations committed to developing high-quality guidelines (http://www.g-i-n.net/index.cfm?fuseaction=about). However, most of these guidelines are not appraised for quality, and it would be useful to develop skills in appraising them for validity and importance prior to deciding on implementation. Criteria for assessing guideline validity are discussed in Chapter 2.3.

What should we do next: how do we search large databases?

If we cannot find a summary of the evidence in the sources listed or if we need original study results we go to such databases as Medline, the large bibliographic health care database that emphasizes medicine or CINAHL for material important to nursing and allied health professions. The Bzdel Resource Guide [3] describes other databases and resources important to KT. Librarians can help with searching or provide search training. Many online tutorials also exist. For example, the tutorial for PubMED, the easy-to-use, free Medline searching system, is located at http://www.nlm.nih.gov/bsd/disted/pubmedtutorial/.

Searching for articles on KT interventions or KT theory or frameworks is difficult. We are currently developing search filters to more easily identify KT material in Medline and CINAHL. These filters retrieve only material that deals with KT in relation to your choice of content (e.g., improving cancer screening rates or hand-washing programs). Filters currently exist as PubMed Clinical Queries that retrieve other content such as randomized controlled trials (http://www.ncbi.nlm.nih.gov/entrez/query/static/clinical.shtml) or qualitative studies and health services research (http://www.nlm.nih.gov/nichsr/hedges/search.html). Watch the KT clearinghouse Web site (www.ktaclearinghouse.ca) for this searching innovation by early 2009.

Should we search the Internet?

The Internet can provide access to technical reports and other nonjournal material related to KT. Google and its companion site, Google Scholar (which includes more scholarly documents than full Google), are good places to start. A summary of other non-Google search engines is located at http://searchenginewatch.com/showPage.html?page=2156221. Some Web sites allow you to search in multiple databases and resource collections with one searchwindow. One such resource that consolidates information that is useful to KT practitioners and researchers is the TRIP—Turning Research into Practice Web site: http://www.tripdatabase.com/index.html.

What are some existing collections of KT material?

Several sites collect and present KT material that is relevant to researchers and practitioners. These sites are described in Table 2.4.1.

How do we search the grey literature?

Grey literature is information that is not under the jurisdiction of commercial publishers. This material is often published by all levels government, academic centers, and businesses in electronic or paper format and is difficult to identify and obtain. Grey literature is especially important to those involved in public health KT. University of British Columbia describes how to search for unpublished literature (http://toby.library.ubc.ca/subjects/subjpage2 .cfm?id=877), and the New York Academy of Medicine collects grey literature related to health services research and public health (http://www.nyam.org/ library/pages/grey_literature_report). European grey literature is available through SIGLE (System for Information in Grey Literature in Europe, http://opensigle.inist.fr/), and information about searching for grey literature related to HTAs and economics studies is found at the HTAi Vortal: http://216.194.91.140/vortal/.

How can we search for literature about KT?

Several characteristics make searching for material related to KT interventions and theory more difficult. KT is a new field that interrelates with several existing disciplines. This complexity leads to an evolving and varied vocabulary with multiple terms for the same concept. For example, as outlined in Chapter 1.1, Canadian researchers use the term *knowledge translation,*

Table 2.4.1 Sites that provide KT material, tools, or both

Site name and Web location	Material contained
Atlantic Health Promotion Research Centre KT Library, Dalhousie University http://www.ahprc.dal.ca/kt/library.cfm	This is a searchable database for KT-related resources (including information and resources about stroke and how organizational and health systems resources affect an organization's ability to absorb and apply research evidence).
Canadian Health Services Research Foundation http://www.chsrf.ca/knowledge_transfer/index.e.php	This provides tools in this section to help make "linkage and exchange"—the regular sharing of issues and results between researchers and the people who need research—easier. This provides other reports and publications of interest.
Centre for Health & Environment Research KT Database, University of British Columbia http://www.web.cher.ubc.ca/ktdatabase/	This online database is full of knowledge translation resources that have been selected based on their relevance to research in environmental and occupational health and health policy.
Cochrane Effective Practice and Organisation of Care Group, University of Ottawa http://www.epoc.cochrane.org/en/index.html	The focus of EPOC is on reviews of interventions designed to improve professional practice and the delivery of effective health services. This includes various forms of continuing education, quality assurance, informatics, financial, organisational and regulatory interventions that can affect the ability of health care professionals to deliver services more effectively and efficiently.
Institute of Knowledge Transfer, UK— The Institute of Knowledge Transfer (IKT) is an independent, democratic, and not-for-profit professional body, established to promote the interests of the profession and the practice of "knowledge transfer" (KT). http://www.ikt.org.uk/index.aspx	A library is planned for 2008.

KT+, McMaster University http://plus.mcmaster.ca/kt/Default.aspx

"KT+ provides access to current evidence on "T2" knowledge translation (i.e., research addressing the knowledge-to-practice gap), including published original articles and systematic reviews on health care quality improvement, continuing professional education, computerized clinical decision support, health services research, and patient adherence. Its purpose is to inform those working in the knowledge translation area of current research as it is published."

KU-UC (Knowledge Utilization—Utilisation des Connaissances), Laval Université http://kuuc.chair.ulaval.ca/english/index.php

"The KU-UC Bibliography search engine allows you to find bibliographic references on innovation and smart practices, dissemination and utilization of social sciences research, knowledge dissemination and utilization in health services, and utilization of evaluation research."

U.S. National Center for the Dissemination of Disability Research library http://www.ncddr.org/ktinfocenter/

"The KT Library is designed to provide information to NCDDR grantees and interested members of the public about a wide spectrum of knowledge translation and evidence-based resources." (disability research KT)

Research Transfer Network of Alberta (RTNA) Alberta Heritage Foundation for Medical Research http://www.ahfmr.ab.ca/rtna/index.php

This group collects and makes available its publications including conference reports, proceedings, and water cooler discussions.

Table 2.4.1 (*Continued*)

Site name and Web location	Material contained
Research Utilization Support and Help (RUSH) Southeastern Educational Developmental Laboratory, Austin TX http://www.researchutilization.org/index.html	This site has a KT tool box of resources associated with disabilities and rehabilitation. Also a nice list of demonstration projects.
CIHR KT Clearinghouse, University of Toronto http://www.k2a.utoronto.ca/ktclearinghouse/home	Another site of tools for all areas of KT practice and research.
National Coordinating Centre for Methods and Tools. Public Health Agency of Canada http://www.nccph.ca/index.php?pid=18	A set of tools and methods concentrating on public health in Canada and elsewhere.
Keenan Research Centre—Research Programs Joint Program in Knowledge Translation—Literature http://www.stmichaelshospital.com/research/ktliterature.php	"RDRB (Research and Development Resource Base) is a literature database focusing specifically on continuing education, continuing professional development, and knowledge translation in the health disciplines." This resource is comprehensive and covers many years.
Program in Policy Decision-Making at McMaster University, Canada http://www.researchtopolicy.ca/whatisnew/	"Through a partnership between McMaster University's Program in Policy Decision-Making and the Canadian Cochrane Network and Centre, we have created an inventory of systematic reviews of governance, financial, and delivery arrangements within health systems from two sources: (1) a manual search of the Cochrane Library (Issue 3, 2007), and (2) an overview of reviews being led by members of the Cochrane Collaboration's Effective Practice and Organization of Care (EPOC) review group (with the search completed up to February 2004 and an updated search currently in progress)."

whereas US and UK researchers may use the terms *research utilization, implementation,* or *diffusion.* Those in business use terms related to marketing, advertising, and change management, whereas engineers speak of technology transfer. Individual clinicians deal with adoption of new techniques and evidence-based practice, whereas policy makers speak of evidence-informed decisions. Table 2.4.2 provides a list of KT-related terms hat we have identified in our attempt to develop a search filter for KT material. The terms themselves are useful for search strategies. A wiki (http://whatiskt.wikispaces.com/) includes these terms and their definitions and we invite you to enhance this site with your knowledge and experience. Bzdel et al. [3] provide insight on searching for KT theories and frameworks. Additionally, named theories can be searched on the Internet and in large databases. The KT filters project will help identify these papers.

Future research

The main areas of research involved in the searching for material relevant to KT researchers and practitioners include production of searching filters for Medline and CINAHL. We need more data on proven retrieval methods for Internet-based resources. A related matter is the need to find consensus on definitions and mapping of terms across disciplines (e.g., Is technology transfer in engineering equivalent to translational research for the U.S. National Institutes of Health or knowledge translation for CIHR?). We also may be able to develop search engines that can search effectively across the many KT resources and sites (Table 2.4.1).

Summary

Searching for existing knowledge is a major foundation of KT. Producing and summarizing existing evidence from multiple sources to address knowledge or action gaps is one of the first tasks of KT. Once this is done, those involved in KT work need to learn about methods and tools used in previous KT projects, how best to build new programs, and the theoretical constructs of KT. Searching for evidence to summarize existing summaries in various formats and for knowledge about KT programs and theory is difficult for many reasons, including vocabulary and its multidisciplinary nature. Using the resources in this chapter, as well as contacting librarians and others experienced in searching, will help you on your road to successful searching.

Table 2.4.2 Terms used by various stakeholder groups for KT activities/components

Applied dissemination	Knowledge synthesis
Applied health research	Knowledge to action
Best practices adoption	Knowledge transfer/ transformation/translation
Capacity building	Knowledge uptake/utilization
Change implementation	Knowledge synthesis, transfer, and exchange
Changing provider/physician/doctor behavior	KSTE
Collaborative development	
Competing	Linkage and exchange
Complex interventions	Opinion leaders
Complexity science/studies	Patient education
Continuing (medical/nursing/dental) education	Patient safety
Cooperation	Popularization of research
Co-optation	Professional behavior/behavior change
Crossing the quality chasm	
Diffusion of innovations	Quality assurance/ improvement
Diffusion(s)	Research capacity
Dissemination	Research implementation
Effective dissemination	Research into action/practice
Effectiveness research	Research mediation
Evaluation research	Research transfer/translation
Evidence uptake	Research utilization
Evidence-based medicine/nursing/practice	Science communication
Feedback and audit (audit and feedback)	Teaching
Gap analysis	Technology transfer
Gap between evidence and practice	Third mission
Getting knowledge into practice	Third wave
GRIP	Total quality assurance/quality improvement
Guideline implementation	Transfer of technologies
Impact	Translating research into practice
Implementation	Translation research
Implementation research/science	Translational research
Implementation science interventions/strategies	Transmission
Implementing research evidence	Turning research into practice
Information dissemination and utilization	TRIP
Innovation adaptation/adoption/diffusion	Utilization
Know-do	
Know-do gap	
Knowledge adoption/brokering	
Knowledge communication/cycle	
Knowledge development and application	
Knowledge diffusion/dissemination	
Knowledge exchange/management	
Knowledge mobilization(mobilization)	

References

1 Ely JW, Osheroff JA, Ebell MH, Chambliss ML, Vinson DC, Stevermer JJ, et al. Obstacles to answering doctors' questions about patient care with evidence: qualitative study. *BMJ* 2002;324[7339]:710.
2 Sudsawad, P. Knowledge translation: introduction to models, strategies, and measures. [Web site of the Southwest Educational Development Laboratory, National Center for the Dissemination of Disability Research]. 2008. URL http://www.ncddr.org/kt/products/ktintro/ [accessed March 26, 2008].
3 Bzdel L, Winther C, Graham P. Knowledge Utilization Resource Guide. 2004. URL http://www.nursing.ualberta.ca/KUSP/Resources/KU%20Resource%20Guide/KUResourceGuide.pdf [accessed March 26, 2008].

Section 3
The Knowledge-to-Action Cycle

3.1 **The action cycle**

Sharon E. Straus

Li Ka Shing Knowledge Institute, St. Michael's Hospital, and Department of Medicine, University of Toronto, Toronto, ON, Canada

The action cycle is the process by which knowledge is implemented. The action phases were derived from a review of 31 planned action theories [1]. Planned action theories focus on deliberately engineering change in health care systems and groups (although many policy maker targeted interventions may also focus on facilitating their access to research on short timelines, not just efforts to bring knowledge to their attention and to support action based on this knowledge). Included are the processes needed to implement knowledge in health care settings; namely, identifying problems and the relevant research; adapting the research to the local context; assessing determinants of KT; selecting, tailoring, implementing, monitoring, and evaluating KT interventions; and determining strategies for ensuring sustained knowledge use.

A group may start the knowledge-to-action process by determining the evidence to practice gap (Chapter 3.2). The knowledge relevant to this problem is then adapted to the local context (Chapter 3.3). Adapting the knowledge to local context extends to assessing barriers and facilitators to knowledge implementation (Chapter 3.4). The action cycle continues with selecting, tailoring, and implementing the KT intervention (Chapter 3.5). Strategies for monitoring knowledge use and evaluating its impact on relevant outcomes must then be developed (Chapter 3.6) along with a plan for sustained knowledge use. (Chapter 3.7). It must be noted that the action cycle is a dynamic and iterative process—with each phase informing the others, and the knowledge creation funnel potentially informing each phase.

Reference

1 Graham ID, Logan J, Harrison MB, Straus SE, Tetroe J, Caswell W, et al. Lost in knowledge translation: time for a map? *J Contin Ed Health Prof* 2006 Winter;26[1]:13-24.

Knowledge Translation in Health Care: Moving from Evidence to Practice. Edited by S. Straus, J. Tetroe, and I. Graham. © 2009 Blackwell Publishing, ISBN: 978-1-4051-8106-8.

3.2 Identifying the knowledge-to-action gaps

Alison Kitson[1] and Sharon E. Straus[2]

[1] Templeton College, University of Oxford, Oxford, UK
[2] Li Ka Shing Knowledge Institute, St. Michael's Hospital, and Department of Medicine, University of Toronto, Toronto, ON, Canada

---

KEY LEARNING POINTS

- Identifying the knowledge-to-action gap is the starting point of knowledge implementation and should involve rigorous methods and relevant stakeholders.

- Strategies for needs assessments depend on the purpose of the assessment, the type of data, available resources, and whether the needs are subjectively versus objectively measured.

- Needs assessments can occur from the perspective of the population, the provider organization, or the health care provider.

What is a "gap"?

One of the first steps in knowledge implementation is assessing the need for knowledge or measuring the "gap" between evidence and practice or policy making [1]. By evidence, we mean the best available research evidence [2]. Ideally, this evidence should come from high-quality practice guidelines or systematic reviews.

Quality indicators can be used as a basis for assessing gaps [3]. The Institute of Medicine's work on patient safety [4], as well as studies highlighting inadequate quality of care [5], have stimulated interest in quality indicators. Quality indicators are measures that monitor, assess, and improve quality of care and organizational functions that affect patient outcomes. Donabedian proposed a framework for quality of care that separates quality into structure, process, and outcome that can be used to categorize quality indicators [6]. Important components of a quality indicator include a descriptive statement, a list of data elements that are necessary for constructing and reporting this measure, detailed specifications on how data elements are to

---

Knowledge Translation in Health Care: Moving from Evidence to Practice. Edited by S. Straus, J. Tetroe, and I. Graham. © 2009 Blackwell Publishing, ISBN: 978-1-4051-8106-8.

be collected, the population on whom the indicator is constructed, the timing of data collection and reporting, the analytic models used to construct the measure, the format in which the results will be presented, and the evidence in support of its use [7]. As with any measurement tool, quality indicators should be valid, reliable, and feasible. Although many countries have instituted national strategies to collect quality indicators for benchmarking in a performance measurement setting [8], there is little agreement on optimal quality indicators across countries.

Quality indicators should be developed through careful consideration of the best available evidence, such as evidence from systematic reviews and the use of an appropriate rating process. Investigators at RAND Health modified the Delphi method to develop quality indicators [9]. Their process involves rounds of anonymous ratings on a risk–benefit scale and an in-person discussion between rounds [3,10]. The goal is to include all relevant stakeholders, and this is probably a key factor in successfully developing quality indicators. This process should be followed by testing of the indicator in real practice settings [10]. A similar process for developing quality indicators is through the use of evidence-based practice guidelines. In this method, a panel of relevant stakeholders develops indicators based on the guidelines.

Although many practice and policy-making gaps can be identified in various settings, it is important to establish a process for selecting which ones to target [10]. Strategies include considering the burden of disease, such as morbidity, mortality, quality of life, and cost. These discussions should involve all relevant stakeholder groups. A modified Delphi process can facilitate this process. Box 3.2.1 provides an example of how a clinician or manager can identify a practice gap. Box 3.2.2 illustrates a gap assessment exercise performed at an organizational level by an acute care hospital [11].

How can we measure the gap?

Needs assessments are a systematic process for determining the size and nature of the gap between current and more desirable knowledge, skills, attitudes, behaviors, and outcomes. Needs assessment strategies depend on the purpose of the assessment, the type of data, and the resources that are available. Needs classification includes felt needs (what people say they need), expressed needs (expressed through action), normative needs (defined by experts), and comparative needs (group comparisons) [14]. We can consider this issue from the perspective of the population, the provider organization, or the health care provider and whether needs are subjectively or objectively measured [15].

Box 3.2.1 Identifying a gap at the practice level

Emily was a newly appointed manager in a unit specializing in caring for people with severe learning and physical disabilities. She discovered that a routine had developed on the unit in which the night nursing staff distributed the morning medications to the clients at 6 a.m. rather than at the prescribed times. Emily knew that the staff was colluding with each other to sign for dispensing medications, at times identified in the paperwork but not followed. When she asked the night duty staff about this issue, staff members said they were doing it to help the day staff and they did not see anything wrong with this practice. Emily's view was that this was a potentially unsafe practice and needed to be altered immediately. She informed her immediate line manager about this practice and told her she was going to change the behavior. Initially, Emily met with hostility from the nursing staff. It was perceived that she was an outsider and had no "right" to change a practice that worked well and was valued by all the nursing staff.

Emily gathered a range of documents on safe practice, on professional standards, and on the safe and effective administration of medications and shared this with her colleagues. She told them she was changing the practice with immediate effect because, in her professional judgment, it was unsafe. She organized training sessions where she took charge of the medication round and demonstrated how to dispense medications at the allotted time.

In this case, the gap was discovered by an outsider to the system who saw it with fresh eyes. The identification of the problem by an outsider was both an advantage and a disadvantage. Advantageous in that Emily was able to assess routine practices and offer a judgment about them; disadvantageous in that her "outsider" status alienated her from the group norms and processes.

Measuring the gap at the population level

At the population level, we can consider the needs of the population by using epidemiological data—objective assessment measures. Administrative databases are sometimes called claims databases. They are a byproduct of administering and reimbursing health care services [16]. Typically, they include information on diagnosis (International Classification of Diseases, 10th Revision, Clinical Modification or ICD-10), procedures, laboratory investigations, billing information, and demographic information. Many administrative databases that can be used for this purpose exist. They range from regional databases (e.g., the Ontario Ministry of Health and Long-term Care [17]) to national databases (e.g., Medicare Provision and Analyses Review [MedPAR] Files). These databases have been used to identify

Box 3.2.2 Identifying gaps at an acute care hospital

In a project aimed at improving the experience of older people in an acute care hospital in Australia, the "gaps" in the service had been identified by many national reports and clinical guidelines on the management of delirium, continence, functional assessment, and pain management. The author (AK) developed an exploratory study to involve interdisciplinary teams in prioritizing a set of clinical areas where, following a structured assessment of the gaps between actual practice and best practice standards (based on the best available evidence), a set of action plans would be drawn up and implemented following a standard quality improvement methodology. The process involved an initial 2-day stakeholder workshop targeted at all the unit and ward managers in the acute care hospital. Staff were invited to share "patients' accounts of care" (both positive and negative), respond to local data on performance of nursing activities such as hydration, nutrition, continence, mobility compared with evidence based standards, and review trends in these data over 3 years. Participants completed a prioritization exercise using a template (Table 3.2.1) to agree on seven clinical interventions to improve patient care. Participants voted for the top seven areas and requests for volunteer "leads" and "deputy leads" for each topic were put forward. Fourteen volunteers were involved in a number of training workshops in these topic areas and were supported to lead a process of identifying the problem or gaps in practice, setting the standard (based on best available evidence), developing the protocol, undertaking the baseline audit, developing the implementation plan, doing the repeat audit, and reporting and disseminating the results. Methods used to help the group identify the gaps in current practice included standard quality improvement techniques such as affinity diagrams (Figure 3.2.1). In addition to these tools, other techniques such as direct observation of patient care and patient storytelling [12,13] were used.

In this project, the chronic problems faced by older people, which were well known by the nursing staff, had a legitimate cause for action because they were part of a national policy and were supported by the senior management team in the hospital. The gaps and needs in the system therefore had a route through which they could be identified in a positive way, and there was commitment from management to support actions to improve the situation.

undertreatment of cardiovascular risk factors in diabetes patients [18] and overuse of benzodiazepines in elderly patients [19]. However, limitations of these databases must be considered. First, they were not developed for research and thus may not contain all the information that will be useful for

Definition

An affinity diagram is used for gathering and organising ideas, opinions, or issues into common themes and to summarize information into manageable and structured components. A problem can be better understood by collating ideas into a broad framework that illustrates the problem being examined.

Purpose

An affinity diagram may be used for:
• Providing structure to a large or complicated issue. This is useful when identifying the central issues involved in developing a new service or product.
• Dividing a complicated issue into broad categories. This is useful when identifying the major steps for completion of a complex project.
• Gaining agreement on an issue or situation, such as needing to identify the direction to be taken in achieving a goal and for achieving consensus.

Method

Steps in constructing an affinity diagram:
1 Start with a clear statement of the problem or issue to be explored.
2 Brainstorm ideas and record these on individual cards or adhesive notes.
3 Group the ideas according to common themes by placing the cards or notes on a table, whiteboard, or butchers paper and move them to positions that the group thinks fit best. Continue to sort until team members are satisfied with the groupings. If there are some issues that do not seem to fit into any group, leave these cards to one side.
4 Create short, descriptive statements that best illustrate the theme for each group of ideas and use these as title cards through group discussion and consensus.
5 Items can be moved from one group to another if consensus emerges during discussion.
6 Consider additional brainstorming to capture new ideas using the group titles to stimulate thinking.
7 Large groupings can be further divided into subgroups by creating subtitles.
8 When the number of ideas has been reduced into manageable groupings, draw the affinity diagram connecting all the title cards with their grouping of ideas.
9 Discuss and prioritize the issues according to their relative importance and the potential impact on current performance.

RAH Safety, Quality & Risk Resource—Affinity Diagram Toolkit, October 2006, with permission [11].

Figure 3.2.1 Affinity diagram (example of a process to identify gaps in routines).

gap analysis, including severity of illness data [20]. Second, coding may be incomplete because there may be limited space for secondary diagnoses [16]. Third, only events for which there are codes can be found [16]. Fourth, the databases may not include the entire population. For example, the Medicare files include only those patients eligible for Medicare, which includes people 65 years and older, some people under 65 with disabilities, and all people with end-stage renal disease, who require renal replacement therapy.

Clinical databases can also be used to perform gap analyses. Clinical databases include registries of patients who have undergone specific procedures or who have certain diagnoses. Examples include the National Cardiac Surgical, Vascular, and Colorectal cancer databases in the United Kingdom [21]. These registries may have data that complement data in administrative databases, including more information on secondary diagnoses and comorbidities. Therefore, clinical databases can sometimes be used in combination with administrative databases to provide additional detail on practice gaps [21]. However, some studies have shown a lack of agreement between administrative and clinical databases [22]. These databases have limitations, including lack of information accuracy.

Measuring the gap at the organization level

Needs assessments at the organization level may be done at the hospital or clinical level. Hospitals in many countries are required by accreditation bodies (e.g., the Joint Commission on the Accreditation of Health Care Organisations [JCAHO]) to collect information on infection control, mortality, and restraint use [23]. This data source could be used to collect information on gaps. With the growing use of computerized health care records in hospitals and community settings, these tools can also extract data for gap assessment [24]. Chart audits can be done to review and assess health records using preset standardized criteria. In chart audits, documented clinical care is measured against review criteria, which is defined as "a systematically developed statement that can be used to assess the appropriateness of specific health-care decisions, services and outcomes" [25]. Ideally, review criteria should be based on valid evidence for the quality indicator and include objective measures, such as target levels of blood pressure and blood glucose in patients at elevated risk of a vascular event.

The Donabedian framework for considering quality of care, which separates quality into structure, process, and outcome, can also be used when considering a chart audit [6]. For example, if we want to look at the issue of prophylaxis against deep vein thrombosis (DVT) in patients admitted to the intensive care unit, structural measures include the availability of DVT prophylaxis (e.g., low molecular weight heparin) at the institution. Process

Table 3.2.1 Criteria for identifying gaps in practice [26]

Criteria for topic selection (identifying gaps in practice):
Yes   No   N/A

Instructions:
For each clinical topic area your group has identified, go through the following questions and answer yes, no, or N/A (not applicable). Identify the top five topics with the most "yes" responses.

Is it an area of clinical concern?

Is it an area of concern to older people?

Do guidelines/best practice sheets/standards/evidence exist that you could use?

Is baseline data available to indicate what performance is like currently?

Is there sufficient interest from the multidisciplinary team to support work on this topic?

Does the topic have a local ward champion?

Does the topic have support from management?

Would doing something be:

   Feasible

   Practical

   Achievable

   Desirable

Would the work apply to all in-patient areas?

---

measures include DVT prophylaxis prescriptions, such as heparin, in the critical care unit. Outcome measures include DVT risk in these patients. Assessing frequency of DVT in these patients would require a larger sample size than would be required if we looked at process measures. This highlights one of the advantages of process measures. Other strategies when completing a chart audit are available from NorthStar, a European initiative focused on quality improvement [26]. Table 3.2.1 shows an approach we can consider when completing a baseline measurement.

Paper health records remain more common than electronic health records, but they may not be as accurate. Rethans found that although paper health records commonly report information on diagnostic tests, they often omit counseling details [27]. Moreover, paper records are prone to lack of standardization and illegibility [28]. Computerized health records may have more accurate data on medications and diagnostic tests [29]. Finally, a key issue to consider when planning a chart audit is privacy and security of health information. Privacy regulations for data from health records vary regionally

Table 3.2.2 Questions to consider when beginning a chart audit

Questions about comparing actual and desired clinical practice	Yes / No / Not sure

Before you measure

- Have you secured sufficient stakeholder interest and involvement?
- Have you selected an appropriate topic?
- Have you identified the right sort of people, skills, and resources?
- Have you considered ethical issues?

What to measure

- Should your criteria be explicit or implicit?
- Should your criteria relate to the structure, process, or outcomes of care?
- Do your criteria have sufficient impact to lead to improvements in care?
- What level of performance is appropriate to aim for?

How to measure

- Is the information you need available?
- How are you identifying an appropriate sample of patients?
- How big should your sample be?
- How will you choose a representative sample?
- How will you collect the information?
- How will you interpret the information?

Reproduced from NorthStar (www.rebeqi.org) [26].

and nationally. Some institutions consider an audit part of standard care, thus it is not subject to institutional review requirements. The need for an ethics review of the audit process should be determined before any project is started.

Measuring the gap at the care provider level

At the care provider level, several strategies can be used for needs assessment, including chart audits, observation, competency assessment, and reflective practice. Direct observation of provider performance can be completed using standardized patients [30] or videorecording [31]. Similarly, competency assessments, including knowledge questionnaires, can be completed. These can be done as certification requirements for the American Board of Internal Medicine [32] or by completing clinical vignettes [33]. Finally, reflective practice, in which clinicians highlight learning opportunities or portfolios using their own experiences, can be considered [34]. However, these more subjective forms of assessment are less accurate for determining needs. Sibley and colleagues observed that clinicians tend to pursue education around topics they already know, while avoiding areas in which they are deficient. This has also been found in systematic reviews of self-assessment by physicians [35,36]. Although surveys, interviews, and focus groups can form needs assessments, they are more subjective and may not accurately reflect true gaps in practice.

Why do gaps exist?

Although audits are a method for obtaining information about practice gaps, be cautioned that it is easy to use practice gaps to blame clinicians. However, evidence of action gaps often reflect systems issues and not solely provider performance [27]. For this reason, we need to look beyond the evidence of a practice gap to determine the "why." Van de Ven [37] argues that in our quest to develop knowledge and translate it into practice, we underestimate what we already know about human behavior; namely, that human beings have problems in paying attention to nonroutine tasks. Also, it is well established that most individuals find dealing with complexity and remembering complex information challenging [38,39]. By contrast, most individuals are efficient processors of routine tasks. They do not concentrate on repetitive tasks once they master them. Skills for performing repetitive tasks are repressed in our subconscious memory, allowing us to pay attention to things other than the performance of the repetitive task [40]. The consequence is that what most individuals do most frequently is what they think about the least. If they do not have ways of evaluating the impact of these routine tasks, then imagine the "drift" that could occur in terms of performance to acceptable standards, norms, and knowledge bases.

March and Simon [41] argue that dissatisfaction with existing conditions stimulates people to seek improved conditions and that they will stop searching when they find a satisfactory result. Satisfactory results are conceptualized as a function of a person's aspiration level (i.e., their internal value system) and the culmination of all past successes and failures they bring to bear on their work experiences [42]. Another problem must be addressed from the social and cognitive psychological literature—the individual's tendency to unconsciously adapt to slowly changing environments, which leads him to tolerate extreme (and possibly dangerous) variations in a process without becoming aware of it [41]. This unconscious adaptation to deteriorating conditions is a feature of all systems, including workers' thresholds for tolerating discomfort (moral or physical). Dissatisfaction (with relationships, behaviors, attitudes, self-worth) is exacerbated to a point where individuals do not move to correct or alleviate their situation because they can no longer see how far they have drifted from their original starting point. Opportunities for new ideas or the introduction of new knowledge are not recognized, problems become critical situations and at the extreme, catastrophes are the inevitable consequence of a system that has drifted far away from its ability to get feedback on routine tasks [43].

At the group and organizational levels, the problems of inertia, conformity, and incompatible preferences are added to the range of individual limitations [43]. Processes and systems within large organizations become the "rules" against which teams working within these organizations evaluate their behavior. If no one in the hierarchy objects to the behavior, the declining status quo is legitimized. Such stark descriptions of the entropic nature of organizations are becoming more commonplace and accepted within organizational theory literature [44,45]. However, in the professionally driven health care system, we may not be aware of the pervasive and potentially negative effects of routinized thinking and our inability to think creatively and objectively about our everyday procedures. We should acknowledge three realities:
- Most people (professionals included) operate on "automatic pilot," spending the least amount of reflective thinking time on tasks they spend most of their time doing.
- Most individuals will unconsciously adapt to worsening conditions or tolerate a gradual lowering of standards to a "lowest common denominator" situation effect. Unchecked, this phenomenon can lead to unsafe and unethical practices condoned by people in a system, who are unaware that their actions and behaviors have shifted into a potentially dangerous zone.
- Active strategies must be put into place to counter these natural trends— namely, acknowledging that task routinization leads to uncritical activity and that within an uncritical, unquestioning working climate individuals and teams will unconsciously adapt to worsening conditions.

Future research

An obvious area for further research is testing how routine data can stimulate the identification of gaps in service delivery, in monitoring changes to practice, and in introducing new practices in a reliable and valid way [46]. Also, understanding how local teams can be more autonomous and self-directing to keep vigilant over routine matters is important. Also important is being clearer about how we identify knowledge-to-action gaps in the health care system [47].

Summary

Identifying gaps in care is a starting point for knowledge implementation. When people in systems are given more freedom to get involved in local problem solving and in making autonomous decisions, they more actively engage in finding creative solutions to routine problems [12,13,48] and in implementing knowledge in care settings. The next articles in this series will move forward in the knowledge implementation cycle to address how to adapt knowledge to local context and how to understand barriers and facilitators to knowledge implementation. Finally, we will address how to select, implement, and evaluate strategies for knowledge implementation.

References

1 Graham ID, Logan J, Harrison MB, Straus SE, Tetroe J, Caswell W, et al. Lost in knowledge translation: time for a map? *J Cont Ed Health Prof* 2006;26:13–24.

2 Straus SE, Richardson WS, Glasziou P, Haynes RB. *Evidence Based Medicine: How to Practice and Teach It.* Edinburgh: Elsevier; 2005.

3 Wenger NS, Roth CP, Shekelle P, and the ACOVE Investigators. Introduction to the assessing care of vulnerable elders-3 quality indicator measurement set. *J Am Geriatr Soc* 2007;55:s247–52.

4 Institute of Medicine. *To Err Is Human.* Washington, DC: National Academy Press; 1999.

5 McGlynn EA, Asch SM, Adams J, Keesey J, Hicks J, DeCristofaro A, et al. The quality of health care delivered to adults in the United States. *New Engl J Med* 2003;348:2635–645.

6 Donabedian A. The quality of care. How can it be assessed? *JAMA* 1988;260:1743–8.

7 Lambie L, Mattke S, and the Members of the OECD Cardiac Care Panel. Selecting indicators for the quality of cardiac care at the health systems level in OECD countries. OECD Technical Paper. 2004. URL http://www.oecd.org/dataoecd/28/35/33865450.pdf [accessed June 20, 2008].

8 Organisation for Economic Cooperation and Development. 2008. URL www.oecd.org [accessed June 20, 2008].

9 Shekelle P. The appropriateness method. *Med Dec Making* 2004;24:228–31.

10 Rosengart MR, Nathens AB, Schiff MA. The identification of criteria to evaluate prehospital trauma care using the Delphi technique. *J Trauma* 2007;62:708–13.

11 The Birthday Party. Royal Adelaide Hospital. Safety, Quality & Risk Resource–Affinity Diagram Toolkit. October 2006.

12 Cunningham G, Kitson A. An evaluation of the RCN Clinical Leadership Development Programme: Part 1. *Nurs Stand* 2000;15:34–37.

13 Cunningham G, Kitson A. An evaluation of the RCN Clinical Leadership Development Programme: Part 2. *Nurs Stand* 2000;15:37–39.

14 Gilliam SJ, Murray SA. *Needs Assessment in General Practice*. London: Royal College of General Practitioners; 1996 (occasional paper 73).

15 Lockyer J. Needs assessment: lessons learned. *J Cont Educ Health Prof* 1998;18: 190–2.

16 Zhan C, Miller MR. Administrative data based patient safety research: a critical review. *Qual Saf Health Care* 2003;12[Suppl II]:ii58–ii63.

17 Institute for Clinical Evaluation Services. URL http://www.ices.on.ca.

18 Shah BR, Mamdani M, Jaakkimainen L, Hux JE. Risk modification for diabetic patients. *Can J Clin Pharmacol* 2004;11:239–44.

19 Pimlott NJ, Hux JE, Wilson LM, Kahan M, Li C, Rosser WW. Educating physicians to reduce benzodiazepine use by elderly patients. *CMAJ* 2003;168:835–9.

20 Feinstein AR. ICD, POR, and DRG: unsolved scientific problems in the nosology of clinical medicine. *Arch Intern Med* 1988;148:2269–74.

21 Aylin P, Bottle A. Use of administrative data or clinical databases as predictors of risk of death in hospital: comparison of models. *BMJ* 2007;334:1044–8.

22 Gorelick MH, Knight S, Alessandrini EA, Stanley RM, Chamberlain JM, Kuppermann N, et al. Lack of agreement in pediatric emergency department discharge diagnoses from clinical and administrative data sources. *Acad Emerg Med* 2007;14:646–52.

23 URL http://www.jointcommission.org [accessed June 20, 2008].

24 Rubenfeld GD. Using computerized medical databases to measure and to improve the quality of intensive care. *J Crit Care* 2004;19:248–56.

25 Institute of Medicine. *Guidelines for Clinical Practice. From Development to Use*. Washington DC: National Academy Press; 1992.

26 URL http://www.rebeqi.org [accessed June 20, 2008].

27 Rethans J, Martin E, Metsemakers J. To what extent to clinical notes by general practitioners reflect actual medical performance? A study using simulated patients. *Br J Gen Pract* 1994;44:153–6.

28 Jennett P, Affleck L. Chart audit and chart stimulated recall as methods of needs assessment in continuing professional health education. *J Cont Educ Health Prof* 1998;18:163–71.

29 Linder JA, Bates DW, Williams DH. Acute infections in primary care: accuracy of electronic diagnoses and electronic antibiotic prescribing. *J Am Med Inform Assoc* 2006;13:61–6.

30 Peabody JW, Luck J, Glassman P, Dresselhaus TR, Lee M. Comparison of vignettes, standardized patients and chart abstraction. *JAMA* 2000;283:1715–22.

31 Shah SG, Thomas-Gibson S, Brooker JC, Suzuki N, Williams CB, Thapar C, et al. Use of video and magnetic endoscopic imaging for rating competence at colonoscopy: validation of a measurement tool. *Gastrointest Endosc* 2002;56:568–73.

32 URL http://www.abim.org/exam/moc [accessed June 2008].

33 Dresselhaus TR, Peabody JW, Luck J, Bertenthal D. An evaluation of vignettes for predicting variation in the quality of preventive care. *J Gen Intern Med* 2004;19:1013–8.

34 Dornan T, Carroll C, Parboosingh J. An electronic learning portfolio for reflective continuing professional development. *Med Educ* 2002;36:767–9.

35 Sibley JC, Sackett DL, Neufeld V, Gerrard B, Rudnick KV, Fraser W. A randomised trial of continuing medical education. *N Engl J Med* 1982;306:511–5.

36 Davis DA, Mazmanian PE, Fordis M, Van Harrison R, Thorpe KE, Perrier L. Accuracy of physician self-assessment compared with observed measures of competence: a systematic review. *JAMA* 2006;296[9]:1094–102.

37 Van de Ven A. Central problem in the management of innovation. *Management Science* 1985;32[5]:590–607.

38 Johnson PE. The expert mind: a new challenge for the information scientist. In MA Bemmelmans (Ed.), *Beyond Productivity: Information Systems Development for Organisational Effectiveness.* Netherlands: North Holland Publishing; 1983.

39 Van de Ven A, Hudson R. Managing attention to strategic choices. In J Pennings (Ed.), *Strategic Decision Making in Complex Organisations.* San Francisco: Jossey-Bass; 1983.

40 Lewin KT et al. Level of aspiration. In J McV Hunt (Ed.), *Personality and the Behavior Disorders.* New York: Ronald Press; 1944.

41 March JG, Simon H. *Organisations.* New York: Wiley; 1958.

42 Helson H. Current trends and issues in adaptation level theory. *American Psychologist* 1964;19:23–68.

43 Van de Ven A. Problem solving, planning and innovation: part 2. Speculations for theory and practice. *Human Relations* 1980;33:757–79.

44 Argyris C, Schon D. *Organisational Learning: A Theory of Action Perspective.* Reading, Mass: Addison-Wesley; 1978.

45 Miller E. *From Dependency to Autonomy. Studies in Organisation and Change.* London: Free Association Books; 1993.

46 Grol R, Berwick DM, Wensing M. On the trail of quality and safety in health care. *BMJ* 2008;336:74–76.

47 Greenhalgh T, Robert G, MacFarlane F, Bate P, Kyriakidou O, Peacock R. Diffusion of innovations in service organisations: a systematic review and recommendations. *Millbank Q* 2004;82[4]:581–629.

48 Catchpole KR, de Leval MR, McEwan A, Pigott N, Elliott MJ, McQuillan A, et al. Patient handover from surgery to intensive care: using Formula 1 pit-stop and aviation models to improve safety and quality. *Paediatr Anaesth* 2007;17:470–8.

3.3 Adapting knowledge to a local context

Margaret B. Harrison[1], Ian D. Graham[2], and Béatrice Fervers[3]

[1]Practice and Research in Nursing (PRN) Group, Queen's University, Kingston, ON, Canada

[2]Canadian Institutes of Health Research, and School of Nursing, University of Ottawa, Ottawa, ON, Canada

[3]French Federation of Cancer Centers, Centre Leon Berard, and Universite Lyon, France

---

KEY LEARNING POINTS

- To avoid duplication of efforts and to optimize use of existing resources, clinical practice guidelines can be adapted to local circumstances and settings.
- The ADAPTE process provides an approach to adapting a guideline to a local context through an explicit, participatory process involving relevant decision makers, including clinicians, managers, researchers, and policy makers.

Why should we adapt clinical practice guidelines for local use?

Using the best available evidence is a fundamental aspect of quality health care, and clinical practice guidelines (Chapter 2.3) are an important tool to inform evidence-based practices. Good quality guidelines are seen as valuable tools to improving quality of care. Guidelines provide synthesized evidence that have been translated into specific practice recommendations. Over the past decade, governments and professional organizations have promoted and supported guideline production. Many countries have infrastructure at the national and/or regional level dedicated to synthesizing evidence and producing guidelines and incentives designed to support practices guided by current guideline recommendations [1]. The background and goals of these initiatives differ depending on political context and the health care system. For instance, in the United Kingdom, the National Health Service (NHS) has infrastructure and incentives built to deliver care guided by current guideline recommendations. National bodies such as NICE (National Institute for Health and Clinical Excellence) in the United Kingdom are dedicated to synthesizing evidence and producing guidelines for use within the NHS. To assess uptake and adherence to guideline-driven care, there are auditing

---

Knowledge Translation in Health Care: Moving from Evidence to Practice. Edited by S. Straus, J. Tetroe, and I. Graham. © 2009 Blackwell Publishing, ISBN: 978-1-4051-8106-8.

functions utilized across Trusts (or regions) in the NHS. Despite these efforts, evaluating implementation strategies shows that overall practice conformity lags behind expectations [2].

Although guidelines may be seen as necessary, they are clearly not *sufficient* to ensure practices and decisions are evidence based. The uptake of evidence at the point of care is a complex and challenging endeavor. It does not occur with simple information dissemination but requires a substantive proactive effort and additional translation for use at the point of decision making [3]. Based on this evidence, the gap between valid guideline recommendations and care delivery may be widened by numerous factors. For example, health care providers may not have the requisite skills and expertise to implement a recommended action, or the setting may not have the mandatory equipment or staff time to deliver a guideline's recommendation [3]. Other challenges include factors such as recommendations not being acceptable to the local patient population or providers due to cultural or other factors. Although guidelines provide evidence in a more usable form for practitioners and health settings than a plethora of primary studies, an important and additional necessary step is the adaptation of the guideline to the context of use.

Although national and international bodies have made major efforts to improve the quality and rigor of guidelines [4,5], less investment is made in understanding how guidelines can better target the local context of care. Customizing a clinical practice guideline for a particular organization may help improve acceptance and adherence. Active involvement of targeted guideline end users in this process has been shown to lead to significant changes in practice [6–8]. As a consequence, the local–regional adaptation of (inter)national evidence-based practice guidelines has become mandatory for cancer care in France [9]. For many regions and provincial/territorial jurisdictions, *de novo* guideline development is not feasible because of lack of time, expertise, and resources. Thus, it makes sense to take advantage of existing high-quality guidelines [10–12].

Adapting existing high-quality guidelines for local use is an approach to reduce duplication of effort and enhance applicability. National guidelines often lack applicability and description of the changes in the organization of care required to implement the recommendations [13]. Most important, the guideline adaptation process is a first step in implementing evidence in practice and one that promotes local uptake of evidence through a sense of ownership by targeted end users. It is an action-oriented and concrete element of facilitating evidence implementation. However, customizing a guideline to local conditions runs the risk that the adapted guideline will depart from its evidence base, putting into question the quality and validity of the recommendations. This chapter outlines a systematic, participatory approach for evaluating and adapting available guidelines to a local context of use while ensuring the quality and validity of the guideline. Whether evidence is provided in the form of knowledge syntheses, patient decision aids, or clinical practice guidelines, end users must consider how it should be adapted to the local context, and the same principles can be applied to ensure local factors are considered prior to the implementation of the evidence.

How do we adapt clinical practice guidelines for local use?

Through an active process, existing guidelines are evaluated and customized to fit local circumstances. This process must preserve integrity of the evidence-based recommendations, albeit supported by the same body of evidence because there may be differences in organizational, regional, or cultural circumstances that could legitimately lead to important variations in guideline recommendations [4,5,10–12,14]. In the process of adapting guideline-specific health questions relevant to a local context of use, specific needs, priorities, legislation, policies, and resources in the targeted setting are considered and addressed.

Ideally, guideline adaptation is a systematic and participatory approach to evaluating and adapting existing guidelines. External evidence is assessed with local data and circumstances such as the size and characteristics of the population, the scopes of practice within health services, and the fit with existing delivery models and services. This local "evidence" is instrumental in promoting improved uptake and guideline use.

With the exception of a few Canadian studies [6,12], no validated process for guideline adaptation has been documented [14]. Recently, Canadian work [11] in this area was integrated with an international initiative known as the ADAPTE collaboration (www.ADAPTE.org) [14]. It is a group of researchers, guideline developers, implementers, and users whose aim is to enhance the use of research evidence through more efficient development and implementation of practice guidelines. A vital activity has been the production of a Web-based resource toolkit to guide the process of adaptation built on collective experience.

The ADAPTE process was developed to facilitate creation of efficient, high-quality adapted guidelines likely to be implemented. The process engages end users in the guideline adaptation process to address specific health questionsrelevant to its use. The goal is to establish a transparent, rigorous, and replicable standard based on the following core principles:
• Respect for evidence-based principles in guideline development [6];
• Use of reliable and consistent methods to ensure the quality of the adapted guideline [5];

- Participation of key stakeholders to foster acceptance and ownership of the adapted guideline, and ultimately to promote its use [9];
- Consideration of context during adaptation to ensure relevance for local practice and policy [15];
- Transparent reporting to promote confidence in the recommendations of the adapted guideline [4,16];
- Use of a flexible format to accommodate specific needs and circumstances [1,17];
- Respect for and acknowledgment of source guideline materials.

What is the ADAPTE process?

The ADAPTE process consists of three main phases, including planning and setup, adaptation, and development of a final product (Table 3.3.1). ADAPTE process users are encouraged to identify the modules and steps most relevant to their situation and context. The *setup phase* outlines the necessary tasks to be completed prior to beginning the adaptation process, including identifying necessary skills and resources and designing the panel. The panel should include relevant end users of the guideline such as health care professionals, managers, and patients. The *adaptation phase* helps in moving from topic selection to identification of specific clinical questions; in searching for, retrieving, and assessing guidelines; in decision making around adaptation; and in preparing the draft-adapted guideline. Assessing retrieved guidelines involves evaluation of their *quality* (using the AGREE instrument [18]), *currency* (how up-to-date they are), and *consistency* (coherence of the recommendation with the underlying evidence). Assessment also consists of the examination of the *acceptability* (to providers and consumers) and *applicability* (feasibility of applying recommendations) of the guidelines' recommendations within the proposed context of use. The evaluation to be conducted in this phase provides an explicit basis for informed and transparent decision making around the selection and modification of source guidelines. This process can result in different alternatives, ranging from adopting a guideline that was produced elsewhere, to language translation and format adaptation, to modifying and updating single recommendations, and to the production of a customized guideline based on various source guidelines. The *finalization phase* includes external review, feedback from relevant stakeholders, and consultation with the developers of source guidelines. Establishing a process for updating the adapted guideline and writing the final document are the last stages.

The ADAPTE process is supported by tools including a Web site (www.ADAPTE.org) that provides a manual and toolkit. For each phase, the

Table 3.3.1 Guideline adaptation with ADAPTE: phases, modules, and steps

---

PHASE I—SETUP

Preparation module

STEP 1   Establish an organizing committee and working panel, resource team.
This group will determine scope, terms of reference, and working plan.

STEP 2   Select a topic using criteria.
Criteria can include prevalence of disease; evidence of underuse, overuse, or misuse of interventions; existence of a good guideline.

STEP 3   Check if adaptation is feasible.
Determine if any guideline is available.

STEP 4   Identify necessary resources and skills.
Resources include consideration of commitment from the panel, meeting costs, and project management. Necessary skills include content expertise and expertise in critical appraisal, information retrieval, implementation, and policy.

STEP 5   Complete tasks for setup phase including terms of reference, declaration of conflicts of interest, consensus process, endorsement bodies, guideline authorship, dissemination, and implementation strategies.

STEP 6   Write the adaptation plan.
This may include the topic area, panel membership, declaration of competing interests, and proposed timeline.

PHASE II—ADAPTATION

Scope and purpose module

STEP 7   Determine/clarify the health questions using PIPOH.
Population; intervention: professions guideline is targeted to outcomes and health care setting.

Search and screen module

STEP 8   Search for guidelines and other relevant documentation.
Search for relevant guidelines and for systematic reviews and health technology assessment reviews published since the guideline.

STEP 9   Screen retrieved guidelines—record characteristics/content.
Perform a preliminary screening to determine if the guidelines are relevant to the topic.

STEP 10   Reduce a large number of retrieved guidelines using AGREE instrument.
Use the rigor dimension of the AGREE tool to assess guideline quality and include only those of highest quality for further assessment.

(Continued)

Table 3.3.1 (*Continued*)

	Assessment module—using tools provided
STEP 11	Assess guideline quality. Use the AGREE instrument to assess quality. Suggest two to four raters; do this independently.
STEP 12	Assess guideline currency. Review the search and publication dates of the guideline and ascertain whether the most current evidence has been included. This will require input from an information scientist and content experts.
STEP 13	Assess guideline content. Can be considered in two formats: recommendations provided and grouped by guideline; recommendations grouped by similarity (e.g., topic covered).
STEP 14	Assess guideline consistency. Assess the search strategy and selection of evidence supporting the recommendations; the consistency between selected evidence and how developers summarize and interpret the evidence; and consistency between interpretation of the evidence and the recommendations.
STEP 15	Assess acceptability and applicability of recommendations.
	Decision and selection module
STEP 16	Review assessments. Provide panel with all documents summarizing the review including AGREE results and recommendations.
STEP 17	Select between guidelines and recommendations to create an adapted guideline. Consider the following options: reject the whole guideline; accept the whole guideline including evidence summary and recommendations; accept the evidence summary; accept specific recommendations; modify specific recommendations.
	Customization module
STEP 18	Prepare draft-adapted guideline. Prepare a draft document respecting the needs of the end users and providing a detailed explanation of the process.
	PHASE III—FINALIZATION
	External review and acknowledgment module
STEP 19	External review—target audiences of the guideline. Include target users of the guideline such as clinicians, managers, and policymakers. Ask if they agree with recommendations, if there are any gaps, if the guideline is acceptable, and if it has any resource implications.

Table 3.3.1 (*Continued*)

STEP 20	Consult with endorsement bodies. Engage relevant professional organizations and societies to endorse the guidelines.
STEP 21	Consult with source guideline developers. Send the adapted guideline to the developers, especially if changes were made to the recommendations.
STEP 22	Acknowledge source documents. Reference all source documents in the final document and ensure that any necessary copyright permissions are obtained.
	Aftercare planning module
STEP 23	Plan for aftercare of the adapted guideline. Decide on a review date and a plan for repeat search and modification.
	Final production module
STEP 24	Produce final guideline document. Include details on implementation tools including care paths and patient information materials. The final document should be easily accessible to end users.

manual provides a detailed description of the aims and tasks, the products and deliverables, and the skills and organizational requirements necessary to undertake the tasks. An example (adaptation of guidelines for cervical cancer screening) is provided throughout the modules. In the toolkit, 19 tools or instruments help structure the process and collect necessary information for decision making. For example, Tool #2 offers a comprehensive search strategy to help identify existing guidelines by searching Web sites of guideline sources (e.g., guideline clearinghouses, known developer's sites, specialty organizations) and MEDLINE. Tool #6 helps a group convert the guideline topic into a set of clear and focused key questions prior to the adaptation process. And Tool #15 proposes a series of structured questions and criteria to guide the assessment and discussion on whether a guideline recommendation is applicable and acceptable in the planned context of use and to identify organizational changes that may be needed to deliver the recommendation. Steps and tools are flexible and have been designed to allow for alteration in the sequence in which they are used to fit with user time or resource restraints.

Future research

Although many current research initiatives focus on implementing guidelines and assessing factors influencing knowledge use in health care practices, many challenges that will need to be addressed by rigorous research remain. First, there is a need to validate the ADAPTE process to determine its impact on guideline implementation. Second, tools to assess implementability of adapted guidelines need to be developed and validated.

Summary

This chapter describes the process for adapting guidelines to the local context. The same principles could be used when considering implementation of knowledge syntheses or patient decision aids. The ADAPTE process offers an approach to this and includes a step-by-step map, whereby clinical, health service, and administrative decision-makers can adapt existing guidelines for local use. A significant benefit of the ADAPTE process is that it breaks down a complicated process into discrete and manageable phases. Notably this participatory approach promotes the adoption of the best evidence-based recommendations *along with* consideration of local needs and circumstances. As an organization works through guideline evaluation and adaptation, an additional benefit is the development of consensus among relevant stakeholders including practitioners, policymakers, and others. The process itself may be a nonthreatening, instructive, and updating experience for those involved in reviewing existing guidelines or providing feedback on the local draft guideline. Adaptation, using a method such as ADAPTE, helps avoid departures from the evidence base and stresses the process of aligning evidence to local context. It directs users to identify potential local barriers in applying research evidence to clinical or policy practice. By actively engaging the targeted users in reviewing guideline recommendations and in discussing any required organizational changes, an environment for communication and collaboration among health professionals, managers, and decision-makers is fostered. This culture is crucial to overcome barriers to implementation.

References

1 Burgers JS, Grol R, Zaat JO, Spies TH, van der Bij AK, Mokkink HG. Characteristics of effective clinical guidelines for general practice. *Br J Gen Pract* 2003;53[486]:15–19.

2 Grimshaw J, Thomas RE, MacLennan G, Fraser C, Ramsay CR, Vale L, et al. Effectiveness and efficiency of guideline dissemination and implementation strategies. *Health Technol Assess* 2004;8[6]:iii–iv, 1–72.

3 Toman C, Harrison MB, Logan J. Clinical practice guidelines: necessary but not sufficient for evidence-based patient education and counseling. *Patient Educ Couns* 2001;42[3]:279–87.

4 GRADE Working Group. Grading quality of evidence and strength of recommendations. *BMJ* 2004;328[7454]:1490–7.

5 The AGREE Collaboration. Development and validation of an international appraisal instrument for assessing the quality of clinical practice guidelines: the AGREE Project. *Qual Safe Health Care* 2003;12[1]:18–23.

6 Harrison MB, Graham ID, Lorimer K, Friedberg E, Pierscianowski T, Brandys T. Leg-ulcer care in the community, before and after implementation of an evidence-based service. *CMAJ* 2005;172[11]:1447–52.

7 Ray-Coquard I, Philip T, Lehmann M, Fervers B, Farsi F, Chauvin F. Impact of a clinical guidelines program for breast and colon cancer in a French cancer centre. *JAMA* 1997;278[19]:1591–5.

8 Ray-Coquard I, Philip T, de Laroche G, Froger X, Suchaud JP, Voloch A, et al. A controlled before and after study: impact of a clinical guidelines programmed and regional cancer network organisation on medical practice. Prototype for a regional cancer network: Impact of clinical guidelines program on medical practice. *Br J Cancer* 2002;86[3]:313–21.

9 Fretheim A, Schunemann HJ, Oxman AD. Improving the use of research evidence in guideline development: 3. Group composition and consultation process. *Health Res Policy Syst* 2006 Nov 29;4:15.

10 Graham ID, Harrison MB, Brouwers M, Davies BL, Dunn S. Facilitating the use of evidence in practice: evaluating and adapting clinical practice guidelines for local use by health care organizations. *J Obstet Gynacol Neonatal Nurs* 2002;31[5]:599–611.

11 Graham ID, Harrison MB, Brouwers M. Evaluating and adapting practice guidelines for local use: a conceptual framework. In S Pickering & J Thompson (Eds.), *Clinical Governance in Practice.* London: Harcourt; 2003, pp. 213–29.

12 Graham ID, Harrison MB, Lorimer K, Piercianowski T, Friedberg E, Buchanan M, et al. Adapting national and international leg ulcer practice guidelines for local use: the Ontario Leg Ulcer Community Care Protocol. *Adv Skin Wound Care* 2005;18[6]:307–18.

13 Burgers JS, Cluzeau FA, Hanna SE, Hunt C, Grol R. Characteristics of high quality guidelines: evaluation of 86 clinical guidelines developed in ten European countries and Canada. *Int J Technol Assess Health Care* 2003;19[1]:148–57.

14 Fervers B, Burgers JS, Haugh M, Latreille J, Mlika-Cabanne N, Paquet L, et al. Adaptation of clinical guidelines: a review of methods and experiences. *Int J Health Care* 2006;18[3]:167–76.

15 Verkerk K, Van Veenendaal H, Severens JL, Hendriks EJ, Burgers JS. Considered judgement in evidence-based guideline development. *Int J Qual Health Care* 2006;18[5]:365–9.

16 Shiffman RN, Shekelle P, Overhage JM, Slutsky J, Grimshaw J, Deshpande AM. Standardized reporting of clinical practice guidelines: a proposal from the conference on guideline standardization. *Ann Intern Med* 2003;139[6]:493–8.

17 Grol R, Dalhuijsen J, Thomas S, Veld C, Rutten G, Mokkink H. Attributes of clinical guidelines that influence use of guidelines in general practice: observational study. *BMJ* 1998;317[7162]:858–61.

18 The AGREE Collaboration. International assessment of quality clinical practice guidelines in oncology using the Appraisal of Guidelines and Research and Evaluation Instrument. *J Clin Oncol* 2004;22:2000–7.

3.4 Assessing barriers and facilitators to knowledge use

France Légaré

Centre de Recherche, Hospital St. François-d'Assise, and Department of Family Medicine, Universite Laval, Quebec, Canada

---

KEY LEARNING POINTS

- Both barriers and facilitators to knowledge use must be considered by those interested in knowledge implementation.
- Taxonomies for barriers and facilitators have been developed and should be used when developing a knowledge-to-action project.
- These identified taxonomies should be further evaluated in other settings and contexts.

The need for effective knowledge transfer and exchange in clinical practice is essential if we are to address the following challenges: (1) expanded availability of health information [1]; (2) extended role of patients in clinical decision making [2]; (3) management of expectations regarding new treatments and technologies [3]; and (4) enhanced patient safety [4]. However, to date, there is a consensus among the implementation research community that most efforts in knowledge translation and exchange at the clinical level have met with little success [5]. Although each phase of the knowledge-to-action cycle is important for ensuring effective knowledge translation and exchange, this chapter aims to highlight specific challenges associated with the assessment of barriers and facilitators to knowledge use. The content reported in this chapter is based on a search of the following specialized source: the Literature Database of the LiKaShing Knowledge Institute—Joint Program in Knowledge Translation—(http://www.stmichaelshospital.com/research/ktliterature.php).

The first section of this chapter addresses the relevance of using conceptual models when assessing barriers and facilitators to knowledge use in health care by briefly presenting the evolution of one of the most often cited models in this field, the Clinical Practice Guidelines Framework for Improvement [6], developed by Cabana and colleagues (1999). The next section addresses

---

Knowledge Translation in Health Care: Moving from Evidence to Practice. Edited by S. Straus, J. Tetroe, and I. Graham. © 2009 Blackwell Publishing, ISBN: 978-1-4051-8106-8.

the measurement of barriers and facilitators to knowledge use by reviewing three relevant instruments: (1) the Attitudes Regarding Practice Guidelines tool [7]; (2) a questionnaire for perceived barriers to change [8]; and (3) the BARRIERS Scale for assessing research use by nurses [9]. The lessons learned from the various cited research initiatives provide valuable insight for implementation researchers, educators, policymakers, and clinicians on how to address barriers and facilitators to knowledge use in health care contexts. The last section of the chapter identifies areas needing further research.

What are the key concepts and conceptual models for assessing barriers and facilitators to knowledge use?

Conceptual models represent sets of concepts (words describing mental images of phenomena) and propositions (statements about the concepts) that integrate the former into a meaningful configuration [10].They may include general guidelines for research, practice, and education. Conceptual models are rarely static, and many evolve as new evidence emerges. Thus, an established worldview engenders a theory that has a narrower focus and can be experimentally refuted [11]. In the context of barriers and facilitators to knowledge use in health care, it is expected that relevant conceptual frameworks would help researchers identify research questions, generate testable hypotheses, assess outcomes with valid and reliable instruments, and make valid inferences from their study results. This framework ensures that researchers can elaborate on theory-based interventions that have the potential for increasingly effective implementation of knowledge into clinical practice [12].

One of the most often cited conceptual frameworks regarding barriers to knowledge use in health care is the Clinical Practice Guidelines Framework for Improvement [6]. This framework was based on an extensive search of the literature of barriers to physician adherence to clinical practice guidelines and was organized according to knowledge, attitudes, or physician behavior [13]. Based on a systematic approach to evidence [14],clinical practice guidelines are defined as systematically developed statements to assist practitioners and patients make decisions about appropriate health care for specific circumstances [15]. Of a total of 5658 potentially eligible articles, Cabana and his colleagues (1999) identified 76 published studies describing at least one barrier to adherence to clinical practice guidelines. Taken together, the included articles reported on 293 potential barriers to physician guideline adherence, including awareness of the existence of the guideline (i.e., ability to correctly acknowledge the existence of shared decision making) ($n = 46$), familiarity with guideline recommendations (i.e., ability to correctly answer questions about the guideline content) ($n = 31$), agreement with the recommendations (i.e., consenting to the recommendations) ($n = 33$), self-efficacy (i.e., feeling one is able to carry out the recommendations) ($n = 19$), outcome expectancy (i.e., perception that one's performance following the use of the recommendations will lead to improved patient outcome or process outcome) ($n = 8$), ability to overcome inertia of previous practice (i.e., feeling one is able to modify his/her routine) ($n = 14$), and absence of external barriers to following recommendations (i.e., perception of factors external to oneself that would impede the use of the recommendations) ($n = 34$) [6].

Following focus group interviews with Norwegian general practitioners on factors affecting adherence to clinical practice guidelines with regard to image-ordering for back pain, Espeland and Baerheim (2003) proposed a revised and extended classification of barriers based on the Clinical Practice Guidelines Framework for Improvement [16]. Newly identified barriers were lack of expectancy that adherence to guidelines will lead to desired health care process, emotional difficulty with adherence, improper access to actual/alternative health care services, and pressure from health care providers and organizations [16].

More recently, the Clinical Practice Guidelines Framework for Improvement was extended. In a study identifying barriers and facilitators to implementing shared decision making in clinical practice, a specific definition was identified for each type of barrier [17]. The study's intention was to help standardize the reporting of barriers and facilitators to knowledge use in the health care context across different studies. Barriers were defined as factors that would limit or restrict implementation of shared decision making in clinical practice [6]. More important, the Clinical Practice Guidelines Framework for Improvement was extended to include a list of potential facilitators of knowledge use in clinical practice [17]. Facilitators were defined as factors that would promote or help implement shared decision making in clinical practice. This is an important development because we tend to forget that the same factor may sometimes be identified as both a barrier and facilitator to knowledge use, demonstrating the importance of developing a more comprehensive and integrated understanding of barriers and facilitators [18,19]. Also, in this more recent study, the Clinical Practice Guidelines Framework for Improvement was further extended with the attributes of innovation as proposed by the Diffusion of Innovation theory [20]. As a result, except for the barrier "lack of awareness" (i.e., the inability of health professionals to state that shared decision making exists) and the facilitator "awareness" (i.e., the ability of health professionals to state that shared decision making exists), the range of factors initially proposed by the Clinical Practice Guidelines Framework for Improvement by Cabana and colleagues (1999) was identified as potential barriers or facilitators. However, one new barrier was identified and added to the list: forgetting (i.e., inadvertently not attending to something).

This revised version of the Clinical Practice Guidelines Framework for Improvement was used in a systematic review of barriers and facilitators to implementing shared decision making in clinical practice [21]. It was successfully applied in extracting data from 31 publications covering 28 unique studies [21]. Table 3.4.1 presents the corresponding definition of each potential barrier and facilitator to knowledge use in the health care context. This list can be a guide when we attempt to consider local barriers and facilitators to knowledge use. For example, it can be used to guide a content analysis of individual interviews or focus groups collected during qualitative studies on research utilization.

What are some tools for assessing barriers and facilitators to knowledge use?

To clearly identify barriers and facilitators to knowledge use in health care practices, there is a need to assess them in a valid and reliable fashion. In this context, there presently is considerable interest in instruments for valid and reliable assessment of barriers and facilitators to knowledge use that can be used by various end users who are trying to implement knowledge.

Based on the Clinical Practice Guidelines Framework for Improvement, a tool for assessing barriers to adherence to hand hygiene guidelines was developed and tested on a group of 21 infectious disease clinicians [7]. The tool uses a 6-point Likert scale and has two sections: attitudinal statements about practice guidelines in general, and specific statements regarding the Hand Hygiene Guideline. The survey was administered twice, at 2-week intervals. The Attitudes Regarding Practice Guideline tool was found to have a test–retest reliability coefficient of 0.86 and a standardized Cronbach alpha of 0.80 [7]. However, the authors concluded that their tool needed to undergo further testing and adaptation as a measure of potential barriers to adherence to clinical practice guidelines in general [7].

Wensing and Grol reported the development of another instrument designed to assess barriers and facilitators to knowledge use [8]. This instrument was applied to 12 different implementation studies in the Netherlands [8]. First, they used literature analyses and focus groups with implementation experts to identify possible barriers to change. Second, they performed validation studies to test psychometric characteristics of the questionnaires. Questions pertained to characteristics of the innovation (i.e., clinical practice guidelines), care provider characteristics, patient characteristics, and context characteristics. In a study on cardiovascular disease prevention in

Table 3.4.1 Taxonomy of barriers and facilitators and their definitions

Knowledge

Lack of awareness	Inability to correctly acknowledge the existence of shared decision making (SDM)
Lack of familiarity	Inability to correctly answer questions about SDM content, as well as self-reported lack of familiarity
Forgetting	Inadvertently omitting SDM [26]

Attitudes

Lack of agreement with specific components of shared decision making

Interpretation of evidence	Not believing that specific elements of SDM are supported by scientific evidence

Lack of applicability

Characteristics of the patient	Lack of agreement with the applicability of SDM to practice population based on the characteristics of the patient
Clinical situation	Lack of agreement with the applicability of SDM to practice population based on the clinical situation
Asking patient about his/her preferred role in decision making	Lack of agreement with a specific component of SDM, such as asking patients about their preferred role in decision making
Asking patient about support or undue pressure	Lack of agreement with a specific component of SDM, such as asking patients about support and/or undue pressure
Asking about values/clarifying values	Lack of agreement with a specific component of SDM, such as asking patients about values
Not cost-beneficial	Perception that there will be increased costs if SDM is implemented
Lack of confidence in the developers	Lack of confidence in the individuals who are responsible for developing or presenting SDM

Lack of agreement in general

"Too cookbook"—too rigid to be applicable	Lack of agreement with SDM because it is too artificial
Challenge to autonomy	Lack of agreement with SDM because it is a threat to professional autonomy
Biased synthesis	Perception that the authors were biased
Not practical	Lack of agreement with SDM because it is unclear or impractical to follow
Overall lack of agreement with using the model (not specified why)	Lack of agreement with SDM in general (unspecified)

Lack of expectancy

Patient's outcome	Perception that performance following the use of SDM will not lead to improved patient outcome

Table 3.4.1 (*Continued*)

Health care process	Perception that performance following the use of SDM will not lead to improved health care process
Feeling expectancy	Perception that performance following the use of SDM will provoke difficult feelings and/or does not take into account existing feelings
Lack of self-efficacy	Belief that one cannot perform SDM
Lack of motivation	Lack of motivation to use SDM or to change one's habits

Behavior

External barriers

Factors associated with patient

Preferences of patients	Perceived inability to reconcile patient preferences with the use of SDM

Factors associated with shared decision making as an innovation

Lack of triability	Perception that SDM cannot be experimented with on a limited basis
Lack of compatibility	Perception that SDM is not consistent with one's own approach
Complexity	Perception that SDM is difficult to understand and to put into use
Lack of observability	Lack of visibility of the results of using SDM
Not communicable	Perception that it is not possible to create and share information with one another in order to reach a mutual understanding of SDM
Increased uncertainty	Perception that the use of SDM will increase uncertainty (for example, lack of predictability, of structure, of information)
Not modifiable/way of doing it	Lack of flexibility to the extent that SDM is not changeable or modifiable by a user in the process of its adoption and implementation

Factors associated with environmental factors

Time pressure	Insufficient time to put SDM into practice
Lack of resources	Insufficient materials or staff to put SDM into practice
Organizational constraints	Insufficient support from the organization
Lack of access to services	Inadequate access to actual or alternative health care services to put SDM into practice
Lack of reimbursement	Insufficient reimbursement for putting SDM into practice
Perceived increase in malpractice liability	Risk of legal actions is increased if SDM is put into practice
Sharing responsibility with Patient*	Using SDM lowers the responsibility of the health professional because it is shared with patient

*Only for the facilitator assessment taxonomy.

general practice involving 329 physicians, they reported that the self-reported barriers that were identified using their questionnaire explained 39% of the self-reported performance. This instrument is available in Dutch and English.

In nursing clinical practice, the BARRIERS Scale was developed to assess barriers to research utilization based on four key dimensions: (1) nurse,(2) setting, (3) research, and (4) presentation [9]. The scale consists of 29 items and is presented in Table 3.4.2. The scale consists of four subscales that map four key dimensions. Each subscale is labeled in accordance with the theory of diffusion of innovation: (1) characteristics of the adopter (i.e., the nurse's research values, skills, and awareness); (2) characteristics of the organization (i.e., setting barriers and limitations from the environment); (3) characteristics of the innovation (i.e., qualities of the research); and (4) characteristics of the communication (i.e., presentation and accessibility of the research). The BARRIERS Scale has been translated into Swedish [22,23]. Interestingly, the group of researchers who translated this scale in Swedish added an additional item that covers the English language as a barrier for Swedish nurses, thus acknowledging the need for cultural adaptation of a barriers assessment tool.

Future research

Although there are many current research initiatives that focus on assessing factors influencing knowledge use in health care practices, many challenges remain that will need to be addressed by rigorous research. First, there is a need to standardize the reporting of barriers and facilitators to translating research into clinical practice [6,24,25]. Researchers may want to consider using existing models that have been tested, such as the Clinical Practice Guidelines Framework for Improvement, to conduct barrier assessment studies [6]. Second, it will be necessary to address barriers as well as facilitators to knowledge use because one factor can be perceived as both a barrier and a facilitator. Therefore, there might be some value in using the revised version of the Clinical Practice Guidelines Framework for Improvement that addresses both barriers and facilitators to knowledge use [21]. Third, we briefly reported on existing instruments with known psychometrics for assessing barriers to knowledge use. We recognize that there may be added value in enhancing the knowledge base of implementation science by encouraging implementation researchers to use standardized, valid, and reliable instruments in assessing barriers and facilitators to knowledge use. However, there is a need to adapt existing instruments to the assessment of facilitators of knowledge, and there is a need to test them in diverse clinical and cultural contexts. Also, implementation researchers might consider addressing the following

Table 3.4.2 Items of the BARRIERS Scale [9]

Nurse
• The nurse is isolated from knowledgeable colleagues with whom to discuss the research.
• There is not a documented need to change practice.
• The nurse does not feel capable of evaluating the research.
• The nurse sees little benefit for self.
• The nurse does not see the value of research for practice.
• The nurse feels the benefits of changing practice will be minimal.
• The nurse is unaware of the research.
• The nurse is unwilling to change/try new ideas.

Setting
• The facilities are inadequate for implementation.
• The nurse does not have time to read research.
• There is insufficient time on the job to implement new ideas.
• Other staff are not supportive of implementation.
• The nurse does not feel she/he has enough authority to change patient care procedures.
• Physicians will not cooperate with implementation.
• The nurse feels results canno be generalized to own setting.
• Administration will not allow implementation.

Research
• The research has not been replicated.
• Research reports/articles are not published fast enough.
• The literature reports conflicting results.
• The nurse is uncertain whether to believe the results of the research.
• The research has methodological inadequacies.
• The conclusions drawn from the research are not justified.

Presentation
• The relevant literature is not compiled in one place.
• Research reports/articles are not readily available.
• Implications for practice are not made clear.
• The statistical analyses are not understandable.
• The research is not reported clearly and in a readable format.
• The research is not relevant to the nurse's practice.

The respondents are asked to rate to what extent they perceived each item as a barrier to the use of research findings on a 4-point scale: 1 = to no extent, 2 = to a little extent, 3 = to a moderate extent, and 4 = to a great extent.

research questions: (1) How should we measure barriers and facilitators to research use to infer what the collective is thinking? (2) Should we collect data from individuals to make sense of the group's thinking? (3) If we do, should we use the mean or the median to represent the group or should we focus on the variation or only on the outliers? (4) How many individuals in a group have to perceive something is a barrier before we decide to address it with an intervention? (5) Is the perception of the opinion leader the most important one? Last, even if these questions are answered, there remains a need for more research on how to choose the right intervention to address a specific barrier and/or facilitator. Only then will the gap between research and practice be adequately addressed.

Summary

Instruments exist to assess barriers and facilitators to knowledge use in health care practices. They can be used to improve the reporting of barrier assessment studies by practitioners attempting to implement knowledge. However, existing instruments may need to be adapted to accommodate the assessment of facilitators to knowledge use. They may also need to be further tested in diverse clinical and cultural contexts. Finally, there can be added value for completion of a systematic review of all instruments specifically designed to assess barriers and facilitators to knowledge use.

References

1 Woolf SH, Chan EC, Harris R, Sheridan SL, Braddock CH, III, Kaplan RM, et al. Promoting informed choice: transforming health care to dispense knowledge for decision making. *Ann Intern Med* 2005;143:293–300.

2 Kiesler DJ, Auerbach SM. Optimal matches of patient preferences for information, decision-making and interpersonal behavior: Evidence, models and interventions. *Patient Educ Couns* 2006;61:319–41.

3 van Steenkiste B, van der Weijden T, Timmermans D, Vaes J, Stoffers J, Grol R. Patients' ideas, fears and expectations of their coronary risk: barriers for primary prevention. *Patient Educ Couns* 2004;55:301–7.

4 Mighten AL. Shared clinical decision making: a model for enhancing patient safety and quality care. *Kansas Nurs* 2007;82:10–11.

5 Grimshaw JM, Thomas RE, MacLennan G, Fraser C, Ramsay CR, Vale L, et al. Effectiveness and efficiency of guideline dissemination and implementation strategies. *Health Technol Assess* 2004;8:iii–iv, 1–72.

6 Cabana M, Rand C, Powe N, Wu A, Wilson M, Abboud P, et al. Why don't physicians follow clinical practice guidelines? A framework for improvement. *JAMA* 1999;282:1458–65.

7 Larson E. A tool to assess barriers to adherence to hand hygiene guideline. *Am J Inf Control* 2004;32:48–51.

8 Wensing M, Grol R. Methods to identify implementation problems. In R Grol, M Wensing, & M Eccles (Eds.), *Improving Patient Care: The Implementation of Change in Clinical Practice*. Oxford: Elsevier Butterworth Heinemann; 2005, 109–21.

9 Funk SG, Champagne MT, Wiese RA, Tornquist EM. BARRIERS: the barriers to research utilization scale. *Appl Nurs Res* 1991;4:39–45.

10 Fawcett J. *Conceptual Models and Theories. Analysis and Evaluation of Conceptual Models of Nursing.* 2nd ed. Philadelphia: F.A. Davis Company; 1989, 1–40.

11 Popper K. *The Logic of Scientific Discovery.* London: Routledge Classics; 2002 reprint.

12 Eccles M, Grimshaw J, Walker A, Johnston M, Pitts N. Changing the behavior of healthcare professionals: the use of theory in promoting the uptake of research findings. *J Clin Epidemiol* 2005;58:107–12.

13 Ajzen I. *Attitudes, Personality and Behavior.* United Kingdom: Open University Press; 1988.

14 Burgers JS, Grol RP, Zaat JO, Spies TH, van der Bij AK, Mokkink HG. Characteristics of effective clinical guidelines for general practice. *Br J Gen Pract* 2003;53:15–19.

15 Field MJ, Lohr KN. Guidelines for clinical practice: from development to use. Washington, DC: Institute of Medicine; 1992.

16 Espeland AA, Baerheim AA. Factors affecting general practitioners' decisions about plain radiography for back pain: implications for classification of guideline barriers—a qualitative study. *BMC Health Serv Res* 2003;24[3]:8.

17 Legare F, O'Connor AM, Graham ID, Saucier D, Cote L, Blais J, et al. Primary health care professionals' views on barriers and facilitators to the implementation of the Ottawa Decision Support Framework in practice. *Patient Educ Couns* 2006;63:380–90.

18 Graham ID, Logan J, O'Connor A, Weeks KE, Aaron S, Cranney A, et al. A qualitative study of physicians' perceptions of three decision aids. *Patient Educ Couns* 2003;2055:1–5.

19 Kennedy T, Regehr G, Rosenfield J, Roberts SW, Lingard L. Exploring the gap between knowledge and behavior: a qualitative study of clinician action following an educational intervention. *Acad Med* 2004;79:386–93.

20 Rogers EM. *Diffusion of Innovations.* 4th ed. New York: The Free Press; 1995.

21 Gravel K, Legare F, Graham ID. Barriers and facilitators to implementing shared decision-making in clinical practice: a systematic review of health professionals' perceptions. *Implement Sci* 2006;9[1]:16.

22 Kajermo KN, Nordstrom G, Krusebrant A, Bjorvell H. Perceptions of research utilization: comparisons between health care professionals, nursing students and a reference group of nurse clinicians. *J Adv Nurs* 2000;31:99–109.

23 Bostrom AM, Kajermo KN, Nordstrom G, Wallin L. Barriers to research utilization and research use among registered nurses working in the care of older people: does the BARRIERS Scale discriminate between research users and non-research users on perceptions of barriers? *Implement Sci* 2008;3:24.

24 Davis DA, Taylor-Vaisey A. Translating guidelines into practice. A systematic review of theoretic concepts, practical experience and research evidence in the adoption of clinical practice guidelines. *CMAJ* 1997;157:408–16.

25 Saillour-Glenisson F, Michel P. Individual and collective facilitators and barriers to the use of clinical guidelines by physicians: a literature review. *Revue Épidémiologique de Santé Publique* 2003;51:65–80.

26 Holmes-Rovner M, Valade D, Orlowski C, Draus C, Nabozny-Valerio B, Keiser S. Implementing shared decision-making in routine practice: barriers and opportunities. *Health Expect* 2000;3:182–91.

3.5 Selecting KT interventions

3.5.1 Selecting, tailoring, and implementing knowledge translation interventions

Michel Wensing, Marije Bosch, and Richard Grol

Scientific Institute for Quality in Healthcare, Radboud University Nijmegen Medical Centre, Nijmegen, The Netherlands

---

KEY LEARNING POINTS

- Knowledge translation (KT) interventions need to be tailored to specific barriers for change, similar to a clinical treatment tailored to a diagnosed health problem.
- Research evidence on KT interventions can provide guidance but not decisively show what intervention is recommended.
- The selection of KT interventions remains an "art," which can be supported by structured methods for choice of objectives, identification of barriers for change, and linkage of KT interventions to these barriers.
- Tailored KT interventions have not been consistently effective partly because tailoring methods vary across studies.
- Multicomponent KT interventions are not consistently effective either partly because the definition of what is a multicomponent KT intervention is fuzzy.

Major variations in chronic heart failure treatment have been repeatedly found. For instance, beta-blocker use in primary care ranged from 10% to 50% between countries, and use of angiotensin-converting enzyme inhibitors (ACE-I) ranged from 50% to 75% [1]. Differences in national guideline recommendations were not sufficient to explain this variation [2]. Comorbidity explained some of the variation in treatment, but 14% of prescriptions were related to patient characteristics not in line with evidence [3]. A study of barriers to adherence to heart failure guidelines found that many family

---

Knowledge Translation in Health Care: Moving from Evidence to Practice. Edited by S. Straus, J. Tetroe, and I. Graham. © 2009 Blackwell Publishing, ISBN: 978-1-4051-8106-8.

physicians found it difficult to change treatment initiated by a cardiologist. Titrating the ACE-I dose was seen as difficult, and initiating ACE-I in patients already using a diuretic or stable on their current medication was seen as a barrier [4]. Suppose these findings can be generalized to any clinical setting: How would we try to improve primary care for chronic heart failure? How would we select interventions to translate knowledge from practice guidelines and research into practice?

We may think of interventions to facilitate uptake of research as training for physicians (e.g., to learn about titrating ACE-I dose) or use of opinion leaders to influence prescribing patterns of cardiologists. We may also consider providing financial incentives to physicians for each heart failure patient who is treated according to guideline recommendations. Or, we could better inform the patient and his family about appropriate heart failure care, hoping that they will ask for this treatment in future consultations with health professionals. Ideally, selection of the KT intervention should be guided by research evidence on the effectiveness and efficiency of various interventions. However, this evidence cannot not explicitly guide our decisions in all situations and circumstances, and so in addition to "science" we will need some "art" to choose or design the KT intervention (Box 3.5.1.1) [5].

It is beyond the scope of this chapter to review the evidence and, instead, we summarize other syntheses [5,6]. Many KT interventions have not been well-evaluated in rigorous studies. For those interventions that have been evaluated, research evidence suggests that their impact is variable and, on average, effect size is moderate. Thus, current research evidence on the effectiveness of KT interventions cannot completely guide the implementer on the best choice of intervention. The following general conclusions can be drawn from the literature:

- Available research evidence focuses mainly on professional interventions, such as various educational programs, feedback, and reminders. The methodological quality is variable but overall is only moderate. The overall absolute change of professional performance is usually not more than 10% on selected outcomes, but such change can be clinically or economically relevant.
- Passive educational interventions, such as written guidelines, lectures, and conferences, are unlikely to change professional behavior if used alone. Active educational interventions, such as outreach visits and quality circles of professionals, are more likely to induce change. Active self-study materials or Web sites (e.g., for distance learning) can be effective as well.
- Professional interventions that bring information close to the point of decision making, such as reminders and decision support, are likely to be effective, particularly in the areas of prevention and test ordering.

> **Box 3.5.1.1** A lifestyle program "Lively Legs" [19]
>
> This project aimed to develop a lifestyle program designed for patients with ulcus cruris who visit dermatology departments of Dutch hospitals. A core feature of the program was the availability of a specialized nurse who had a counselling role and helped the patients identify options for lifestyle improvements. The researchers used intervention mapping to develop the program, a technique from the health promotion field. Because preliminary results of the effects of the program were promising, the researchers anticipated wide-ranging implementation and decided to invite the steering group for a brainstorming session to identify possible obstacles to the implementation of the program on Dutch dermatology wards and to develop strategies to overcome these. Two sessions were held and these included six people of varying disciplines who were involved with this patient group. Sessions lasted an hour and a half. Participants were asked to individually consider possible relevant factors at several levels: the level of the patient, the level of the nurses, the level of social interaction, the level of the organization, and, finally, the level of broader structures such as legislation using a prestructured sheet. After all factors were collected on the blackboard, targets were formulated for the factors considered most important and modifiable. To define which factors were considered most important, participants divided three points among the factors. Examples of factors considered important were the lack of knowledge about ulcus cruris among nurses and the poor communication between nurses and support services. Subsequently, participants brainstormed to identify implementation strategies that looked most promising to overcome the barriers selected and, thereby, to achieve the targets chosen. Although both groups identified targets at varying levels, educational strategies were predominantly chosen to address these factors.

- Patient-directed interventions, such as preconsultation questionnaires or decision aids, can support quality improvement in some cases, but insight into the effects of interventions on quality of care is limited.
- Organizational interventions, such as revision of professional roles and multidisciplinary teams, can influence clinical outcomes and efficiency in some cases. But their impact on knowledge translation is unclear and they seem particularly to improve efficiency and patient satisfaction.
- Financial interventions for patients or professionals influence volumes of health care use, which may be relevant for quality improvement (e.g., volume of preventive services). Their effect on appropriateness of clinical decisions and practice patterns is less clear. Moreover, evidence on the sustainability of these interventions is limited.

This "art" of selecting a KT intervention can use structured procedures, at least partly. Many implementation experts suggest that a structured approach at various levels is needed to address professionals, patients, teams, organizations, and wider systems [6]. Structured approaches for planning change have been developed in various scientific disciplines and include, for instance, intervention mapping, marketing, precede/proceed, quality cycle, change management, organizational development, community development, and health technology assessment [7]. Whether these structured approaches result in better knowledge uptake, and which of their constituent components are most relevant, remains unproven. Interestingly, planning models for change propose more or less the same steps or stages, although their number of steps varies widely [8,9]. The aim of this chapter is to provide an overview and guidance on structured methods to select KT interventions.

Getting started: what are the objectives for KT?

An important step in the selection of KT interventions is the choice of specific objectives for the KT program. Goal setting can contribute to effective behavioral change [10]. Ultimately, the objectives should be related to outcomes for patients, populations, and society. For instance, the objectives for improving heart failure treatment could include higher survival rates (e.g., resulting from better use of ACE-inhibitors and beta-blockers) and lower health care costs (e.g., resulting from fewer hospital admissions). Many KT objectives have been defined in terms of specific changes in treatments or other aspects of health care delivery (e.g., more prescribing of ACE inhibitors and beta-blockers). The expectation is that such changes result in better outcomes. Ideally, strong research evidence supports this expectation, but in reality such evidence is not always available. For instance, much of the evidence on effectiveness of heart failure treatment is based on hospital patients and may not be fully applicable to heart failure patients in primary care.

Several methods can be used to select the objectives for KT, such as a Delphi procedure [11]. For instance, a study showed that about 30% of children seen in primary care with diagnosed urinary tract infections had not received antibiotics treatment [12]. Therefore, we invited nine family physicians to consider what aspects of primary care for these patients needed to be targeted in a KT program. A Delphi procedure, in which they first received a written questionnaire on 22 potential objectives, was used. They were asked to rate the clinical relevance of these objectives and to comment in their own words on the objectives. In a second round we reported the results of the first round and offered a number of revised objectives. This procedure resulted in a final set of seven objectives, including "all children aged less than six months old with a (suspected) UTI are referred to secondary care for treatment" and "all children with a UTI have to have a follow-up contact within three to five days after finishing the antibiotic treatment, in which the urine is tested by using a dipstick or urine culture."

What are the indicators that can be used to measure implementation?

The objectives need to be defined in terms of specific indicators that are used to measure degree of implementation. Clinical guidelines or other recommended practices can be analyzed to identify such indicators. The indicators should have good measurement properties, support from key stakeholders, and high feasibility in use. The science and practice of indicator development is evolving quickly. Current best practice is a structured Delphi procedure with panels of stakeholders who review available evidence, followed by a test in real practice [8]. Research of practice variation and quality assessment has provided many methods for such tests including chart audits, patient surveys, video observations, and secondary analysis of routine data. For example, a European project on cardiovascular risk management in primary care used a two-stage Delphi procedure to select indicators [13]. One-hundred one family physicians from nine countries (80% of those invited) were involved in both rounds of this procedure. From an initial list of 650 indicators, 202 indicators were derived, of which 44 were rated as valid (22%). These indicators covered lifestyle (8), clinical performance (27), and organizational aspects (9) of care. Different instruments were developed for measurement: abstraction tools for medical record audits in patients with cardiovascular disease and in patients with high risk for cardiovascular disease, a questionnaire, and an interview guide for family physicians.

What are potential barriers to change?

Once the objectives have been identified, most planning models suggest that each chosen objective with respect to barriers for change be analyzed. For instance, reducing inappropriate use of proton pump inhibitors may be hampered by resistance in patients to change their routines, lack of knowledge in physicians (e.g., about their side effects), organizational routines such as automatic delivery of repeat prescriptions, and financial incentives (e.g., more prescriptions translate into higher income for pharmacies) [14]. It is usually not possible to analyze and address each objective in much detail, so a prioritization of objectives has to be done.

There is a wide range of methods for identifying barriers to change [8], and these are discussed in Chapter 3.4. Briefly, they can be broadly divided into three categories. A first category comprises methods to identify barriers for change as reported by professionals, patients, and others: interviews, questionnaires, and group methods. This can be done relatively simply or more scientifically, but a disadvantage is that the reported barriers may in reality have little or no impact on KT. An example was the study of barriers for changing heart failure treatment, described above, which was based on semistructured questionnaires [4]. This study found that family physicians perceived on average four barriers in prescribing ACE inhibitors or optimizing ACE inhibitor dose. However, no significant relationships were found between barriers perceived and ACE inhibitorprescribing.

A second category comprises the analysis of practice variation with respect to its determinants. This approach requires large observational datasets and statistical methods for analyzing variation in health care delivery across patients. The study of variation in heart failure treatment in relation to comorbidity was a good example of this [3]. A third category of methods consists of methods to analyze determinants of effectiveness of KT interventions. This approach requires longitudinal datasets and advanced quantitative methods. An example is an explorative metaregression analysis of guideline implementation studies in hospital settings, which found evidence for the influence of organizational factors on the effectiveness of KT interventions [15]. The latter two categories of methods provide insight into the impact of specific factors, but a limitation to their use is that usually only a few potential determinants of change can be examined in a single study.

How can we link KT interventions to these barriers?

Once objectives have been chosen and barriers for change have been identified, the next step is to link specific KT interventions to these barriers. This process is similar to a clinical treatment that is tailored to a diagnosed health problem [6]. For instance, a project that aimed to reduce inappropriate long-term use of proton pump inhibitors in patients with dyspepsia focused on one specific barrier: the routine provision of repeat prescriptions, without evaluating and discussing their usefulness with the patient. We developed and successfully tested in a randomized trial a discontinuation letter for patients [16]. Another study found that some patients with nonspecific low back pain resisted advice to stay physically active and avoid passive physiotherapy. Therefore, we developed and tested a training session for physicians that included communication skills training. A randomized trial showed that this had positive effects on professional behavior and patient satisfaction with care but not on functional status and sick leave [17].

Linking KT interventions to barriers is probably the most creative step in the design of KT programs because it is challenging to provide clear guidance on how to proceed. Both exploratory and theory-inspired methods can be used. Exploratory methods try to avoid implicit assumptions on what would work but instead advocate using an "open mind." In many cases, some sort of brainstorming in a group is used to identify as many solutions as possible to a problem [18]. Box 3.5.1.1 provides an example of this approach [19]. An alternative to traditional brainstorming is electronic brainstorming using Internet platforms to allow members to enter their ideas anonymously while providing for anonymous distribution of ideas to all participants. Our experience is that the type of implementation interventions suggested by participants can be unsurprising—they tend to mention what they know, such as continuing professional education and information technology solutions. The involvement of a wide range of stakeholders in this process could contribute to the success of the KT program.

Alternatively, theory is used to understand the factors that determine practice variation and change [20,21]. Box 3.5.1.2 provides an example of this approach [22]. A "common sense" use of theories would be to consider the chosen objectives and decide what interventions various theories suggest to influence determinants for change. This decision can be taken in a group so that this method is actually close to the exploratory method described above.

Box 3.5.1.2 Tailored interventions to implement guidelines on depression [22]

This study aimed to determine whether methods tailored to overcome barriers to change using psychological theories are more effective than dissemination alone in the implementation of guidelines for depression among general practitioners. To test this hypothesis, 1239 general practitioners in England were invited to take part in the study. The practices of those who agreed to take part were divided into intervention and control practices. Each practitioner in the intervention group participated in an in-depth interview 6 weeks after disseminating the guidelines to identify their obstacles to implementing them. Interviews were recorded and transcribed. For every comment related to obstacles to change, a psychological theory explaining aspects of individual behavior change was suggested by the reviewer and discussed among the researchers until consensus was reached about what specific theory best explained the observed obstacle. The theory was then used to select the implementation method. For example:

"If a general practitioner reported anxiety about assessing suicide risk and uncertainty about the form of question to use, the theory identified would be self-efficacy. In this case, the implementation method might include the provision of scripts of questions for assessing suicide risk for the general practitioner to use in consultations." If a practitioner faced several obstacles she also received several implementation methods. The theories most commonly found to explain observed barriers were preparedness to change (many practitioners had not given thought to the need to change performance) and self-efficacy (which referred to the fact that practitioners did not feel able to ask about suicide risk or to discuss compliance with medication). In the case of factors related to preparedness to change, feedback was given on the stage of contemplation that the practitioner was in. In the case of factors related to self-efficacy, educational outreach visits were organized and feedback was given as well as quotations from practitioners who felt able to discuss suicide risk. Further, factors related to social influence theory were addressed through small group discussions with peers, educational outreach by an expert clinician as well as feedback to enable performance comparison with others. Factors related to cognitive dissonance theory were addressed by educational outreach visits and feedback accompanied by a reminder of the evidence. Finally, organizational obstacles were mentioned (although the researchers did not ask for them) but could not be addressed in this study. The intervention did not increase adherence to all guideline recommendations.

Table 3.5.1.1 suggests which KT interventions could be linked to a number of theory-based factors [23]. There is no firm research evidence to suggest either exploratory or theory-based approaches. We suggest combining explorative and theory-based methods to select and tailor interventions. Explorative methods may help consider issues that were not anticipated beforehand. The use of theory, however, might help broaden the scope of factors considered and would therefore reduce the chance of overlooking important issues.

What factors should we consider when deciding to use a single or multicomponent KT intervention?

One important decision concerns the use of a single KT intervention or multifaceted KT intervention. Whereas early research suggested that multi-component interventions for KT are most effective [49], later research has raised doubts about this claim [5]. The assumption was that multicomponent

Table 3.5.1.1 KT interventions linked to objectives, barriers for change, and theory

Objectives refer to (or target of the intervention)	Barriers for change	Theory	KT interventions (examples)
1. Cognitive factors			
Information behavior needs to provide brief description of each of these concepts for the reader as "information behavior" may not be self-explanatory to everyone—this comment applies to almost everything in this column	Learning style, learning conceptions, innovation adoption behavior, use of communication channels	Cognitive theory on learning [24]	Use various information delivery methods or adapt to individual needs
Domain knowledge	Domain knowledge, professional knowledge, complexity of the innovation, intelligence, cognitive competences	Cognitive theory on learning [24]	Change the mix of professional skills in the organization

2. Motivational factors

Motivation	Intention goal setting, stages of change, persuasion	Theory on motivation for learning [25] Theory on stages of change [26] Theory on adopter characteristics [27]	Provide information, social influence, action planning according to needs
Beliefs about consequences	Outcome expectancies, attributions of behavior, impact, centrality, duration of the innovation	Social cognitive theory [28] Theory on innovation characteristics [27]	Provide education and feedback, adapt the innovation to improve consequences
Attitudes	Attitudes, utilities, advantage, costs, risks of the innovation	Theory of planned behavior [29]	Provide education on consequences
Perceived subjective norms	Perceptions of other behavior, social, professional role, compatibility, visibility of the innovation, social comparison	Theory of planned behavior [29]	Organize social influence
Beliefs about capabilities	Perceived behavioral control, self-confidence	Social cognitive theory [28] Theory of planned behavior [29]	Provide skills training
Emotion	Satisfaction with performance, attractiveness of the innovation	Theory on motivation for learning [25]	Provide feedback; Provide education and counseling to change individual standards (*Continued*)

Table 3.5.1.1 (*Continued*)

Objectives refer to (or target of the intervention)	Barriers for change	Theory	KT interventions (examples)
3. Behavioral factors			
Behavioral regulation	Coping behaviors, observational learning, central/peripheral route	Social cognitive theory [28] Coping theory [30]	Provide feedback and reminders to enable self-regulation; Provide education and counseling to change individual standards
Skills	Competence, behavioral capability, flexibility, divisibility, triability of the innovation	Cognitive theory on learning [24]	Provide education to improve competency; Use decision support systems
4. Interaction in professional teams			
Team cognitions	Objectives, group vision, task orientation, group norms	Theory on team effectiveness [31] Theory on group decisions [32]	Change team members or decision processes
Team processes	Group composition, participation safety	Theory on team effectiveness [31] Theory on group decisions [32]	Training to change group processes

5. Structure of professional networks

Leadership and key individuals	Change agents, opinion leaders, source of the message	Theory on persuasion [33] Theory on leadership [34]	Identify and involve formal and informal leaders
Social network characteristics	Range, density, multiplexity, weak ties, etc.	Social support theory [35] Theory on social comparison [36] Theory on diffusion of innovations [27]	Involve change agents to transfer information; Develop networks to create more "weak" linkages

6. Organizational structures

Specification	Clinical protocols, benchmarking, systems perspective	Disease management systems [37] Theory on organizational innovativeness [38]	Implement integrated care systems, e.g., chronic care model
Flexibility	Flexible delivery system, minimum specification, formalization, fragmentation, operational variety	Complex adaptive systems [39] Theory on organizational innovativeness [38]	Redesign specific services in the organization
Leadership structure	Constancy of purpose, management in different stages, centralization, management attitudes/tenure, administrative intensity	Theory on quality management [40] Theory on organizational innovativeness [38]	Recruit and train to have specific types of leaders

(Continued)

Table 3.5.1.1 (*Continued*)

Objectives refer to (or target of the intervention)	Barriers for change	Theory	KT interventions (examples)
Specialization	Differentiation, professionalism	Theory on organizational innovativeness [38]	Change the mix of professional skills in the organization
7. Organizational processes			
Continuous improvement	Training of professionals, talent-developing programs, process mindedness, continuous education, concern for measurement, experimental mindset	Theory on quality management [40] Theory on organizational learning [41]	Create teams for improvement
External communication	Customer mindedness, reactiviness, scanning imperative, complexity, external influence, suppliers as partners	Theory on quality management [40] Theory on organizational innovativeness [38]	Undertake patient satisfaction activities
Internal communication	Climate of openness, generative relationships, involvement of nonmedical professionals, employee mindedness, cooperation focus, multiple advocates, ownership, cultural diversity, involvement of target group	Theory on quality management [40] Theory on organizational innovativeness [38] Theory on organizational learning [41] Theory on knowledge management [42] Theory on organizational culture [43]	Undertake care provider satisfaction activities; Use ICT for transfer of information

8. Organizational resources			
Technical knowledge	Competence base, organizational intelligence, creativity, knowledge information systems	Theory on organizational innovativeness [38]	Change the mix of professional skills in the organization
Organizational size	Size of teams	Theory on organizational innovativeness [38]	Merge/split organizations or departments
9. Societal factors			
Professional development	Education and legal protection related to body of knowledge	Theory on professional development [44]	Revise professional roles
Priority on societal agenda	Public relations, political action	Theory on agenda building [45]	Undertake activities to influence policymakers
10. Financial incentives			
Positive incentives	Rewards, simple attractors, resources, structures for rewards, slack resources, support for innovation, provider utility function	Theory on financial reimbursement [46]	Change the provider reimbursement and patient copayment
Provider and patient financial risk sharing	Budgets, capitation, etc., supplier induced demand	Theory on financial reimbursement [46]	Change the provider reimbursement and patient copayment

(Continued)

Table 3.5.1.1 (*Continued*)

Objectives refer to (or target of the intervention)	Barriers for change	Theory	KT interventions (examples)
Transaction costs	Cost improvement, switching costs related to innovation	Theory on contracting [47]	Change the financial system for health care
Competition intensity	Maturity of the market	Theory on competition and innovation [48]	Introduce market characteristics, such as financial risk and improved information for users
11. Regulations			

interventions addressed a larger number of barriers for change and therefore were more effective. However, research evidence did not clearly support this claim. A complicating factor is that the definition of what is a "single intervention" is difficult. For instance, outreach visits that include instruction, motivation, planning of improvement, and practical help hardly comprise a single intervention. A multicomponent intervention that combines different types of professional education (e.g., lectures, materials, and workshops) still only addresses lack of knowledge. We suggest that multicomponent interventions could be more effective than single interventions if they address different types of barriers for change. As these tend to require more resources, the efficiency (and feasibility and sustainability) of multicomponent interventions needs to be evaluated.

Future research

How comprehensive and systematic the analysis of determinants of change has to be remains to be seen. The added value of tailoring KT interventions has yet to be proven. A systematic review on the effectiveness of tailored versus nontailored interventions could not show the added value of tailoring interventions to barriers identified [50]. However, the main reason for this conclusion was the lack of sufficient details concerning how assessed barriers influenced the choice of interventions in the included papers. An explorative review that included some of the same studies [51] found that many KT interventions chosen focused on a few cognitive factors in health professionals, such as knowledge gaps, although a much wider range of barriers for change was considered in studies of change determinants.

Many KT projects are pragmatic activities in busy and complex environments and, therefore, they should deliver an optimal effect at the lowest possible cost. KT interventions should not just aim to improve health care delivery, they should also aim to sustain improvements. Practitioners and managers have every reason to be critical about systematic, resource-consuming methods. More research is needed on how to design KT programs and particularly on the linkage between barriers for change and choice of KT interventions. A challenge for researchers is to define testable hypotheses, even in situations that are to some extent unique and in complex KT programs that address multiple issues and stakeholders. Health policymakers face short-term needs for improvement in health care delivery and therefore design pragmatic KT programs. They should also invest in KT research to enhance the sustained impact of KT interventions [52,53].

Specific areas requiring research include the effectiveness and efficiency of systematic KT intervention development compared to pragmatic, simple methods for choosing KT interventions. Another issue is how different stake-holders, including patients, are best involved in KT intervention development. In some situations, stakeholder involvement might have more impact on the effectiveness of a KT intervention than the specific procedure for developing it or the type of intervention. At a more fundamental level, continued research is needed on determinants of improvement in health care so that knowledge on such determinants can guide the choice of KT interventions.

Summary

The choice of KT interventions remains an "art" informed by science, meaning that practice-based experience and creativity are important in selecting KT interventions. We suggest that the use of a stepwise approach and structured methods helps take a comprehensive and balanced approach. Also, research evidence on KT interventions can provide some guidance, if only to show which interventions need to be avoided.

References

1 Cleland JG, Cohen-Solal A, Aguilar JC, Dietz R, Eastaugh J, Follath F, et al. Management of heart failure in primary care (the IMPROVEMENT of Heart Failure Programme): an international survey. *Lancet* 2002;360:1631–39.

2 Sturm HB, Van Gilst WH, Swedberg K, Hobbs FDR, Haaijer-Ruskamp FM. Heart failure guidelines and prescribing in primary care across Europe. *BMC Health Serv Res* 2005;5:57.

3 Sturm HB, Haaijer-Ruskamp FM, Veeger NJ, Baljé-Volkers CP, Swedberg K, Van Gilst WH. The relevance of comorbidities for heart failure treatment in primary care: a European study. *Eur J Heart Failure* 2006;8:31–37.

4 Kasje WN, Denig P, De Graeff PA, Haaijer-Ruskamp FM. Perceived barriers for treatment of chronic heart failure in general practice: are they affecting performance? *BMC Fam Med* 2005;6:19.

5 Grimshaw J, Thomas RE, Maclennan G, Fraser C, Ramsay CR, Vale L, et al. Effectiveness and efficiency of guideline dissemination and implementation strategies. *Health Technology Assessment* 2004;8:6.

6 Grol R, Grimshaw J. From best evidence to best practice: effective implementation of change in patients' care. *Lancet* 2003;362:1225–30.

7 Grol R, Bosch M, Hulscher M, Eccles M, Wensing M. Planning and studying improvement in patient care: the use of theoretical perspectives. *Milbank Quarterly* 2006;85:93–138.

8 Grol R, Wensing M, Eccles M. *Improving Patient Care. The Implementation of Change in Clinical Practice.* New York: Elsevier; 2004.

9 Graham ID, Tetroe J, KT Theories Research Group. Some theoretical underpinnings of knowledge translation. *Acad Emerg Med* 2007;14[11]:936–44.

10 Locke EA, Latham GP. *A Theory of Goal Setting and Task Performance.* Englewood Cliffs, NJ. Prentice Hall; 1991.

11 Linstone HA, Turoff M. *The Delphi Method: Techniques and Applications.* Reading, MA: Addison-Wesley; 1975.

12 Harmsen M, Wensing M, Braspenning JCC, Wolters R, Van der Wouden JC, Grol R. Management of children's urinary tract infections in Dutch family practice: a cohort study. *BMC Fam Pract* 2007;13[8]:9.

13 Campbell S, Ludt S, Van Lieshout J, Wensing M, Grol R, Roland M. Quality indicators for the prevention and management of cardiovascular disease in primary care in nine European countries. *Eur J Cardiovasc Prev Rehab* 2008 (provisionally accepted).

14 Krol N, Spies T, Van Balen J, Numans M, Muris J, Wensing M, et al. Dyspepsia in general practice: medical care and its determinants. *Qual Prim Care* 2003;1: 173–80.

15 Dijkstra R, Wensing M, Thomas R, Akkermans R, Braspenning J, Grimshaw J, et al. The relationship between organisational characteristics and the effects of clinical guidelines on medical performance in hospitals, a meta-analysis. *BMC Health Serv Res* 2006;6:53.

16 Krol N, Wensing M, Haaijer-Ruskamp F, Muris J, Numans M, Van Balen J, et al. Patient-directed strategy to reduce prescribing for patients with dyspepsia in general practice: a randomised trial. *Alim Pharm Therap* 2004;19;917–22.

17 Engers AJ, Wensing M, Van Tulder MW, Timmermans A, Oostendorp R, Koes BW, et al. Implementation of the Dutch low back pain guideline for general practice: a randomized trial. *Spine* 2005;30:595–600.

18 Osborn AF. *Applied imagination: Principles and Procedures of Creative Problem Solving.* 3rd ed. New York: Charles Scribner's Sons; 1963.

19 Heinen MM, Bartholomew LK, Wensing M, Van de Kerkhof P, Van Achterberg T. Supporting adherence and healthy lifestyles in leg ulcer patients: systematic development of the Lively Legs program for dermatology outpatient clinics. *Pat Educ Counsel* 2006;61:279–91.

20 Eccles M, Grimshaw J, Walker A, Johnston M, Pitts N. Changing the behaviour of healthcare professionals: the use of theory in promoting the uptake of research findings. *J Clin Epidemiol* 2005;58:107–12.

21 Sales A, Smith J, Curran G, Kochevar L. Models, strategies, and tools. Theory in implementing evidence-based findings in health care practice. *J Gen Intern Med* 2006;21:S43–49.

22 Baker R, Reddish S, Robertson N, Hearnshaw H, Jones B. Randomised controlled trial of tailored strategies to implement guidelines for the management of patients with depression in general practice. *Br J Gen Pract* 2001;51[470]:737–41.

23 Wensing M, Bosch M, Foy R, Van der Weijden T, Eccles M, Grol R. *Factors in Theories on Behaviour Change to Guide Implementation and Quality Improvement.* Radboud University Nijmegen Medical Centre, Centre for Quality of Care Research; 2005.

24 Norman G. Research in medical education: three decades of progress. *BMJ* 2002;324:1560–2.

25 Newman P, Peile E. Valuing learner's experience and supporting further growth: educational models to help experienced adult learners in medicine. *BMJ* 2002;325:200–2.

26 Prochaska JO, Velicer WF. The transtheoretical model of health behavior change. *Am J Health Promotion* 1997;12:38–48.

27 Rogers EM. *Diffusion of Innovations.* 4th ed. New York: The Free Press; 1995.

28 Bandura A. *Social Foundations of Thought and Action.* Englewood Cliffs, NJ: Prentice Hall; 1986.

29 Ajzen I. The theory of planned behaviour. *Organ Behav Hum Decis Process* 1991;50:179–211.

30 Lazarus RS, Folkman S. *Stress Appraisal and Coping.* New York: Springer; 1984.

31 De Dreu CKW, Weingart LR. Task versus relationship conflict, team performance, and team member satisfaction: a meta-analysis. *J Applied Psychology* 2003;88: 741–9.

32 Turner ME, Pratkanis AR. Twenty-five years of groupthink theory and research: lessons from the evaluation of a theory. *Organ Behav Hum Decis Making* 1998; 73[2–3]:105–15.

33 Petty RE, Wegener DT, Fabrigar LR. Attitudes and attitude change. *Annu Rev Psychol* 1997;48:609–48.

34 Yukl G. *Leadership in Organisations.* 4th ed. Englewood Cliffs, NJ: Prentice Hall; 1998.

35 Hogan B, Linden W, Najarian B. Social support interventions. Do they work? *Clin Psychol Rev* 2002;2:381–440.

36 Suls J, Martin R, Wheeler L. Social comparison: why, with whom, and with what effect? *Curr Dir Psychol Sci* 2002;11[5]:159–63.

37 Hunter DJ. Disease management: has it a future? It has a compelling logic, but it needs to be tested in practice. *BMJ* 2000;320:530.

38 Damanpour F. Organizational innovation: a meta-analysis of effects of determinants and moderators. *Acad Manage J* 1991;34:535–90.

39 Plesk PE, Greenhalgh T. Complexity, leadership, and management in healthcare organizations. *BMJ* 2001;323:746–9.

40 Prajogo DI, Sohal AS. TQM and innovations: a literature review and research framework. *Technovation* 2001;21:539–58.

41 Senge, PM. *The Fifth Discipline. The Art and Practice of the Learning Organization.* London: Random House; 1990.

42 Garavelli AC, Gorgoglione M, Scozzi B. Managing knowledge transfer by knowledge technologies. *Technovation* 2002;22:269–79.

43 Scott T, Mannion R, Davies H, Marshall MN. Implementing culture change in health care: theory and practice. *Int J Qual Health Care* 2003(b);15[2]:111–18.

44 Freidson E. *Profession of Medicine.* New York: Dodds, Mead; 1970.

45 Walters TN, Walters LM, Gray R. Agenda building in the 1992 presidential campaign. *Public Relations Review,* 1996;22[1]:9–24.

46 Sonnad SS, Foreman SE. An incentive approach to physician implementation of medical practice guidelines. *Health Economics* 1997;6:467–77.

47 Chalkley M, Malcomson JM. Contracting for health services when patient demand does not reflect quality. *J Health Econ* 1998;17:1–19.

48 Funk P. Induced innovation revisited. *Economica* 2002;69:155–71.

49 Wensing M, Van der Weijden T, Grol R. Implementing guidelines and innovations in primary care: which interventions are effective? *Br J Gen Pract* 1998;48:991–7.

50 Shaw B., Cheater F., Baker R., Gillies C., Hearnshaw H., Flottorp S., et al. Tailored interventions to overcome identified barriers to change: effects on professional practice and health outcomes. *The Cochrane Database of Systematic Reviews* 2008. Issue 3. Art. No.: CD 005470. DOI:10.1002/14651858.CD005470.

51 Bosch M, Van der Weijden T, Wensing M, Grol R. Tailoring quality improvement interventions to identified barriers: a multiple case analysis. *J Eval Clin Pract* 2007;13:161–8.

52 Grol R, Berwick DM, Wensing M. On the trail of quality and safety in health care. *BMJ* 2008;336:74–6.

53 Tetroe JM, Graham ID, Foy R, Robinson N, Eccles M, Ward J, et al. Health research funding agencies' support and promotion of knowledge translation: an international study. *Milbank Quarterly* 2008 (in press).

3.5.2 **Educational interventions**

Dave Davis[1] *and Nancy Davis*[2]

[1] Association of American Medical Colleges, Washington, DC, USA
[2] National Institute for Quality and Education, Pittsburgh, Pennsylvania, USA

KEY LEARNING POINTS

- Education is a broad and holistic word; the acronym "CME" conveys a gestalt of short courses, whereas effective education of physicians can be seen as an intervention, often with predisposing, enabling, and reinforcing strategies.
- Large group sessions, the mainstay of traditional CME, can also be made more effective by paying attention to rigorous needs assessments and by increasing interactivity and engagement in the learning process.
- Other interventions also show promise: small group learning, communities of practice, and distance education.
- Finally, self-directed learning is increasingly better understood and may be assisted by the addition of portfolio learning and self-assessment exercises.

The term "education" has many broad meanings, though its gestalt—especially in continuing medical education (CME), where education implies a large group session often held in a hotel or conference setting—is one that demonstrates little evidence of effect on clinician performance or health care outcomes. "Education" is a broad and holistic phrase. The American Medical Association (AMA) defines CME as "any and all ways by which physicians learn and maintain their competence"—clearly a more fulsome construct than attending a short course [1]. This section describes educational interventions designed to promote the incorporation of best evidence into the practices of health professionals. It describes more common educational interventions while ensuing chapters build on the overview provided in Chapter 3.5.1 and describe other knowledge translation (KT) interventions such as academic detailing, reminders, audits, and feedback. This section will address a theoretical basis for physician* learning and education; an outline of effective large group methods; innovations in formal education employing high- (and low-) tech strategies; and finally, future trends in CME and health professional education.

What are the purposes of education?

The question of *why* health professionals learn is driven by many external forces. These include the knowledge explosion, specialty society interest in CME, the use of CME "credit" to document knowledge and skills maintenance, and a large interest among pharmaceutical and other commercial interests that recognize CME as a means of influencing physician practice. There are many internal forces at work as well—including an innate sense of professionalism on the part of most health care workers.

The question of *"how"* physicians learn has been examined. For example, Fox and his colleagues asked over 300 North American physicians what practices they had changed and what forces had driven that change [2]. Physicians undertaking any change widely described an image of that change—for example, the general physician needing to be more comfortable with an ethnic population. The forces for change were varied. Although changes arose from traditional educational experiences, many more were intrapersonal (e.g., a recent personal experience) or from changing demographics (e.g., aging or changing populations and patient demands). Finally, changes varied from smaller "adjustments" or accommodations (e.g., adding a new drug to a regimen within a class of drugs already known and prescribed) to much larger

---

*In this section, reference is made most frequently to physician education because the majority of studies in this area have employed physicians. Where possible, reference is made to other health professionals.

"redirections," such as adopting an entirely new method of practice. Schon describes the internal process of learning and "reflection," suggesting that a potent learning mechanism is secondary to self-appraisal and awareness built from clinical experiences. This leads to the building of a new and expanded competency or "zone of mastery" [3]. Candy's description of the traits of the self-directed learner also deserves elaboration [4]. These traits include discipline and motivation; analytic abilities; ability to reflect and be self-aware; curiosity, openness, and flexibility; independence and self-sufficiency; well-developed information-seeking and retrieval skills; good general learning skills. Clearly, these are desirable—if not always fully achievable—attributes.

Over the years, many authors have suggested steps in the change process [5]. Rogers [6] referred to this as the decision-innovation process, and Prochaska and Velicer [7] referred to it as the transtheoretical model. Specifically focusing on physicians, Pathman [8] used the model—awareness-agreement-adoption-adherence—to describe the process. Here, the physician becomes aware of a new finding or practice,proceeds with the process of agreeing with it, and then to an irregular adoption of it. Finally, the physician adheres to the practice, conforming to guideline recommendations whenever indicated. These "stages" of learning are important when considering the effect of educational interventions. A more complete discussion of educational theories is provided in Chapter 4.3.

What is the process for education?

Education is a means to effect performance change and to improve practice outcomes, thereby achieving KT. Green's PRECEED model [9], which incorporates elements that are characterized as predisposing, enabling, and reinforcing, helps conceptualize education as an intervention. In this model, predisposing elements include mailed guidelines, didactic lectures, conferences, and rounds that may *predispose* toward change in knowledge uptake; patient education materials and other tools (e.g., flowcharts) that may *enable* the change; and finally *reinforcing strategies* including reminders or audits and feedback, useful to solidify a change already made. One systematic review supports this construct [10] and allows us to consider aligning educational interventions to the stage of learning as shown in Table 3.5.2.1.

Portraying the characteristics of educational intervention and the process through which the learner adheres to a new practice provides a rough framework to highlight educational interventions using the four steps in the Pathman model as an organizing principle. First, several systematic reviews have identified that most didactic conferences [10,11] or mailed materials [12], employing only one technique, are infrequent producers of performance

Table 3.5.2.1 Alignment: placing educational intervention in the context of health professional learning

Learning/change continuum	Awareness	Agreement	Adoption	Adherence
Elements of change:	*Predisposing elements:*	*Enabling*	*strategies;*	*Reinforcing elements:*
Possible roles for educational interventions	Conferences, lectures, rounds, print materials	Small group learning activity; Interactivity in lectures	Workshops; Materials distributed at conferences; Audit and feedback	Audit and feedback; Reminders

change. This finding, however, may be "unfair" to such traditional modalities because they may play a crucial role in predisposing to change. For example, where health professionals are unaware of new evidence, conferences, print materials, and rounds may predispose to change. Second, if learners are aware of a new finding or guideline but do not agree with it, small group learning or increased interactivity in the conference setting exposes the learner to peer influence [13], a strong predictor of increased discussion and consensus. Third, if the issue is one of adoption of a new manual or communication skill or complex care algorithm, more in-depth workshops or on-line learning experiences may facilitate the change [13]. Finally, once the process has been adopted, system-based interventions such as reminders or audits and feedback may be considered to facilitate sustainability [14].

What educational interventions can we use to effect KT?

Large group sessions

Educational events for relatively large numbers of learners are commonplace, although evidence indicates this type of educational intervention produces little, if any, performance change. However, several studies [10,11,15,16] have outlined relatively useful and effective strategies within the large group model to increase the impact on performance and health care outcomes. These strategies include needs assessment [15], increased interactivity [16], and variation in the educational method [11].

Determining needs and setting objectives

There is ample evidence that not only the needs of learners but also their patients or health care system should drive CME [11]. Health systems frequently use only objectively determined needs (e.g., the clinical care "gap") to drive the educational agenda, a process that misses an understanding of the learning process and that may fail to lead to benefit. In contrast, CME planners frequently use subjective needs assessments, despite evidence that clinicians may be poor self-assessors [17,18] and that objectively determined gaps may more closely link the CME process to demonstrable outcomes. Subjective needs assessment strategies include questionnaires, focus groups, structured individual interviews, and diaries or log books, described in more detail in Chapter 3.2. To offset the self-assessment deficiencies inherent in these methods and to create a more holistic needs assessment strategy, objective tools can be used including standardized assessments of knowledge and/or skills, chart audits, peer review, observation of health professional practice, and reports of practice patterns and physician performance data [19].

Results of these needs assessments can produce objectives for educational activities. CME—along with undergraduate and graduate education—has shifted from conceiving of these as learning objectives (what the learner should know or be able to do at the end of the activity) to behavioral objectives (what the learner should be expected to do as a result of what has been learned).

Formatting the large group session

Several strategies can enhance delivery of effective formal, large group CME. They include increasing the interactivity of the sessions, employing multiple methods within the framework of the activity, and using other strategies to increase reach and impact [11].

Multiple methods

As discussed in Chapter 3.5.1, there is no clear evidence suggesting a benefit of multicomponent interventions over single-component interventions. However, there are suggestions that multicomponent interventions could be more effective than single interventions if they address different types of barriers for change. Within the context of the formal CME event, most recent evidence demonstrates that multiple methods used in the context of the activity may promote uptake and translation into practice [11]. The methods may be characterized in several ways. First, formal sessions may use a variety of presentation media (e.g., audio tapes to present heart sounds; actual or standardized patients or videotapes; panel discussions to present conflicting perspectives on one topic; debates to highlight issues where agreement lacks; quizzes to determine learning needs or outcomes). Second, given that knowledge is a necessary but not sufficient condition for performance change, practice enablers may be distributed and used during a standard CME event—examples include patient care reminders, protocols and flow sheets, patient education materials, wall charts, and other measures that may be used in the practice setting after the activity concludes [11]. Third, CME activities may use clinical scenarios and vignettes to increase relevance and applicability of educational material. Vignettes are frequently derived from actual clinical cases and modified to ensure patient confidentiality and to exemplify history, diagnosis, or management details [20]. They promote reflection and interaction. There are many methods to present such cases or clinical stories. Short paper cases can use prompts to discuss diagnosis or management; standardized patients can present highly credible clinical findings and histories;video and audio cases, role playing, and sophisticated simulation techniques may add relevance and increase learning potential [11]. Staging a multimethod learning experience so it is interrupted shows evidence of increased effect [11]. Two workshops of 3 hours each, for example, held a month apart, allow the learners to absorb information from the first event, apply it in the work setting, and then discuss the process with reinforcement of learning during the second event. An example of this interrupted learning process is the opportunity afforded by the weekly or monthly recurrence of clinical rounds.

Interactivity

With fairly clear evidence for effect [16], interactivity increases the interplay between audience members or between participants and the presenter. There are a number of ways in which this can be accomplished:

- Interaction between the presenter and participants: Planners may increase the question and answer sessions of lectures, divide lectures into 10-minute periods followed by questions and answers [20], and/or use an audience response system [21]. The last may use technology to poll the audience for responses to projected questions or use low-tech options (although not anonymous) to employ color-coded cards.
- Interaction between participants: buzz groups: Described by the noise they make in a normally quiet audience, these groups allow participants to engage neighboring audience members in conversation. Pyramiding or snowballing builds on interactions between pairs of participants to groups of four or six, eventually involving all participants. An example is "think-pair-share." This begins with practice reflection (e.g., a quiet moment for participants to think of a particular case), followed by a discussion with a neighboring participant, then with the larger audience.

Small group learning

Small group learning in CME is one of many innovations created by the growth in problem-based learning methods in undergraduate medical education. This method uses groups of 5–10 individuals and employs many of the principles of effective CME (e.g., case vignettes, group discussion, and high degree of interactivity). Groups meet regularly, usually without an expert, and are led by one of their own membership who acts as facilitator. Common in Canada and Europe, these groups demonstrate impact on competence and performance—most likely a combination of their concentration on evidence-based materials and on their heavy reliance on peer pressure and influence [13,22]. Whereas some groups are informal and self-organizing, many others are a part of national maintenance of competence and CME programs, such as professional licensing bodies [23].

Distance education techniques

Although in-person CME remains a primary knowledge delivery vehicle, there are other ways in which KT may be accomplished. For example, visiting speaker programs may use Web, video, or audiocasts. Not unlike their live "cousins," these activities must be interactive to engage the learner and improve impact and may employ interactive cases and other methods to stimulate the learner to use critical thinking and problem solving. Recent studies have shown increases in physician knowledge and knowledge retention following participation in on-line CME courses [24], and if appropriately designed, they may be superior to live activities in effecting physician behavioral changes [25].

On-line communities of practice [26] are another potential KT intervention: groups of learners experience audio conferences, case discussions, and follow-up or support by electronic means using reminders, cases, and other means to promote networking and consulting among peers. These groups can help evaluate the effectiveness of the education as well as determine needs for new activities and can build both a community and shared knowledge base.

Self-directed learning

Some health professionals possess a learning style preference or logistical need for more self-directed choices. These include traditional sources such as textbooks, monographs, clinical practice guidelines, and journals that provide clinical information. Important developments to aid self-directed learning have included the advent of printed or computerized self-assessment programs, which provide learners with feedback about their competence as they read materials and answer questions, receiving feedback.

Portfolio-based learning [27,28] is also an important tool in self-directed learning, derived from the concept of the artist's or photographer's collection of his or her work. More complex than a simple accumulation of exemplary work, the portfolio is intended to document educational activities undertaken by the clinician, quality documentation (chart reviews done or achievement of performance milestones), identified learning gaps, examples of learning plans and objectives and resources used to meet them, and other data related to performance and health care outcomes. Portfolios can be used for self-reflection, self-assessment, and learning, or they may be used in an educational manner—providing grist for conversation with a peer or other mentor or applied to questions of relicensure, recertification, and other needs.

What are some current trends in CME?

There are many trends and challenges in the construction, delivery, and use of CME leading to a more holistic and integrated understanding of this last and longest phase of clinicians' learning. They include:

- The changing construct of "CME": from traditional understanding of CME as an information transfer vehicle to a more complete understanding of the learning process and the complex health care world in which this occurs.
- An increasing focus on health care outcomes and performance using performance measures, moving CME planners to increase attention at Levels 4–6 of the Moore [29] evaluation schema (Table 3.5.2.2) rather than its previous occupation with lower levels.
- New and emerging disease states: Here the need for rapid response educational technologies exists in the face of serious SARS-like, pan-flu, and bioterrorism issues, and they speak to the need for technologies such as SMS texting, fax networks, e-mail, and other means including the concept of "push" technologies.
- Chronic disease management: Health researchers have outlined the need for improved management of chronic diseases, many with comorbidities, in an aging population. These needs show promise in driving the educational aspects of KT—creating interprofessional education initiatives, disseminating and incorporating complex care algorithms, point of care learning resources, and other methods.
- Maintenance of licensure and certification: The traditional notion of credit, linked to mandatory CME participation, at least for physicians, is increasingly questioned by licensing boards and specialty societies and boards. The traditional credit hour documents CME participation but falls short in demonstrating translation to maintained competence or improved performance. With the movement toward more self-directed, practice-based learning, critics have argued for a relative value system that provides higher value credit for activities that demonstrate improved practice. This notion is incorporated into the movement toward maintenance of licensure and recertification in the United States and Canada [30,31].

Table 3.5.2.2 Outcomes for continuing education/continuing professional development [29]

Level	Outcome	Metrics or indicators
1	Participation	Attendance
2	Satisfaction	Participant satisfaction
3	Learning	Changes in knowledge, skills, or attitude
4	Performance	Changes in practice performance
5	Patient health	Changes in patient health status
6	Population health	Changes in population health status

Future research

There are many research directions in which CME plays a significant role. Of these, several become important in an era of accountability and movement toward demonstrated competence and performance as a result of CME participation. They include questions about the learner (Are self-assessment and self-directed learning core character logic traits or can they be taught? If the latter, how can this best be accomplished?); the communication vehicles (What knowledge transmission vectors work best? PDA-mediated educational messages vs. traditional educational ones); the context of learning (e.g., the seeing of learning, its remuneration pattern, its linkage to IT resources); and the effect on learning and uptake. Finally, a large question for CME research is the uptake of information in which the variables include questions about the nature, complexity, compatibility, and level of evidence to be adopted.

References

1 American Medical Association. 2008. URL http://www.ama-assn.org/ [accessed March 2008].
2 Fox RD, Mazmanian PE, Putnam W. *Changing and Learning in the Lives of Physicians.* New York: Praeger; 1994.
3 Schön, D. A. *The Reflective Practitioner: How professionals Think in Action.* London: Temple Smith; 1983.
4 Candy, PC. *Self-Direction for Lifelong Learning.* San Francisco: Jossey-Bass; 1991.
5 Grol R, Wensing M, Eccles M. *Improving Patient Care. The Implementation of Change in Clinical Practice.* London: Elsevier; 2005.
6 Rogers E. *Diffusion of Innovations.* 5th ed. New York: Free Press; 2003.
7 Prochaska JO, Velicer WF. The transtheoretical model of health behaviour change. *Am J Health Promot* 1997;12:38–48.

8 Pathman DE, Konrad TR, Freed GL, Freeman VA, Koch GG. The awareness-to-adherence model of the steps to clinical guideline compliance. The case of pediatric vaccine recommendations. *Med Care* 1996;34:873–89.

9 Green LW, Kreuter MW. *Health Promotion Planning: An Educational and Ecological Approach.* 4th ed. New York: McGraw-Hill; 2005.

10 Davis DA, Thomson MA, Oxman AD, Haynes RB. Changing physician performance. A systematic review of the effect of continuing medical education strategies. *JAMA* 1995;274:700–5.

11 Marinopoulos SS, Dorman T, Ratanawongsa N, Wilson LM, Ashar BH, Magaziner JL, et al. Effectiveness of continuing medical education. *Evid Rep Technol Assess* 2007;[149]:1–69.

12 Wagner TH. The effectiveness of mailed patient reminders on mammography screening: a meta-analysis. *Am J Prev Med* 1998;14:64–70.

13 Peloso PM, Stakiw KJ. Small-group format for continuing medical education: a report from the field. *J Cont Educ Health Prof* 2000;20:27–32.

14 Jamtvedt G, Young JM, Kristoffersen DT, O'Brien MA, Oxman AD. Audit and feedback: effects on professional practice and health care outcomes. *Cochrane Database of Systematic Reviews* 2006[2]: CD000259.

15 Davis DA, Thomson O'Brien MA, Freemantle N, Wolf F, Mazmanian P, Taylor-Vaisey A. Impact of formal continuing medical education: do conferences, workshops, rounds and other traditional continuing education activities change physician behaviour or health outcomes? *JAMA* 1999;282[9]:867–74.

16 Thomson O'Brien MA, Freemantle N, Oxman AD, Wolf F, Davis DA, Herrin J. Continuing education meetings and workshops: effects on professional practice and health care outcomes. *Cochrane Database of Systematic Reviews* 2001, Issue 2.

17 Sibley JC, Sackett DL, Neufeld V, Gerrard B, Rudnick KV, Fraser W. A randomised trial of continuing medical education. *N Engl J Med* 1982;306[9]: 511–5.

18 Davis DA, Mazmanian PE, Fordis M, Van Harrison R, Thorpe KE, Perrier L. Accuracy of physician self-assessment compared with observed measures of competence: a systematic review. *JAMA* 2006;296[9]:1094–102.

19 Lockyer J. Needs assessment: lessons learned. *J Cont Educ Health Pfor* 1998;18: 190–2.

20 Brose JA. Case presentation as a teaching tool: making a good thing better. *J Am Osteopath Assoc* 1992;92:376–8.

21 Gagnon RJ, Thivierge R. Evaluating touch pad technology. *J Cont Educ Health Prof* 1997;20–26.

22 The Foundation for Medical Practice Education. 2008. URL http://www.fmpe.org/en/about/background.html [accessed March 2008].

23 Ontario College of Family Physicians. 2008. URL http://www.ocfp.on.ca/English/OCFP/CME/default.asp?s=1 [accessed March 2008].

24 Casebeer LL, Kristofco RE, Strasser S, Reilly M, Krishnamoorthy P, Rabin A, et al. Standardizing evaluation of on-line continuing medical education: physician

knowledge, attitudes and reflection on practice. *J Contin Educ Health Prof* 2004; 24[2]:68–75.

25 Fordis M, King JE, Ballantyne CM, Jones PH, Schneider KH, Spann SJ, et al. Comparison of the instructional efficacy of Internet-based CME with live interactive CME workshops: a randomized controlled trial. *JAMA* 2005;294[9]: 1043–51.

26 Wenger EC, Snyder WM. Communities of practice: the organisational frontier. *Harvard Business Review* 2000;Jan:139–45.

27 Parboosingh J. Learning portfolios: potential to assist health professionals with self-directed learning. *J Cont Educ Health Prof* 1996;16:75–81.

28 Campbell C, Parboosingh J, Gondocz T, Babitskaya G, Lindsay E, De Guzman RC, et al. Study of physicians' use of a software program to create a portfolio of their self-directed learning. *Acad Med* 1996;71[10]:S49–51.

29 Moore DL. A framework for outcomes evaluation in the continuing professional development of physicians. In D Davis et al. (Eds.), *The Continuing Professional Development of Physicians*. Chicago: AMA Press; 2003.

30 American Board of Internal Medicine. URL www.abim.org/exam/moc.

31 The Royal College of Physicians and Surgeons of Canada. 2008. URL http://rcpsc .medical.org/opd/index.php [accessed March 2008].

3.5.3 **Linkage and exchange interventions**

Martin P. Eccles and Robbie Foy

Institute of Health and Society, Newcastle University, Newcastle upon Tyne, UK

KEY LEARNING POINTS

- Opinion leaders and outreach visitors can produce small but worthwhile changes in health care professional behavior, but their cost-effectiveness is not well-understood.
- The effectiveness of knowledge brokers is unclear.

Mittman and colleagues [1] noted that health care professionals work within peer groups that share common beliefs, assumptions, and group norms, and that individual behavior can be strongly influenced by these factors. They identified a number of strategies to facilitate the implementation of research findings by using these social influences, a phenomenon that comes from literature on the diffusion of innovations. The strategies of educational outreach (also known as academic detailing), opinion leaders, and knowledge brokers are linked by the fact that they are designed to achieve their effect by using the interpersonal relationships between health care practitioners.

What linkage and exchange activities can be used to effect KT?

Educational outreach visits

O'Brien and colleagues [2] reviewed studies of educational outreach. They state that the term educational outreach describes a personal visit by a trained person to health professionals in their own settings. This type of "face-to-face" visit has been referred to as university-based educational detailing, public interest detailing, and academic detailing. Originally described as a multicomponent process, key principles include surveys of practitioners to determine barriers to appropriate practice and the subsequent development of an intervention tailored to address those barriers using simple messages; targeting of practitioners with low compliance; and the delivery of the intervention by a respected person. The intervention often included feedback on existing practice.

Within the review, the authors identified 34 comparisons of educational outreach visits versus no intervention. They found that the median absolute improvement in compliance with desired practice was 5.6% (interquartile range [IQR] 3.0–9.0%). These improvements were highly consistent for prescribing (median 4.8%, IQR 3.0–6.5% for 17 comparisons) but varied for other types of professional performace (median 6.0%, IQR 3.6–16.0% for 17 comparisons). The authors could not find compelling explanations for the observed variation.

Opinion leadership

Opinion leadership is the degree to which an individual can influence other individuals' attitudes or overt behavior informally in a desired way with relative frequency [3]. This informal leadership is not a function of the individual's formal position or status in the system; it is earned and maintained by the individual's technical competence, social accessibility, and conformity to the system's norms. When compared to their peers, opinion leaders tend to be more exposed to all forms of external communication, have somewhat higher social status, and are more innovative [3]. However, the most striking feature of opinion leaders is their unique and influential position in their system's communication structure; they are at the center of interpersonal communication networks—interconnected individuals who are linked by patterned flows of information.

Within research studies, opinion leaders have usually been identified by either a sociometric instrument or a self-designating instrument. Grimshaw and colleagues [4], studying different methods of opinion leader identification across different groups of health care workers and settings within the United Kingdom NHS, concluded that the feasibility of identifying opinion leaders with an off-the-shelf sociometric instrument was variable across different professional groups and settings within the NHS. Although it is possible to identify opinion leaders using a self-designating instrument, the effectiveness of such opinion leaders has not been rigorously tested in health care settings. Opinion leaders appear to be monomorphic (different leaders for different issues).

Within a systematic review of the effectiveness of opinion leadership, Doumit and colleagues [5] reviewed 12 studies and found that opinion leader interventions produced changes in compliance, with desired practice ranging from absolute improvement of 25% to a worsening of 6%. The overall median improvement was 10%.

Knowledge brokers

Driven by the poor linkages between researchers and policymakers [6,7] and the realization that the results of research studies should not be viewed as an end but a stage in a process, there is an emerging interest in the role of individuals who can continue the translation process, from researchers to policymakers. They differ from outreach visitors and opinion leaders, in as much as these have mainly been used with health care professionals as their target. The expectation is that knowledge brokering will result in better incorporation of research into policy and practice. Such individuals are called knowledge brokers; the conceptual underpinning of knowledge brokering is unclear as it is defined by a role rather than a set of core attributes. The Canadian Health Services Research Foundation defines knowledge brokering as "all the activity that links decision makers with researchers, facilitating their interaction so that they are able to better understand each other's goals and professional cultures, influence each other's work, forge new partnerships, and promote the use of research-based evidence in decision-making." Systematic knowledge brokering is much more recent than either opinion leaders or educational outreach, and so its effectiveness is unclear because it has not been subjected to the same degree of rigorous investigation.

Future research

To advance the field, future research should examine a number of areas, including the role of outreach visitors in a wider range of settings than the prescribing related areas in which they have been mainly used. It would be useful to identify key attributes of clinician/team behaviors or contexts that particularly lend themselves to the use of opinion leaders, knowledge brokers, and educational outreach visits. Clarification of the key conceptual attributes of knowledge brokers and studies of their effectiveness will be useful. Finally, cost-effectiveness of each of these three linkage interventions will substantially advance the field.

Summary

Opinion leaders and educational outreach visitors can produce small but worthwhile changes in health care professional behavior. The cost-effectiveness of these interventions is not well-understood, however. The effectiveness of knowledge brokers is less clear.

References

1　Mittman BS, Tonesk X, Jacobson JD. Implementing clinical practice guidelines: social influence strategies and practitioner behavior change. *Qual Rev Bull* 1992:413–22.

2　O'Brien MA, Rogers S, Jamtvedt G, Oxman AD, Odgaard-Jensen J, Kristoffersen DT, et al. Educational outreach visits: effects on professional practice and health care outcomes. *Cochrane Database of Systematic Reviews* 2007[4]:CD000409.

3　Rogers EM. *Diffusion of Innovations*. 4th ed. New York: Free Press; 1995.

4　Grimshaw JM, Eccles MP, Greener J, Maclennan G, Ibbotson T, Kahan JP, et al. Is the involvement of opinion leaders in the implementation of research findings a feasible strategy? *Implementation Science* 2006;1:3.

5　Doumit G, Gattellari M, Grimshaw J, O'Brien MA. Local opinion leaders: effects on professional practice and health care outcomes. *Cochrane Database of Systematic Reviews* 2007;Jan 24[1]:CD000125.

6　Innvaer S, Vist GE, Trommaid M, Oxman A. Health policy-makers' perceptions of their use of evidence: a systematic review. *J Health Serv Res Pol* 2002;7:239–44.

7　Lormas J. The in-between world of knowledge brokering. *BMJ* 2007;20[334]:129–32.

3.5.4 **Audit and feedback interventions**

Robbie Foy and Martin P. Eccles

Institute of Health and Society, Newcastle University, Newcastley upon Tyne, UK

> **KEY LEARNING POINTS**
>
> - Measuring adherence to clinical practice recommendations can highlight important implementation gaps and inform subsequent priorities for knowledge implementation.
> - Audit and feedback can effectively improve professional practice, although the effects on clinical practice are usually small to moderate.
> - More research is needed on the effects of audit and feedback compared to other interventions and the mechanisms by and contexts in which it works best.

There are recognized gaps and delays in the implementation of evidence-based practice [1,2]. Data from chart audits help confirm or identify these gaps and are commonly incorporated into feedback interventions to promote implementation. Audit and feedback is defined as "any summary of clinical performance of health care over a specified period of time" given in a written, electronic, or verbal format [3].

Chart audits

In chart audits, documented clinical care is measured against a review criterion, defined as "a systematically developed statement that can be used to assess the appropriateness of specific healthcare decisions, services and outcomes" [4]. Review criteria are often derived from clinical guideline recommendations, which ideally should be rigorously developed based on evidence from systematic reviews or from formal consensus processes where strong evidence is lacking, as described in Chapter 2.3.

Review criteria can be explicit or implicit [5,6]. Explicit criteria aim to maximize the reliability and objectivity of measurement. For example, patients newly diagnosed with essential hypertension and who either have persistent high blood pressure of 160/100 mmHg or more, or are at raised cardiovascular risk with persistent blood pressure of more than 140/90 mmHg have a record of being offered drug therapy [7]. Implicit criteria involve peer or expert clinicians making judgments about desired care. They, therefore, tend to be more subjective and less reliable than explicit criteria. Implicit criteria are mainly used to assess complex processes of care or adverse outcomes (e.g., maternal deaths related to childbirth).

Review criteria can relate to the structure of health care delivery (e.g., presence of calibrated devices for measuring blood pressure), health care processes (e.g., prescription of antihypertensive medication), and patient outcomes. The latter can include short-term or surrogate outcomes (e.g., blood pressure levels) or long-term outcomes (e.g., stroke). Structural and process criteria must be valid so that strong evidence exists that their improvement is associated with improvement in outcomes of care. Outcome criteria tend to be less sensitive to detecting changes in practice—because many factors may influence patient outcomes—and generally require more resources, larger sample sizes, and longer follow-up to detect important changes.

Target levels of performance can guide subsequent decisions on whether implementation activities are worthwhile. Given the law of diminishing returns, attempts to improve already high levels of performance may not be as productive as switching attention to alternative priorities. For many clinical actions, there is a "ceiling" beyond which health care systems' and clinicians' abilities to improve performance are limited because they function at or near maximum capabilities [8]. There are other good reasons not to expect 100% adherence to targets. For example, eligible patients may prefer to avoid drug treatment or experience unacceptable adverse effects.

There are a number of practical considerations in planning and conducting chart audits including sampling procedures, sample size, and data collection. An account of these can be found at NorthStar (http://www.rebeqi.org) [9]. One issue worth a brief comment is the underdocumentation of clinical actions in medical records. However, this is becoming less tenable for evidence-based clinical actions considered by professional consensus, included in the development of review criteria, to be important enough to merit documentation.

Audit and feedback

The mechanism by which audit and feedback works is self-evident; demonstrating the gap between actual and desired performance will motivate clinicians or health care systems to address that gap. Self-regulation theory probably is the most closely related theory to this [10]. "Self-regulation" is a process of determining goals and then using these as reference values to bring existing states into line with those goals. The success of any desired change depends on the individual's ability to change hisbehavior (e.g., clinical practice skills) or on external influences on behavior (e.g., organizational factors).

A Cochrane Review of 118 randomized trials concluded that audit and feedback can effectively improve professional practice and that the effects on clinical practice are generally small to moderate [3]. For example, when percentage adherence with desired practice was measured, the effects ranged from a 16% decrease to a 70% increase, with a median improvement of 5%. There are a number of explanations for this variation that mainly relates to the different permutations in the provision of feedback, context, and the nature of targeted clinical behaviors. Delivery of feedback can vary according to:

• Type of format, that is, verbal, paper, or electronic;
• Frequency and duration, for example, as a one-off step or continuously, often over a period of time;
• Source, for example, whether from a supervisor or professional body;
• Content, for example, information on health care processes or patient outcomes, use of identifiers to permit comparisons between individual professionals, teams, or facilities; and
• Use of various sources to deliver feedback, such as supervisors or professional bodies.

Higher-intensity feedback is associated with greater effects, but like other interventions to change professional practice, there is a risk that the higher costs of intensive strategies may outweigh the benefits [11]. It is also uncertain whether combining audit and feedback with other strategies, such as educational meetings, increases effectiveness. Given the relative paucity of head-to-head comparisons of different methods of providing feedback and of comparisons of audit and feedback versus other interventions, it remains difficult to recommend one intervention strategy over another on empirical grounds.

Contextual factors and nature of targeted behaviors may also influence effectiveness. The Cochrane Review of audit and feedback found that the relative effects of audit and feedback were greater when baseline adherence to recommended practice was low [3]. Clinicians' motivation to change practice and their engagement level with feedback intervention (whether they are active or passive recipients) may influence change. Contrary to expectations, there is evidence that the effects of audit and feedback are greater for recommendations perceived by clinicians to be less compatible with current norms [12] and for tasks associated with lower motivation [13].

The broader context also matters. Audit and feedback is primarily used as a means to change the behavior of individual clinicians and teams. However, effective implementation often requires action across different levels of health care systems, such as securing senior leadership commitment to change [14].

Future research

Future research on audit and feedback can usefully focus on three questions. First, by what mechanism or mechanisms does audit and feedback exert its effects? Second, which contextual features (e.g., setting, characteristics of health care professionals) and attributes of targeted clinical behaviors negate or enhance the effects of audit and feedback? Third, how does audit and feedback, by itself or in combination with other interventions, compare against other interventions to change clinical behavior?

Summary

There are only limited insights into how and when audit and feedback can work more effectively [15]. Ultimately, its selection as a KTA intervention is a matter of judgment based upon the current evidence base, a working "diagnosis" of the implementation gap causes, and the availability of supporting resources and skills [16]. In principle, getting the diagnosis right offers a rational basis for choosing an approach to delivering feedback. Hypothetically, if perceived peer pressure is identified as a key determinant of clinicians' practice or motivation to change for a given context, feedback could reasonably incorporate peer comparison [17].

References

1 McGlynn EA, Asch SM, Adams J, Keesey J, Hicks J, DeCristofaro A, et al. The quality of care delivered to adults in the United States. *N Engl J Med* 2003;348: 2635–45.
2 Seddon ME, Marshall MN, Campbell SM, Roland MO. Systematic review of studies of quality of clinical care in general practice in the UK, Australia and New Zealand. *Qual Health Care* 2001;10:152–8.
3 Jamtvedt G, Young JM, Kristoffersen DT, O'Brien MA, Oxman AD. Audit and feedback: effects on professional practice and health care outcomes. *Cochrane Database of Systematic Reviews* 2006[2]: CD000259.
4 Institute of M, Field MJ, Lohr KN. *Guidelines for clinical practice. From development to use.* Washington: National Academy Press; 1992.
5 Naylor CD, Guyatt GH, for the Evidence-Based Medicine Working Group. Users' guides to the medical literature. XI. How to use an article about a clinical utilization review. *JAMA* 1996;27518:1435–9.
6 Campbell SM, Braspenning J, Hutchinson A, Marshall M. Research methods used in developing and applying quality indicators in primary care. *Qual Saf Health Care* 2002;11:358–64.
7 National Institute for Health and Clinical Excellence. *Management of Hypertension in Adults in Primary Care.* London: NICE; 2006.
8 Wyatt JC, Paterson-Brown S, Johanson R, Altman DG, Bradburn MJ, Fisk NM. Randomised trial of educational visits to enhance use of systematic reviews in 25 obstetric units. *BMJ* 1998;317:1041–6.
9 Akl EA, Treweek S, Foy R, Francis J, Oxman AD, The ReBEQI Group. NorthStar, a support tool for the design and evaluation of quality improvement interventions in healthcare. *Implementation Sci* 2007;2:19.
10 Carver CS, Scheier M. *Attention and Self-Regulation: a Control-Theory Approach to Human Behavior.* New York: Springer-Verlag; 1981.
11 Mason J, Freemantle N, Nazareth I, Eccles M, Haines A, Drummond M. When is it cost effective to change the behaviour of health professionals? *JAMA* 2001: 2988–92.
12 Foy R, MacLennan G, Grimshaw J, Penney G, Campbell M, Grol R. Attributes of clinical recommendations that influence change in practice following audit and feedback. *J Clin Epidemiol* 2002;55:717–22.
13 Palmer RH, Louis TA, Hsu LN, Peterson HF, Rothrock JK, Strain R, et al. A randomized controlled trial of quality assurance in sixteen ambulatory care practices. *Med Care* 1985;23:751–70.

14 Ferlie EB, Shortell SM. Improving the quality of health care in the United Kingdom and the United States: a framework for change. *Milbank Q* 2001;79[2]: 281–315.

15 Foy R, Eccles M, Jamtvedt G, Young J, Grimshaw J, Baker R. What do we know about how to do audit and feedback? Pitfalls in applying evidence from a systematic review. *BMC Health Serv Res* 2005;5:50.

16 National Institute for Clinical Excellence. *Principles for Best Practice in Clinical Audit.* Abingdon: Radcliffe Medical Press; 2002.

17 Ajzen I. The theory of planned behaviour. *Organizational Behaviour and Human Decision Processes* 1991;50:179–211.

3.5.5 Informatics interventions

Samir Gupta[1] and K. Ann McKibbon[2]

[1]Li Ka Shing Knowledge Institute, St. Michael's Hospital, Toronto, ON, Canada
[2]Department of Clinical Epidemiology and Biostatistics, McMaster University, Hamilton, ON, Canada

---

KEY LEARNING POINTS

- Many informatics applications can be effective knowledge translation (KT) tools, delivering evidence to health professionals, other caregivers, and patients.
- Informatics interventions that speed KT can be found in the areas of patient and physician education; reminder systems; systems to summarize and present data; and decision support. They have been shown to improve education, improve adherence through reminders, efficiently collect and present data from multiple sources, and effectively support decision making. Their effects on health outcomes have been less well-demonstrated.
- Many of these effective informatics applications exist as demonstration projects and/or on a small scale. We have yet to harness the full potential of integrating the KT process with informatics applications.

Knowledge translation (KT) deals with the collecting, summarizing, and packaging of (research) knowledge and its delivery in a timely and appropriate format to those who use it to care for patients and populations. Informatics interventions do the same with (patient) information: collecting, summarizing, packaging, and delivering. Both domains share the theoretical foundation of epistemology: understanding and knowing the limits and validity of knowledge [1,2]. KT and informatics are natural partners that enhance health care by improving the functions of health care providers, patients and their families, and decision-makers. This chapter will focus on how informatics interventions can target KT interventions toward patients and clinicians.

Informatics interventions can improve KT in four overlapping domains:
- Education, especially on-line interactive education and education that is tailored to individual clinicians and patients.
- Lessening the "cognitive load" on clinicians. Cognitive load refers to the amount of information that we can process at any given time. As the load increases, our ability to cope with all pieces of information decreases. Certain information tasks can be managed by technology, leaving the clinician's mind free to process details that truly matter to the patient. For example, reminder systems are efficient for determining if specific actions occurred and for sending reminders if they have not. Examples include periodic testing such as mammographies and blood tests for medication levels. Reminder systems are the best, but not the only, example of informatics interventions that can reduce the cognitive load for clinicians, enhancing their ability to make considered and informed decisions.
- Summarizing data and presenting it in a useful and timely manner as well as in a variety of formats is a pillar of the KT and health care process—computers do this quickly, consistently, and accurately.
- Computerized decision support systems (CDSSs) support clinicians in their decision making with respect to diagnosis and therapy, and decision aids help patients make informed and considered decisions. These tools are probably the most promising informatics interventions to promote best practices.

The remainder of this chapter will discuss examples of projects that have proven useful and effective in these four areas. We recognize that this categorization is arbitrary and many informatics interventions include education, reminding, and decision support components. We have space to mention only a few interventions for each area. We provide citations to systematic reviews of the evidence for informatics interventions that have been most effective in KT.

Education

Traditional educational methods that include reading materials or viewing Web sites may not be the most effective method of transferring knowledge as outlined in Chapter 3.5.2. Curran and Fleet [3] reviewed the literature on Web-based continuing education and found that evidence on effectiveness was either lacking or showed weak positive effects. Similar results are found when evaluating Web-based patient education. Individualized education based on needs assessment leads to more learning and improved practice when compared to static, one-size-fits-all educational modalities [4]. Informatics interventions can thus improve learning by identifying gaps and suggesting "as-needed" content information for patients and clinicians. Also, clinicians can guide patient learning by using existing educational sites, many of which contain excellent, timely content. For example, MedlinePLUS (http://www.nlm.nih.gov/medlineplus/) is one of the most comprehensive and reliable sites developed for patients and is sometimes also used by clinicians. This site contains numerous links to existing health care sites that meet the quality standards of the U.S. National Library of Medicine.

It is interesting to note that high-quality resources for patients may also affect clinician behavior. Saryeddine and colleagues [5] described a comprehensive, evidence-supported patient education site for those having hip or knee total joint replacement. User surveys showed that providers felt that patient use of this site and the information that patients brought to consultations increased the clinicians' knowledge and directed their care decisions toward recommended standards. This same pattern of cross-partner learning was observed in Canadian diabetes care [6].

Reminder systems

Reminder systems can reduce the cognitive load for clinicians. Computers efficiently check data against clinical rules and provide prompts for screening tests, drug interactions, prescription changes, monitoring regimens (especially for toxic drugs), and all aspects of patient and provider adherence. Evidence shows that reminder systems free clinicians to concentrate on the unique needs of each individual patient rather than sorting and processing standard data [7]. However, once reminders are turned off, behavior usually returns to baseline [8]. Patient reminder systems can also be useful, especially in relation to adherence to preventive care actions and chronic disease management. For example, Thomas and colleagues [9] noted improvements in care (higher adherence to guideline recommendations for hemoglobin A1C testing [61.5% vs. 48.1%, $p = 0.01$]) after implementing an audit and feedback system that included reminders for diabetes patients.

Summarizing and presenting data

Computers are excellent at storing, synthesizing, and presenting data in an efficient and user-friendly format. Not only can these interventions be used for formal on-line medical education, but they can also enable informal KT by delivering knowledge embedded within information systems derived from evidence-based guidelines [10]. For example, several groups such as the NICE group in the United Kingdom (described in Chapter 2.3) have developed tagging specifications for guidelines so that content can be "matched" to individual patients in electronic medical records systems (EMRs) [11]. In addition, clinicians can use an on-line self-directed chart audit utility to measure their own performance against evidence-based practice benchmarks to identify and bridge care gaps in their own practices [10].

Hospital clinicians often require immediate access to information while at the bedside [11], and portable computers are particularly well-suited to this task. For example, providing physicians with a handheld computer containing a local antibiotic guideline, local bacterial resistance and susceptibility profiles, current microbiology lab reports, and a pulmonary infection score calculator decreased antibiotic use and length of stay in the intensive care unit in a before and after study [12]. Another KT intervention that collects and summarizes data and delivers it at the point of care is PharmaNet, a British Columbia-wide pharmacy database that provides physicians with prior prescription data for individual patients [13].

Patient self-management with direct patient-to-physician communication and physician-prompting is a potentially powerful tool enabling evidence-based management of chronic diseases and may benefit from information technology to enter, transfer, and present patient data. This has been demonstrated in asthma management, where an Internet-based asthma monitoring tool relaying patient-filled asthma control parameters directly to physicians resulted in superior asthma control (Internet vs. family physician odds ratio 3.26, $p < 0.001$), compared to conventional in-office monitoring [14]. Patients may also use mobile phone technology based on the short message service (SMS) system, information kiosks, and Web videoconferencing tools to relay symptoms directly to a computer interface available to physicians and/or triage nurses.

Clinical decision support systems and patient decision aids

CDSSs generate patient-specific assessments and recommendations for clinicians or patients with software algorithms that match individual patient data to a computerized knowledge database. These systems are superior to paper-based resources because they present the information that providers require "just-in-time," without overloading them with unnecessary data. CDSSs have addressed diagnostic, prevention or screening, drug dosing, or chronic disease management decisions. They may be stand-alone systems functioning in parallel with an existing paper or EMR , or they may be integrated into an EMR, enabling direct and automated patient data import, obviating manual data entry, in many cases without a requirement for user initiation. In a systematic review of the effectiveness of CDSSs, Garg and colleagues [15] reported improved practitioner performance in most studies, particularly when the CDSS automatically prompted users. However, effects on patient outcomes were poorly studied and inconsistent and require further evaluation.

Computerized decision aids are a special subset of CDSSs that are targeted directly to patients. Patient decision aids are described in more detail in Chapter 2.3. Decision aids enable patients to participate in their own health care decisions by providing evidence-based information about various options and outcomes that is relevant to their particular case. For example, Protheroe and colleagues [16] used a randomized controlled trial to demonstrate that a self-directed, interactive computerized decision aid for women with menorrhagia significantly reduced decisional conflict and improved menorrhagia-specific knowledge and quality of life, compared to an information leaflet alone. Furthermore, the decision aid demonstrated applicability and acceptability across a wide range of socioeconomic and educational classes.

Future research

Informatics interventions that are KT tools exist in many forms and locations, facilitating KT and improving health care for clinicians, patients, and families. Many of these interventions, however, are demonstration projects and/or have been implemented only in local settings. Broadening the scope of these interventions remains an area for future research and development. This endeavor will involve many facets and partners, including technology (improving information standards and enhancing system interoperability), social sciences (understanding individual needs and characteristics to design truly useful and easy-to-use interventions), and business (managing system change with financial integrity), in addition to health providers and patients. Also, personal health records is an area of great potential, requiring interdisciplinary research, both qualitative and quantitative, to obtain the best results for all stakeholders. Finally, the most pressing need for future research is in the assessment of the effects of informatics and KT interventions on patient and wellness outcomes. To date, we have a good understanding of the effects of these interventions on process outcomes, but we have little evidence of their benefit on the outcome that matters most: patient health.

Summary

As the volume and breadth of research evidence continues to grow, a wide and advancing range of informatics interventions will assume an increasingly important role in ensuring the effective and timely translation of this new knowledge into clinical practice. However, there are limitations to the use of these interventions, such as limited access to the Internet in some developing countries, inconsistent EMR use in primary, secondary, and tertiary care settings, and a paucity of systems that integrate evidence with clinical data in a user-friendly format. Selection of an informatics KT intervention will thus be limited in certain settings.

References

1 Musen MA. Medical informatics: searching for underlying components. *Methods Inf Med* 2002;41:12–19.

2 Blois MS. *Information and Medicine: The Nature of Medical Descriptors.* Berkeley, CA: University of California Press; 1984.

3 Curran VR, Fleet L. A review of evaluation outcome of web-based continuing medical education. *Med Educ* 2005;39:561–7.

4 Wenghofer EF, Way D, Moxam RS, Wu H, Faulkner D, Klass DJ. Effectiveness of an enhanced peer assessment program: introducing education into regulatory assessment. *J Cont Educ Health Prof* 2006;26[3]:199–208.

5 Saryeddine T, Levy C, Davis A, Flannery J, Jaglal S, Hurley L. Patient education as a strategy for provider education and engagement: a case study using myJointReplacement.ca. *Healthc Q* 2008;11[1]:84–90.

6 Nasmith L, Coté B, Cox J, Inkell D, Rubenstein H, Jimenez V, et al. The challenge of promoting integration: conceptualization, implementation, and assessment of a pilot care delivery model for patients with type 2 diabetes. *Fam Med* 2004;36[1]: 40–5.

7 Dexheimer JW, Sanders DL, Rosenbloom ST, Aronsky D. Prompting clinicians: a systematic review of preventive care reminders. *AMIA Annu Symp Proc* 2005:938.

8 Schriger DL, Baraff LJ, Rogers WH, Cretin S. Implementation of clinical guidelines using a computer charting system. Effect on the initial care of health care workers exposed to body fluids. *JAMA* 1997;278:1585–90.

9 Thomas KG, Thomas MR, Stroebel RJ, McDonald FS, Hanson GJ, Naessens JM, et al. Use of a registry-generated audit, feedback, and patient reminder intervention in an internal medicine resident clinic—a randomized trial. *J Gen Intern Med* 2007;22[12]:1740–4.

10 Ho K, Bloch R, Gondocz T, Laprise R, Perrier L, Ryan D, et al. Technology-enabled knowledge translation: frameworks to promote research and practice. *J Cont Educ Health Prof* 2004;24[2]:90–9.

11 Peleg M, Boxwala AA, Tu S, Zeng Q, Ogunyemi O, Wang D, et al. The InterMed approach to sharable computer-interpretable guidelines: a review. *J Am Med Inform Assoc* 2004;11:1–10.

12 Sintchenko V, Iredell JR, Gilbert GL, Coiera E. Handheld computer-based decision support reduces patient length of stay and antibiotic prescribing in critical care. *J Am Med Inform Assoc* 2005;12:398–402.

13 BC Ministry of Health. *BC Doctors Welcome PharmaNet's Expansion.* Vancouver, BC.

14 Rasmussen LM, Phanareth K, Nolte H, Backer V. Internet-based monitoring of asthma: a long-term, randomized clinical study of 300 asthmatic subjects. *J Allergy Clin Immunol* 2005;115[6]:1137–42.

15 Garg AX, Adhikari NK, McDonald H, Rosas-Arellano MP, Devereaux PJ, Beyene J, et al. Effects of computerized clinical decision support systems on practitioner performance and patient outcomes: a systematic review [see comment]. [Review] [128 refs]. *JAMA* 2005;293[10]:1223–38.

16 O'Connor AM, Stacey D, Entwistle V, Llewellyn-Thomas H, Rovner D, Holmes-Rovner M, et al. Decision aids for people facing health treatment or screening decisions. [update of Cochrane Database Syst Rev. 2001;(3):CD001431; PMID: 11686990]. [Review] [231 refs]. *Cochrane Database of Systematic Reviews* 2003;2:CD001431.

3.5.6 **Patient-mediated interventions**

Annette M. O'Connor

Department of Epidemiology, University of Ottawa School of Nursing, and Ottawa Health Research Institute, Ottawa, ON, Canada

---

KEY LEARNING POINTS

- Patient-mediated interventions aim to actively engage patients to improve their knowledge, experience, service use, health behavior, and health status.
- Patient education and information improve knowledge. Other outcomes improve with interventions that have more specific and personalized information, and that add professional or other social support.
- Research is needed on underlying frameworks, essential elements and duration, cost-effectiveness, and implementation strategies.

A fundamental strategy to reduce knowledge-to-care gaps is an informed, activated patient [1,2]. "Patient-oriented" interventions promote patients' involvement in implementing appropriate, safe, effective, and responsive self-care and health care. This chapter summarizes the state of knowledge and research gaps regarding patient-oriented strategies. Coulter and Ellins' framework [1] is used to classify these strategies into four broad categories according to their intent to improve health literacy, clinical decision making, self-care, and patient safety. Coulter and Ellins conducted a comprehensive review [1,3] and identified 129 reviews of patient-oriented interventions focused on the following patient outcomes:

- Knowledge (knowledge of condition, long-term complications, self-care, treatment options, likely outcomes; comprehension and recall of information);
- Experience (patients' satisfaction, doctor–patient communication, quality of life, psychological well-being, self-efficacy, and involvement and empowerment of patients);
- Use of services and costs (hospital admission rates, length of hospital stay, number of visits to general practitioners, cost-effectiveness, costs to patients, days lost from work or school); and
- Health behavior and status (health-related lifestyles, self-care activities, treatment adherence, severity of disease or symptoms, physical functioning, mental functioning, and clinical indicators).

The numbers of reviews with positive, mixed, or negative results are displayed in Figures 3.5.6.1 to 3.5.6.4. The effects of the four classes of interventions are discussed in detail below.

Health literacy interventions

According to a Canadian Expert Panel on Health Literacy [4], a health-literate person is able to access, understand, evaluate and communicate information as a way to promote, maintain, and improve health in a variety of settings across the life-course. Coulter and Ellins [1,3] reviewed 25 reviews of interventions to improve health literacy including:

- Written health information materials (e.g., brochures);
- Alternative format resources (e.g., Internet);
- Targeted approaches for disadvantaged groups with low health literacy (e.g., using nonwritten media, such as pictograms, videotape, and interactive computer systems); and
- Mass media campaigns (e.g., television, radio, newspapers, posters, leaflets and booklets, interactive mass media applications) to promote specific health behaviors or service use (e.g., screening).

Figure 3.5.6.1 shows health literacy interventions have the most consistent positive effects on knowledge and to a lesser extent on patients' experience and use of health services. Health literacy interventions alone do not have consistent positive effects on behavior and health status.

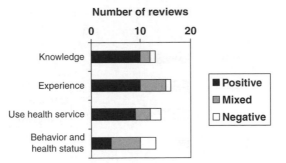

Figure 3.5.6.1 Reviews of health literacy interventions (*n* = 5).

In terms of specific interventions, written materials such as brochures improve knowledge and recall especially if they are personalized. Combined written and oral information can improve patient experience and sometimes the use of health services. Other formats, such as Web sites, improve user satisfaction, and some studies report positive effects on self-efficacy and health behavior. Evaluations of information adapted for disadvantaged populations who lack health literacy skills were mixed. Some studies performed in these populations have shown positive effects on knowledge and health behavior; few studies have examined effects on reducing inequalities in health status. Targeted mass media campaigns increase awareness, at least in the short term (3–4 months). There is some evidence of beneficial effects on use of services (drugs, medical or surgical procedures, diagnostic tests) but less so on health behavior. However, two studies [5,6] showed that the mass media could be effective in influencing smoking behavior among young people.

Clinical decision-making interventions

Coulter and Ellins [1,3] reviewed 22 reviews on interventions to improve clinical decision-making interventions including:
• Training sessions in communication skills for clinicians;
• Question prompts for patients and coaching to develop patients' skills in preparing for a consultation, deliberating about options, and implementing change; and
• Patient decision aids that explain options, clarify values, and provide structured guidance or coaching in deliberation and communication.
As Figure 3.5.6.2 shows, the most consistent positive effect is on knowledge, followed by use of health services. More specifically, the review of reviews of health professional training in communication skills demonstrated effectiveness in improving communication skills. The reviews that examined question

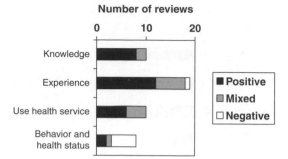

Figure 3.5.6.2 Reviews of clinical decision-making interventions (*n* = 22).

prompts and coaching found that these interventions have positive effects on patients' knowledge, information recall, and participation in decision making. Their effects on satisfaction and treatment outcomes were inconsistent. The reviews of patient decision aids indicate that they improved patients' participation, increased knowledge of their treatment options and outcome probabilities, and improved agreement between patients' values and subsequent treatment decisions. For example, in a review of 11 trials, discretionary surgery decreased in 9 trials without apparent adverse effects on health outcomes [7]. Patient decision aids are described in more detail in Chapter 2.3.

Self-care interventions

Self-care and self-management interventions aim to improve people's practices in maintaining health and managing disease. Coulter and Ellins [1,3] reviewed 67 reviews of these interventions. The specific interventions were:
• Self-management education, which helps people develop skills to cope with their condition (asthma, diabetes, arthritis/rheumatic, hypertension, COPD) and to manage daily problems;
• Self-monitoring and self-administered treatment;
• Self-help groups and peer support;
• Patient access to personal medical information;
• Patient-centered tele-care.
As Figure 3.5.6.3 shows, these interventions generally improve knowledge, patient experience, and health behavior and outcomes. To a lesser extent, they improve use of health services.

Regarding specific interventions, there are mixed effects from self-management education programs, including the widely used Lorig model (a community-based self-management program that provides patients with

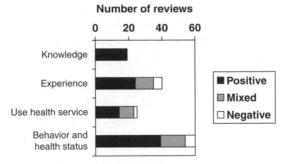

Figure 3.5.6.3 Reviews of self-care and chronic disease self-management interventions (*n* = 67).

the skills needed to manage their chronic health condition). Self-management education programs improve knowledge, coping behavior, adherence, self-efficacy, and symptom management. Programs that include skill development are more effective than those that provide information alone. Health services use and cost are sometimes reduced and quality of life is enhanced. There are short-term beneficial effects on health behavior and health status within 3 to 6 months, which tend to lessen over time. Quality-of-life effects tend to sustain beyond the intervention period.

Considering programs targeted to specific disease conditions, asthma self-management programs when combined with regular practitioner review and patient action plans can improve service use (reduction in hospitalizations: RR 0.64, CI 0.56–0.82; unscheduled visits: RR 0.68, CI 0.56–0.81); quality of life (SMD 0.29, CI 0.11–0.47); and self-efficacy (SMD 0.36, CI 0.15–0.57). Children and adolescents also have moderate improvements in lung function. In contrast, the effects of arthritis self-management education on pain (effect size range 0.12–0.22) and function (effect size range 0.07–0.27) have been small and short-lived. When diabetes self-management education is combined with other disease management strategies, blood glucose control improves and diabetic complications from Type 1 diabetes are reduced. For patients with Type 2 diabetes, group education improves blood glucose and blood pressure.

The most effective elements of self-management education have been difficult to ascertain. Larger effect sizes are associated with programs that focus on specific topics; use participative teaching methods; have multiple components including regular review by health professionals; involve family or other informal caregivers; and last at least 12 weeks.

Compared to self-management education, there are fewer reviews of self-monitoring (8), peer support groups (3), patient-held medical records (4), and patient-centered tele-care (4). Blood glucose self-monitoring in patients with diabetes has not been shown to be effective [8,9]. In contrast, blood pressure and anticoagulant therapy self-monitoring have similar outcomes to those of professionally managed care. In the case of hypertension, self-monitoring is cost neutral; for anticoagulation therapy it is cost saving. Self-help and support groups are viewed positively by participants in terms of information sharing, experiences, and problem solving. In the case of care-giver support groups, they improve confidence, coping, family function, and perceived burden of care. However, self-help and support groups do not affect health behavior or outcomes.

Patients view patient-held records as useful and increasing their sense of control. Recording consultations improve patients' recall, understanding, and uptake of information. However, the effects on health behavior or health status have not been affected by either patient-held records or recording consultations.

Patient-centered tele-care in the home reduces patients' perceived isolation and improves self-efficacy, quality of life, patient empowerment, and psychological outcomes such as depression. There is less evidence of other health status measures, use of services, and cost-effectiveness. However, cost savings are evident when routine care is replaced by "virtual visits."

Patient safety interventions

Patient-oriented interventions whose aim is to improve patient safety include: information about choosing safe providers, patient involvement in infection control, encouraging adherence to treatment regimens, checking records and care processes, and patient reporting of adverse events. Most of the 18 reviews by Coulter and Ellins [1,3] focus on improving safety through better treatment adherence. As Figure 3.5.6.4 shows, safety interventions are effective for improving knowledge and patient experience, and to a lesser extent use of services and health behavior or health status.

The most effective strategy to optimize patients' treatment adherence is to simplify dosing regimens. Relative improvement ranged from 8% to 19.6% in seven of nine trials. Education and information provision are necessary but not sufficient to improve adherence. The long-term effects of treatment adherence interventions are understudied. One review of patient-oriented hospital infection control campaigns concluded that they increased compliance with hand hygiene when hand-washing facilities were provided along with patient encouragement to ask health workers if they washed their hands. There have been no systematic reviews of patient reporting of adverse drug

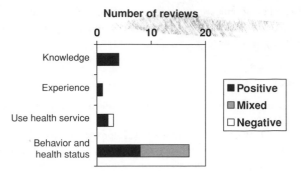

Figure 3.5.6.4 Reviews of safety interventions (*n* = 18).

events. In individual studies, evidence is mixed on the role of patient safety information in preventing adverse events. There are unknown effects of direct patient reporting on adverse event monitoring systems. There is one review on equipping patients for safer health care. There were some beneficial effects on patients' knowledge and confidence from an educational video. Personalized information on drugs had no effect on patients' experience of care. The effects on error rates and adverse events were mixed, so no conclusion can be made. Considering the surgical context, there are no reviews asking patients to mark the site where their surgery will take place; however, single studies show that patients do not always follow through with requests to mark the correct surgical site.

Future research

Research gaps regarding patient-oriented interventions occur at the fundamental and implementation levels. There are fundamental questions about the underlying theoretical frameworks of interventions, essential effective elements, required duration, and adaptation for disadvantaged groups. More focus is needed on cost-effectiveness, long-term outcomes, and health inequalities. In the case of interventions with established efficacy (e.g., professional communication skills training, patient decision aids), research is needed on optimal strategies to address implementation barriers.

Summary

Interventions that actively engage patients can have positive effects on patients' knowledge, experience, service use, health behavior, and health status. Patient education and information improve knowledge. Additional strategies are needed to change other outcomes. These include increasing the specificity and personalization of information, combining interventions with professional or other social support, and extending duration when long-term behavior change is expected.

References

1 Coulter A, Ellins J. Effectiveness of strategies for informing, educating and involving patients. *BMJ* 2007;335:24–7.
2 Bodenheimer T, Wagner EH, Grumbach K. Improving primary care for patients with chronic illness: the chronic care model, Part 2. *JAMA* 2002;288:1909–14.
3 Coulter A, Ellins J. *Patient-focused Interventions: a review of the evidence.* London: Health Foundation; 2006. www.pickereurope.org/Filestore/Publications/ QEI_Review_AB.pdf [accessed May 2, 2008].
4 Expert Panel on Health Literacy. A Vision for a Health Literate Canada: Report of the Expert Panel on Health Literacy. Canadian Public Health Association; 2008.
5 Flynn BS, Worden JK, Secker-Walker RH, Badger GJ, Geller BM. Cigarette smoking prevention effects of mass media and school interventions targeted to gender and age groups. *J Health Educ* 1995;26[2]:45–51.
6 Hafstad A. *Provocative anti-smoking appeals in mass media campaigns. An intervention study on adolescent smoking.* University of Oslo: Institute of General Practice and Community Medicine; 1997.
7 O'Connor AM, Stacey D. *Should patient decision aids (PtDAs) be introduced in the health care system?* WHO Regional Office for Europe's Health Evidence Network (HEN); 2005.
8 Welschen LM, Bloemendal E, Nijpels G, Dekker JM, Heine RJ, Stalman WA, et al. Self-monitoring of blood glucose in patients with type 2 diabetes who are not using insulin. *Cochrane Database of Systematic Reviews* 2005;Apr 18[2]:CD005060.
9 Coster S, Gulliford MC, Seed PT, Powrie JK, Swaminathan R. Monitoring blood glucose control in diabetes mellitus: a systematic review. *Health Technology Assessment* 2000;4[12]:i–iv, 1–93.

3.5.7 **Organizational interventions**

Ewan Ferlie

School of Management, Royal Holloway University of London, Egham, Surrey, UK

KEY LEARNING POINTS

- Internationally, there is slow but cumulative growth of organizational-level research on the implementation of organizational change programs, including knowledge management and knowledge translation (KT).

- This literature draws on social science theories and methods, as well as those connected to the biomedical research tradition.
- Key findings often suggest notions of "emergence," local processes, and limits to top-down control.
- The interface with management practice is problematic, and more attention needs to be paid to getting research into practice.

Health care organizations (e.g., hospital or primary care practice/ organization) typically operate at the middle level, between the micro level of clinical practice and macro level of health policy. The middle level is increasingly important with the move away from traditional clinical dominance over work practices and toward a more corporate perspective, implying stronger management of clinical practice. In publicly funded health care, the middle level is charged by the national policy level with implementing organization-wide interventions to improve service quality. In more market-oriented systems, privately funded hospitals adopt organizational interventions to improve their position in the market. Such intervention cycles have appeared with greater intensity over the last 20 years. Some (but not all) of them have been independently evaluated so that a knowledge base is emerging. This article offers an overview of this expanding field and suggests key messages for implementing knowledge within organizations.

Successive organizational change programs are evident in health care over the last 20 years. We have moved from total quality management [1–2], through business process engineering (BPR) [3] and plan-do-study-act (PDSA) cycles. Change management interventions (e.g., organization development or culture change programs) have been imported, as have clinical practice guidelines. We currently see the attempted redesign of care pathways using the principles of service improvement. These complex interventions seek to improve service quality but often run into implementation barriers.

What do we know about program "implementation" in health care? There is both conceptual and empirical knowledge. The concept of the *implementation process* comes from political science [4] and organizational behavior (OB). Political scientists see health care arenas as a bargaining process between various interest groups with differential power [5]. Organizational behavior scholars study themes of organizational culture and change management, as well as the process of organizational change, seeing it as a combination of "receptive context" [6] and appropriate action. These scholars distinguish between incremental, strategic, and transformational modes of change. Non-incremental forms of change are difficult to achieve in health care, as managers have little power and professionals more. The basic concept of professional dominance is important [7] but subject to contest and revision. Health care displays many colocated professions so innovations that cross the frontier between professions are vulnerable to blockage [8]. An empirical evidence base is developing, with some overviews on service redesign and change management [9–10].

What organizational KT interventions could we consider in health care?

Quality programs

Total quality management was an early organizational intervention that encouraged thinking about quality improvement as well as traditional goals of cost reduction and activity increases, using structured methods of diagnosis, intervention, and reflection. Total quality management was initially used in Japanese manufacturing organizations, crossing into North America and Europe in the 1980s, including into health care settings. These ideas encouraged feedback from patients and rank and file staff upward.

Organizational research suggests only partial success in implementation efforts. Joss and Kogan's [1] UK empirical study of total quality management implementation (see also Shortell et al. [2] for a similar American study) found only moderate impact as the total quality management agenda had greater ownership from nurses than powerful clinicians or senior managers. Ovretveit's [11] international overview of the public service quality improvement field suggests more successful programs are those in which the approach has been tailored to the organization and applied over a number of years. Later examples include business process re-engineering (attempting a more radical form of organizational transformation, although McNulty and Ferlie [3] again found nontransformational impact) and, more recently, service improvement models, including "breakthrough collaboratives" (back to incremental change with higher professional ownership) [12].

Substantial evaluative literature stresses [9] such factors as variation in the level of change ambition between different change programs, the need for sustained effort, local and often disappointing variability in impact, for professional ownership and engagement, and for senior management leadership. Ferlie and Shortell's [13] multitier model recommends reinforcing quality improvement interventions at each level. Shojania and Grimshaw [14] urge the development of a quality improvement evidence base, following the paradigm of evidence-based medicine, suggesting that evidence to guide quality programs is in its infancy.

Organizational change programs

A second important area is change management. As health care organizations move into more turbulent environments, the capacity to manage significant organizational-wide change becomes more important. Interventions include organizational development or culture change programs, empowerment programs and management development programs for clinicians moving into management roles. Empirical studies attempt to unpick the organizational correlates of effective change management (Pettigrew et al.'s UK study [6] suggests a local "receptive context for change") and often use qualitative and case study-based methods. This primary literature has been helpfully reviewed [10] and implications for managers highlighted.

General findings are emerging across various empirical studies in relation to the variable implementation of change programs in health care, given problems of limited organizational change capacity [10] and change overload; the importance of productive interprofessional roles and relationships and also of linkage between professional and managerial blocks; evidence of dispersed rather than individualized or heroic leadership; and of challenges to sustain attention and build up basic organizational change capacity over time.

Implementation of evidence-based practice guidelines

As described in Chapter 2.4, national (e.g., National Institute for Health and Clinical Excellence [NICE] in the UK) and international bodies (e.g., World Health Organization) have been developing practice guidelines or best practices. They are an important summary resource for change agents who wish to access an evidence overview. But how are they implemented in the local organization? Organizational researchers get inside the "black box" of the health care organization and understand how the organization puts evidence in practice and with what success. Lomas [15] recommends multiple and reinforcing interventions rather than one change lever. Dopson and FitzGerald [16] suggest factors correlated with more rapid implementation, such as the presence of a clinical opinion leader, but stress that the overall configuration is crucial. There is also distinctive literature on the uptake of clinical guidelines [17,18] and on interventions that promote greater uptake, which draws more on the perspectives of clinically based research, often including overviews of trials and other "rigourous" studies. Strategies for guideline implementation are further discussed in Chapter 3.5.1.

Organizational knowledge creation and synthesis

This research field is developing a knowledge base, but it is at an early stage. Given the growth in funding for organizational evaluations, more empirical projects have been funded and now reported. However, the dynamics of knowledge production are different in this field than they are in biomedical fields. There are few randomized trials or meta-analyses, and alternative qualitative methods such as comparative case study designs are used. Literature reviews (9,10) are typically structured differently from traditional systematic reviews and may also be narrative based so they are looser than traditional synthesis and require a greater degree of interpretation. Buchanan et al. [19] represents a recent research informed overview for the reflective practitioner.

Future research

How will this field develop over the next decade? What research is now needed? A coming theme is organizational research into knowledge translation (KT) and knowledge management programs themselves. To build a more cumulative knowledge base, they should be seen more generically as another cycle of organizational change programs, so empirical studies should be informed by findings and concepts already generated by prior studies of organizational change in health care (some of which have been reviewed here). We know about how clinicians use research, but we need to know more about how managers use management-related research and, in particular, know the conditions in which they are more likely to use research. (We already know that many managers do not use research; thus, the study of positive outliers is more interesting.) Finally, international comparative studies on knowledge implementation programs are needed to build a more cumulative knowledge base that can examine health system effects.

Summary

Designing organizational systems and interventions to support KT is an increasingly important health policy stream. Such interventions have increasingly been subject to primary evaluative research. Substantial organizational research literature has built up over the last decade—for example, in the field of service improvement. A major finding is that the implementation process is often emergent, uncertain, and affected by the local context and features of action. This literature suggests looser models, concepts, and language (e.g., the implementation "process") that take account of uncertainty or the unintended or perverse effects of interventions. The top's search for control is imperfectly realized in practice as organizational systems have an organic as well as predictable quality.

Knowledge creation and synthesis in this field have distinctive characteristics. Organizational behavior is a form of social rather than natural science. There are fewer uncontested forms of knowledge in this organizational field than in the biomedical domain (e.g., there are few or even no meta-analyses of randomized trials). There is greater use of social science research methods, including qualitative methods. There are relatively few overviews, and those that exist often use looser approaches to review than those found in traditional synthesis in the biomedical domain. The managerial audience that may take a particular interest in this field often has an undeveloped research culture and finds it difficult to locate, read, and interpret primary organizational research.

What are the implications for more reflective managerial practitioners seeking to engage in evidence-informed practice that can support organizational knowledge translation? They will need to identify, review, and discuss relevant implementation literature briefly signaled here. This is not easy in a field where reviews are scarce. They will need to have built-up adequate research methods, appraisal, and interpretive skills to engage with a literature base in which concepts are as important as empirical findings. They should consider the implications of the literature for their local context, customizing or adapting it as appropriate. Within the spirit of reflective practice, they may build in local knowledge production (perhaps, using PDSA or action research methods) and reflection during implementation.

References

1 Joss R, Kogan M. *Advancing Quality: TQM in the NHS*. Buckingham: Open University Press; 1995.
2 Shortell S, Bennet C, Byck G. Assessing the impact of continuous quality improvement on clinical progress: what will it take to accelerate progress? *The Milbank Q* 1998;76:593–624.
3 McNulty T, Ferlie E. *Reengineering Health Care*. Oxford University Press;2002.
4 Pressman J, Wildavsky A. *Implementation*. Berkeley: University of California Press; 1973.
5 Alford R. *Health Care Politics*. London: University of Chicago Press; 1975.
6 Pettigrew A, Ferlie E, McKee L. *Shaping Strategic Change*. London: Sage; 1992.
7 Friedson E. *Professional Dominance: The Social Structure of Medical Care*. New York: Atherton Press; 1970.
8 Abbott A. *The System of Professions*. University of Chicago Press; 1988.
9 Locock L. Health care redesign: meaning, origins and application. *Qual Saf Health Care* 2003;12:53–7.
10 Iles V, Sutherland I. *Organisational change—a review*. London: School of Hygiene and Tropical Medicine, NHS Service Delivery and Organisation Rand D Programme.
11 Ovretveit J. Public service quality improvement. In E Ferlie, L Lynn, & C Pollitt (Eds.), *Oxford Handbook of Public Management*. Oxford: Oxford University Press; 2005:537–62.
12 Berwick D. A primer on leading the improvement of systems. *Br Med J* 1996;312: 619–22.

13 Ferlie E, Shortell S. Improving the quality of health care in the UK and USA: a framework for change. *Milbank Q* 2001;79[2]:281–315.

14 Shojania K, Grimshaw J. Evidence-based quality improvement—the state of the science. *Health Aff (Millwood)* 2005;24[1]:138–50.

15 Lomas J. Retailing research: increasing the role of evidence in clinical services for children. *Millbank Q* 1993;71[3]:459–74.

16 Dopson S, FitzGerald L. (eds.). *Knowledge to Action.* Oxford: Oxford University Press; 2005.

17 Grimshaw J, Campbell M, Eccles M, and Steen I. Experimental and quasi experimental designs for evaluating guideline implementation strategies. *Family Pract* 2000;17:S11–18.

18 Grimshaw JM, Thomas RE, MacLennan G, Fraser C, Ramsay CR, Vale L, et al. Effectiveness and efficiency of guideline dissemination and implementation strategies. *Health Technol Assess* 2004;8[6]:iii–iv, 1–72.

19 Buchanan D, FitzGerald L, Ketley D. *The Sustainability and Spread of Organizational Change.* London: Routledge; 2007.

3.6 Monitoring and evaluating knowledge

3.6.1 Monitoring knowledge use and evaluating outcomes of knowledge use

Sharon E. Straus [1,2], *Jacqueline Tetroe* [3], *and Ian D. Graham* [3,4], *Merrick Zwarenstein* [5], *Onil Bhattacharyya* [2,6]

[1] Department of Medicine, University of Toronto, Toronto, ON, Canada
[2] Li Ka Shing Knowledge Institute, St. Michael's Hospital Toronto, ON, Canada
[3] Knowledge Translation Portfolio, Canadian Institutes of Health Research, Ottawa, ON, Canada
[4] School of Nursing, University of Ottawa, Ottawa, ON, Canada
[5] Sunnybrook Research Institute, University of Toronto, and Institute for Clinical Evaluative Research, Toronto, ON, Canada
[6] Department of Family and Community Medicine, University of Toronto, Toronto, ON, Canada

---

KEY LEARNING POINTS

- Knowledge use can be instrumental (concrete application of knowledge), conceptual (changes in understanding or attitude), or persuasive (use of knowledge as ammunition).
- Whereas knowledge use is important, the impact of its use on patient, provider, and system outcomes is of greatest interest.
- Strategies for evaluating knowledge implementation should use explicit, rigorous methods and should consider qualitative and quantitative methodologies.

Monitoring knowledge use

In the knowledge-to-action cycle, after the knowledge translation (KT) intervention has been implemented (Chapter 3.5), knowledge use should be monitored. This step is necessary to determine how and to what extent

---

Knowledge Translation in Health Care: Moving from Evidence to Practice. Edited by S. Straus, J. Tetroe, and I. Graham. © 2009 Blackwell Publishing, ISBN: 978-1-4051-8106-8.

knowledge has diffused through target decision-maker groups [1]. Measuring and attributing knowledge use is still in its infancy within health research. How we measure knowledge use depends on our definition of knowledge and knowledge use and on the perspective of the knowledge user.

There have been several models or classifications of knowledge use [2–6]. Larsen described conceptual and behavioral knowledge use [2]. Conceptual knowledge use refers to using knowledge to change the way users think about issues. Instrumental knowledge use refers to changes in action as a result of knowledge use. Dunn further categorized knowledge use by describing that it could be done by the individual or a collective [3]. Weiss also described several frameworks for knowledge use including the problem-solving model, which she described as the direct application of study results to a decision [4]. In this model she mentions that research can "become ammunition for the side that finds its conclusions congenial and supportive. Partisans flourish the evidence ... to neutralize opponents, convince waverers and bolster supporters [4]." Beyer and Trice considered this a different form of knowledge use and labeled it symbolic knowledge use, which they added to Larsen's framework [5]. Symbolic use involves the use of research as a political or persuasive tool. More recently, Estabrooks has described a similar framework for knowledge use including direct, indirect, and persuasive research utilization where these terms are analogous to instrumental, conceptual, and symbolic knowledge use respectively [6].

We find it useful to consider conceptual, instrumental, and persuasive knowledge use [1]. As mentioned above, conceptual use of knowledge implies changes in knowledge, understanding, or attitudes. Research could change thinking and inform decision making but not change practice. For example, based on knowledge that self-monitoring of blood glucose in newly diagnosed type 2 diabetes mellitus patients is not cost-effective and is associated with lower quality of life [7,8], we understand a newly diagnosed patient's concern about self-monitoring.

Instrumental knowledge use is the concrete application of knowledge and describes changes in behavior or practice [1]. Knowledge can be translated into a usable form, such as a care pathway, and is used in making a specific decision. For example, a clinician orders deep venous thrombosis (DVT) prophylaxis in patients admitted to the intensive care unit. This type of knowledge could be measured by assessing how frequently DVT prophylaxis is ordered in appropriate patients.

Persuasive knowledge use is also called strategic or symbolic knowledge use and refers to research used as a political or persuasive tool. It relates to the use of knowledge to attain specific power or profit goals (i.e., knowledge as ammunition) [1]. For example, we use our knowledge of adverse events associated with use of mechanical restraints on agitated inpatients to persuade the nursing manager on the medical ward to develop a ward protocol about their use.

How can knowledge use be measured?

There are many tools for assessing knowledge use. Dunn completed an inventory of available tools for conducting research on knowledge use [3]. He identified 65 strategies to study knowledge use and categorized them into naturalistic observation, content analysis, and questionnaires and interviews [3]. He also identified several scales for assessing knowledge use but found that most had unknown or unreported validity and reliability. Examples of available questionnaires to measure knowledge use include the Evaluation Utilization Scale [9] and Brett's Nursing Practice Questionnaire [10]. This latter questionnaire focuses primarily on the stages of adoption outlined by Rogers [11], including awareness, persuasion, decision, and implementation. Most frequently, knowledge utilization tools measure instrumental knowledge use [12]. Often, these measures rely on self-report and are subject to recall bias. For example, an exploratory case study described call center nurses' adoption of a decision support protocol [13]. Participating nurses were surveyed about whether they used the decision support tool in practice. Eleven of 25 respondents stated that they had used the tool, and 22 of 25 said they would use it in the future. The authors identified potential limitations of this study, including recall bias and a short follow-up period (1 month) without repeated observation [13]. In a more valid assessment of instrumental knowledge use, participants also underwent a quality assessment of their coaching skills during simulated calls [14].

Assessing instrumental knowledge use can also be done by measuring adherence to recommendations or quality indicators. For example, Grol and colleagues completed a series of studies involving family physicians in the Netherlands who recorded their adherence to 30 national guidelines [15]. Three hundred forty-two specific adherence indicators were constructed and physicians received educational sessions on how to record performance on these indicators. Computer software was developed to relate actual performance to clinical conditions to assess adherence. They were able to determine that guidelines with lowest adherence scores included those for otitis externa and diagnosis of asthma in adults, whereas those with highest adherence scores were for micturition problems in older men and diagnosis of heart failure [15].

In addition to considering the type of knowledge use, we should also consider who are the targets for knowledge use (i.e., the public, health care professionals, policymakers). Different targets may require different strategies for monitoring knowledge use. Assessing knowledge use by policymakers may require strategies such as interviews and document analysis [16]. When assessing knowledge use by physicians, we could consider measuring use of care paths or ordering relevant medications, often measured through use of administrative or clinical databases. When measuring knowledge use by the public, we can also measure patient attitudes or use of resources through surveys and administrative databases.

What is the target level of knowledge use that we are aiming for? As mentioned in Chapter 3.2, this target will be based on discussions with relevant stakeholders including consideration of what is acceptable and feasible and whether a ceiling effect may exist. If the degree of knowledge use is found to be adequate, strategies for monitoring sustained knowledge use should be considered. If the degree of knowledge use is less than expected or desired, it may be useful to reassess barriers to knowledge use. In particular, the target decision makers can be asked about their intention to use the knowledge. This exploration may uncover new barriers. In the case study of the use of decision support for a nurse call center, it was identified through a survey that use of the decision support tool might be facilitated through its integration in the call center database, incorporating decision support training for staff and informing the public of this service [13].

When should we measure knowledge use versus the impact of knowledge use? If the implementation intervention targets a behavior for which there is strong evidence of benefit, it may be appropriate to measure the impact of the intervention in terms of whether the behavior has occurred (instrumental knowledge) rather than whether a change in clinical outcomes has occurred [17]. For example, we recently completed a study of a strategy to implement the Osteoporosis Canada guidelines in a northern Ontario community setting [18]. The primary outcome of this randomized trial was appropriate use of osteoporosis medications (instrumental knowledge) rather than patient fractures (clinical outcome). We felt that there was sufficient evidence in support of use of osteoporosis medication to prevent fragility fractures that we did not need to measure fractures as the primary outcome. In cases such as this study, outcome measurement at the patient level could be prohibitively expensive, but failure to measure at the patient level does not address whether the intervention improves relevant clinical outcomes.

Evaluating the impact of knowledge use

The next phase of the knowledge-to-action cycle is to determine the impact of knowledge implementation [1]. In this phase we want to determine if the knowledge use impacts health, provider, and system outcomes. Whereas assessing knowledge use is important, its use is of particular interest if it influences important clinical measures such as quality indicators.

Evaluation should start with formulating the question of interest. As mentioned in Chapter 2.3, we find the PICO framework to be useful for this task. Using this framework, the "P" refers to the population of interest, which could be the public, health care providers, or policymakers. The "I" refers to the KT intervention, which was implemented and which might be compared to another group ("C"). The "O" refers to the outcome of interest, which in this situation refers to health, provider, or organizational outcomes.

In the previous section, we described strategies for considering knowledge use that can be used to frame outcomes. Donabedian proposed a framework for quality of care that separates quality into structure, process, and outcome. It can be used to categorize quality indicators and to frame outcomes of both knowledge use and impact of knowledge use [19]. Structural indicators focus on organizational aspects of service provision, which could be analogous to instrumental knowledge use. Process indicators focus on care delivered to patients and include when evidence is communicated to patients and caregivers. These indicators are analogous to instrumental knowledge use. Outcome indicators refer to the ultimate goal of care, such as patient quality of life or hospital admission. For example, if we want to look at the issue of prophylaxis against DVT in patients admitted to the intensive care unit, structural measures would include the availability of DVT prophylaxis (e.g., low molecular weight heparin or intermittent pneumatic compression) at the institution (instrumental knowledge use). Process measures include prescription of DVT prophylaxis such as heparin in the critical care unit (instrumental knowledge use). And outcome measures include risk of DVT in these patients. Table 3.6.1.1 provides a framework for differentiating knowledge use from outcomes.

In a systematic review of methods used to measure outcome change following a KT intervention, Hakkennes and Green grouped measures into three main categories [17], which we have modified to focus on impact of knowledge use:

1 Patient level:
   a. Measurement of an actual change in health status, such as mortality or quality of life;
   b. Surrogate measurement, such as length of stay or attitudes.
2 Health care provider level:
   a. Measurement of provider satisfaction.
3 Organizational or process level:
   a. Measurement of change in health care system (e.g., wait lists) or costs.

Hakkennes and Green found that of 228 studies evaluating strategies for guideline implementation, 93% measured outcomes at the level of clinician, and 13% used surrogate measures at the provider level [17]. Less than one-third of studies used patient-level outcomes.

Table 3.6.1.1 Measures of knowledge use and impact of knowledge use

Construct	Description	Examples of measures	Strategy for data collection
Knowledge use			
• Conceptual	Changes in knowledge levels, understanding, or attitudes	Knowledge attitudes; intentions to change	Questionnaires, interviews
• Instrumental	Changes in behavior or practice	Adherence to recommendations (e.g., change in prescribing, adoption of a new nursing practice, or abandonment of existing practice)	Administrative database or clinical database
Outcomes			
• Patient	Impact on patients of using/applying the knowledge	Health status (morbidity or mortality); health-related quality of life; satisfaction with care	Administrative database, clinical database, questionnaires
• Provider	Impact on providers of using/applying the knowledge	Satisfaction with practice; time taken to do new practice	Questionnaires, interviews
• System/society	Impact on the health system of using/applying the knowledge	Costs; length of stay; waiting times	Administrative database, clinical database

Methods for evaluating KT interventions

After formulating the question, we need to match it to the appropriate evaluation design. When developing an evaluation, we need to consider rigor and feasibility. By rigor, we mean the strategy for evaluation should use explicit and valid methods. Both qualitative and quantitative methodologies could be used. By feasible, we mean the evaluation strategy is realistic and appropriate given the setting and circumstances. As with any evaluation, the strategy should be ethical.

Selection of our evaluation strategy also depends on whether we want to enhance local knowledge or provide generalizable information on the validity of the KT intervention. As mentioned in Chapter 6.1, those interested in local applicability of knowledge (i.e., whether an intervention worked in the context in which it was implemented) should use the most rigorous study designs feasible. These may include observational evaluations where the researcher does not have control over the allocation of study participants to the intervention or a comparable control. Those interested in generalizable knowledge (i.e., whether an intervention is likely to work in comparable settings) should use the most rigorous research evaluation design they can afford, such as randomized trials (or experimental evaluation).

A third form of evaluation to consider is process evaluation. Process evaluation may involve determining the extent to which target decision makers were actually exposed to the intervention or the dose of the intervention. It may also include a description of the experience of those exposed to the intervention and potential barriers to the intervention. For example, a study designed to evaluate the effectiveness of an educational intervention on the use of radiography for diagnosis of acute ankle injuries revealed no impact of the active dissemination of the Ottawa Ankle Rules. However, less than a third of those receiving the intervention were actually physicians with the authority to order x-rays, raising the question of whether the intervention was not effective or simply not direct to the appropriate target decision-makers [20]. This type of evaluation is also useful to allow corrections to the intervention or implementation strategy based on what is revealed. We believe that process evaluation should occur alongside observational and experimental evaluation.

Qualitative evaluation methods can be helpful in exploring the "active ingredients" of a KT intervention and thus are particularly useful in process evaluation. In a randomized trial of a comprehensive, multifaceted guideline implementation strategy for family physicians, no changes in cholesterol testing were noted after a 1-year intervention [21]. This finding led to completion of interviews with family physicians who expressed concern about the extra workload associated with implementation of the guidelines and suggested revisions to the diagnostic algorithm [22]. Triangulation should be considered in qualitative studies where a variety of strategies for data collection (e.g., interviews, surveys, focus groups) are used to enhance validity. Qualitative research can also be useful for identifying unintended impacts of the intervention. For a more comprehensive description of qualitative research methods, we encourage readers to review the textbook by Denzin and Lincoln [23].

Quantitative evaluation methods included randomized and quasi-experimental studies. Randomized trials are more logistically demanding but provide more reliable results than nonrandomized studies. Nonrandomized studies can often be implemented more easily and are appropriate when randomization is not possible. For complete description of these strategies, see Chapter 6.1.

Mixed methods can be used to evaluate KT interventions and are particularly helpful in evaluating complex KT interventions, which are further discussed in Chapter 3.6.2. We propose that the evaluation phase is also an opportunity to explore factors that can contribute to sustainability of the intervention. Both quantitative and qualitative evaluation strategies can help identify factors that influence sustained knowledge use. Sustainability is further discussed in Chapter 3.7.

Future research

There are several areas of potential research outside of instrumental knowledge use, including the development and evaluation of tools for measuring knowledge use. Enhanced methods for exploring and assessing sustained knowledge use should also be developed.

References

1 Graham ID, Logan J, Harrison MB, Straus SE, Tetroe J, Caswell W, et al. Lost in knowledge translation: time for a map? *J Cont Ed Health Prof* 2006;26:13–24.
2 Larsen J. Knowledge utilization. What is it? *Knowledge: Creation, Diffusion, Utilization* 1980;1:421–2.
3 Dunn WN. Measuring knowledge use. *Knowledge: Creation, Diffusion, Utilization* 1983;5:120–33.
4 Weiss CH. The many meanings of research utilization. *Public Administration Rev* 1979;Sept:426–31.
5 Beyer JM, Trice HM. The utilization process: a conceptual framework and synthesis of empirical findings. *Admin Sci Q* 1982;27:591–622.
6 Estabrooks C. The conceptual structure of research utilization. *Res Nurs Health* 1999;22:203–16.
7 Simon J, Gray A, Clarke P, Wade A, Neil A, Farmer A, et al. Cost effectiveness of self monitoring of blood glucose in patients with non-insulin treated type 2 diabetes: economic evaluation of data from the DiGEM trial. *BMJ* 2008;336:1174–7.
8 O'Kane MJ, Bunting B, Copeland M, Coates VE: ESMON Study Group. Efficacy of self monitoring of blood glucose in patients with newly diagnosed type 2 diabetes (ESMON study): randomised controlled trial. *BMJ* 2008;336:1177–80.
9 Johnson K. Stimulating evaluation use by integrating academia and practice. *Knowledge* 1980;2:237–62.
10 Brett JL. Use of nursing practice research findings. *Nurs Res* 1987;36:344–9.
11 Rogers E. *Diffusion of Innovations.* 5th ed. New York: Free Press; 2003.

12 Estabrooks CA, Floyd J, Scott-Findlay S, O'Leary KA, Gushta M. Individual determinants of research utilization: a systematic review. *J Adv Nurs* 2003;43:506–20.

13 Stacey D, Pomey MP, O'Connor AM, Graham ID. Adoption and sustainability of decision support for patients facing health decisions: an implementation case study in nursing. *Impl Sci* 2006;1:17.

14 Stacey D, O'Connor AM, Graham ID, Pomey MP. Randomised controlled trial of the effectiveness of an intervention to implement evidence-based patient decision support in a nursing call centre. *J Telemed Telecare* 2006;12:410–5.

15 Grol R. Successes and failures in the implementation of evidence-based guidelines for clinical practice. *Med Care* 2001;39[Suppl 2]:46–54.

16 Hanney SR, Gonzalez-Block MA, Buxton MJ, Kogan M. The utilization of health research in policy-making: concepts, examples and methods of assessment. *Health Res Policy Sys* 2002;1:2.

17 Hakkennes S, Green S. Measures for assessing practice change in medical practitioners. *Impl Sci* 2006;1:29.

18 Ciaschini P, Straus SE, Dolovich L, et al. Randomised trial of a community-based guideline implementation strategy to optimize appropriate use of osteoporosis medications. (Manuscript submitted.)

19 Donabedian A. The quality of care. How can it be assessed? *JAMA* 1988;260:1743–8.

20 Cameron C, Naylor CD. No impact from active dissemination of the Ottawa Ankle Rules: further evidence of the need for local implementation of practice guidelines. *CMAJ* 1999;160:1165–8.

21 Grol R, Dalhuijsen J, Thomas S, Veld C, Rutten G, Mokkink H. Attributes of clinical guidelines that influence use of guidelines in general practice. *BMJ* 1998;317:858–61.

22 Van der Weijden T, Grol R, Schouten B, Knottnerus A. Barriers to working according to cholesterol guidelines. *Eur J Public Health* 1998;8:113–8.

23 Denzin N, Lincoln YS (eds.). *Handbook of Qualitative Research.* Thousand Oaks, CA: Sage; 2000.

3.6.2 Framework for evaluating complex interventions

Sasha Shepperd
Department of Public Health, University of Oxford, Headington, Oxford, UK

KEY LEARNING POINTS

- The active ingredient(s) of complex interventions can be difficult to identify.
- Stakeholders can inform trialists on which element(s) of a complex intervention are essential to reproduce.

- Other types of evidence can improve the relevance of trials for policy makers.
- The MRC Framework for the Development and Evaluation of Randomised Controlled Trials for Complex Interventions to Improve Health provides a mechanism for formally integrating other types of evidence and supporting the transfer of evidence-based interventions.
- External validity can be strengthened through the involvement of key health care decision makers.

An unbiased summary of research evidence has the potential to inform those making health care decisions to implement, modify, or withdraw an intervention. In theory, this should apply to all health care interventions, whether simple or complex. Although several methods for improving the implementation of evidence for a range of interventions have been tested [1], a relatively neglected area in knowledge translation (KT) is the application of evidence from evaluations of complex interventions.

Framework for evaluating complex interventions

What is a complex intervention? To some extent, all interventions can be seen as complex, with some being more complex than others. The relatively simple act of prescribing a pill is accompanied by a series of steps to ensure adherence, understanding, checking for side effects, and drug interactions. However, the key active ingredient, the pill, is readily identified, and the other actions would not take place without this. For interventions at the more complex end of the spectrum, it is difficult to identify the precise mechanism which may contribute to outcome because these interventions contain a number of different elements that act independently or interdependently [2]. One example of this type of intervention is systems of care for patients recovering from a stroke to optimize health outcomes. Patients who survive a stroke experience varying degrees of disability, which places them, and their families, under considerable stress. The organization of inpatient services plays a major role in both the survival and recovery of these patients. Stroke units, compared with less-organized forms of inpatient care, are effective for improving the survival of patients who have had a stroke and reducing the dependency level experienced by these patients [3]. This evidence is derived from a systematic review, but it is not immediately obvious from the included trials which elements of a stroke unit are associated with a beneficial outcome.

In recent years, complex interventions have been a focus of debate within the research community as empirical evidence demonstrates a beneficial effect for some complex interventions and not for others. This debate has led

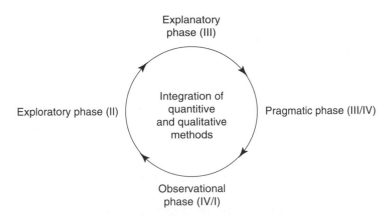

Figure 3.6.2.1 MRC Framework for evaluating complex interventions [2].

researchers, clinicians, and policy makers to question which element(s) of an intervention are essential to reproduce improved outcomes, and also if, as often is the case, a trial has shown no effect, whether due to problems with the study design or conduct. A number of initiatives from the research community attempting to address these methodological and conceptual challenges have been debated. One of the most influential is the Medical Research Council (MRC) Framework for the Development and Evaluation of Randomised Controlled Trials for Complex Interventions to Improve Health [2]. The MRC Framework, which is currently being updated, provides researchers with an iterative step-wise approach to determine the state of knowledge about a complex intervention being evaluated. Current work on the update extends the advice on implementation, or KT, to include involving stakeholders in the choice of research question and design, using a mix of approaches to dissemination and considering how the context of research may relate to local applicability.

Although the focus of the MRC Framework is on randomized trials, the approach can be used with other study designs. The steps include (1) *defining the intervention*, which involves identifying the existing evidence and any theoretical basis for the intervention to describe intervention components; (2) *an exploratory phase*, where the acceptability and feasibility of delivering the intervention and the comparison intervention are assessed and the study design is piloted; (3) *an explanatory phase*, when the final trial design is implemented in a relevant setting with appropriate eligibility criteria, taking into account statistical power and relevant measures of outcome; and finally, (4) *a pragmatic phase*, where implementation of the intervention is examined, with attention paid to the fidelity of the intervention, participants eligible for the intervention, and any possible adverse effects. Although the existing evidence base and type of intervention may make some phases redundant, the final phase is integral and directly relevant to KT.

Knowledge translation, complex interventions, and the iterative loop

The process of translating knowledge and informing policy is complex, with a range of factors to be considered. The MRC Framework, although designed for those evaluating complex interventions, can be used to facilitate the translation and interpretation of evidence by providing a mechanism for formally integrating additional forms of evidence relevant to all decision-makers. Additional evidence, usually qualitative or survey data, has been used within the context of single randomized trials and systematic reviews. In some cases, their use casts light on the most likely mechanism of action. Using the example of stroke units mentioned earlier, it appears from a survey of trialists contributing data to the systematic review [3] that stroke units are a focal point for the organization and coordination of services rather than a center for the provision of intensive rehabilitation. A common feature of stroke units included in the meta-analysis by Langhorne and colleagues was that care was organized and coordinated by a multidisciplinary team of professional staff interested or knowledgeable about stroke. The stroke units also encouraged the involvement of carers in the rehabilitation process [4].

Other outcomes and process variables relevant to KT can be explored through the use of additional evidence. These types of studies can be done iteratively alongside an evaluation, to inform trial development, or retro-spectively. A qualitative study [5] conducted parallel to a trial of intensive case management for people with severe mental illness investigated the active ingredients of the intervention in terms of staff roles, practice, and organizational features. Providing a comprehensive assessment and needs-led service were regarded as the key mechanisms of this intervention, and organizational features, such as an absence of team management, limited the extent to which case managers could make an impact. Finally, the degree to which an intervention has been sustained outside the trial setting can be explored, for example by assessing the volume and type of patients using an "admission avoidance hospital at home" after the completion of a randomized trial [6].

There is a wide scope to include input from policymakers, clinicians, and health care managers at each phase of primary and secondary research on complex interventions, but this is underutilized. Involving decision-makers in shaping the question and defining the intervention can help ensure the relevance of research, but the political context can shift the significance of the evaluation over a relatively short period of time. In addition, input from health care decision makers has the potential to strengthen the external validity of the research. Local applicability is a key factor influencing the use of evidence, and identifying the variables that define the context of the research findings can help health care decision-makers explicitly address this [7].

The importance of the external validity of complex interventions has recently received attention, with the development of standards to improve the quality and relevance of research [8,9]. Not surprisingly these standards focus on contextual variables affecting the delivery of an intervention, which have an obvious bearing on KT. This link between KT and external validity should be further explored to ensure that a number of additional attributes identified as important by health care decision-makers are considered by the research community. These factors include data on accessibility, the risk of adverse events [10], cost-effectiveness, and the sustainability of interventions over time. Relatively little attention has been paid to the sustainability of interventions in contrast with the initial implementation of a KT strategy.

Future research

Using a framework that, at least in theory, systematically addresses factors considered important by stakeholders during the design stage of a complex intervention evaluation should improve subsequent implementation. However, there is little evidence documenting this process. Descriptive research that documents how health care decision-makers are identified and subsequently contribute to key decisions would be valuable. In addition, exploring the areas where it is difficult to reach agreement can be informative and can provide a realistic set of expectations for this type of collaborative research. Clearly, there is a risk that the research process can become overly complicated, and this needs to be guarded against.

Summary

Using a framework that explicitly addresses each stage of evaluating a complex intervention has the potential to support the transfer of evidence-based interventions from both primary and secondary research. This will also help prevent interventions from being unsuccessfully, or inefficiently, implemented and resources being wasted.

References

1 Dopson S, Locock L, Chambers D, Gabbay J. Implementation of evidence-based medicine: evaluation of the Promoting Action on Clinical Effectiveness programme. *J Health Serv Res Policy* 2006;6:23–31.

2 Campbell M, Fitzpatrick R, Haines A, Kinmonth AL, Sandercock P, Spiegelhalter D, et al. Framework for design and evaluation of complex interventions to improve health. *BMJ* 2000;321[7262]:694–6.

3 Stroke Unit Trialists' Collaboration. Organised inpatient (stroke unit) care for stroke. *Cochrane Database Sys Rev* 2007;Art. No.: CD000197.

4 Langhorne P, Pollock A, with the Stroke Unit Trialists Collaboration. What are the components of effective stroke unit care? *Age Ageing* 2002;31:365–71.

5 Weaver T, Tyrer P, Ritchie J, Renton A. Assessing the value of assertive outreach. *Br J Psych* 2003;183:437–45.

6 Wilson A, Parker H, Wynn A, Spiers N. Performance of hospital at home after a randomised controlled trial. *J Health Serv Res Policy* 2003;8:160–4.

7 Lavis J, Davies J, Oxman A, Denis JL, Golden-Biddle K. Towards systematic review that inform health care management and policy-making. *J Health Serv Res Policy* 2005;10:21–34.

8 Green LW, Glasgow RE. Evaluating the relevance, generalization and applicability of research—issues in external validation and translation methodology. *Eval Health Prof* 2006;29:126–53.

9 Glasgow RE, Green LW, Klesges LM, Abrams DB, Fisher EB, Goldstein MG, et al. External validity: we need to do more. *Ann Behav Med* 2006;31[2]:105–8.

10 Glenton C, Underland V, Kho M, Pennick V, Oxman A. Summaries of findings, descriptions of interventions, and information about adverse effects would make reviews more informative. *J Clin Epidemiol* 2006;59:770–8.

3.7 Sustaining knowledge use

Barbara Davies and Nancy Edwards

University of Ottawa School of Nursing, Ottawa, ON, Canada

KEY LEARNING POINTS

- Sustained knowledge use refers to the continued implementation of innovations over time and depends on the ability of workers and organizations to adapt to change.
- Tension exists between the routinization of one innovation and the receptiveness to subsequent innovations.
- There is limited research about sustainability, possibly because of short-term funding periods from most research agencies.
- Key factors found to influence sustainability include the relevance of the issue, attitudes of stakeholders, leadership, financial supports, and political climate.
- Sustainability planning is recommended early in the knowledge-to-action cycle, when interventions are being designed.
- Addressing sustainability requires planning for "scaling up" knowledge use.

What factors determine whether a person will sustain a lifestyle behavior change, a physician will continue to order a specific medication, a hospital will sustain a policy for minimum restraint use for agitated patients, or a health care region will continue to provide mental health community services for vulnerable populations? These questions about determinants of the sustained use of new knowledge to improve the health of populations, to build stronger health care systems, and to better inform government policies are vitally important. Researchers and policy makers are challenged to better understand health determinants and to working toward a health care system "driven by solid, research-informed management and policy decisions" [1]. To achieve timely, evidence-informed decision making, there is a call for increased dialogue and linkages between knowledge producers and knowledge users [1] and a call for "moving research into policy, programs and

---

Knowledge Translation in Health Care: Moving from Evidence to Practice. Edited by S. Straus, J. Tetroe, and I. Graham. © 2009 Blackwell Publishing, ISBN: 978-1-4051-8106-8.

practice" [2]. The issue of sustained knowledge use is a critical component of the science and practice of knowledge translation (KT).

What is sustainability?

Sustainability is "the degree to which an innovation continues to be used after initial efforts to secure adoption is completed" [3] or is "when new ways of working and improved outcomes become the norm" [4]. Despite the apparent simplicity of these definitions, researchers report that sustainability of new innovations in health care is one of the most central and exasperating issues in addressing the gap between knowledge and practice [5]. Perhaps the exasperation lies in the difficulty of determining how and when to maximize factors that will create sustained knowledge use. Sustainability is not a steady, linear process. Rather, multiple determinants interact at variable rates depending on contextual factors. These factors include receptivity to new knowledge and capacity to interpret and apply the new knowledge by the individual, an organization, or a system.

Models for sustainability

Of 31 models about KT, 11 described a step that was separate and subsequent to the step of evaluation, labeled as maintain change or sustain ongoing knowledge use [6]. A specific sustainability model, as well as a leader's guide, is available from the NHS Institute for Innovation and Improvement in the United Kingdom [4,7]. This sustainability model revolves around three core elements of process, staff, and organization. Factors in the process domain are benefits beyond helping patients; credibility of evidence; adaptability; and monitoring progress. For the staff domain, factors are training and involvement; behaviors; senior leaders; and clinical leaders. Finally, for the organization domain, factors are fit with goals and the culture and infrastructure. In addition to this U.K. model, an American report describes perspectives about the "science of spread" [8], and a position paper prepared for the New Zealand Ministry of Health describes an action plan for the spread of proven health innovations [9].

A challenge to sustainability is the tension that exists between the routinization of one idea and the receptivity to a subsequent good idea [10]. Sustainability is not always a desirable outcome when the need for modification is evident. As new knowledge is constantly being produced, sustainability strategies need to build in processes that allow for the integration of new insights emerging from the production of research knowledge and new insights arising as knowledge is applied. Moreover, it is not uncommon for

Table 3.7.1 Terms related to sustainability

Routinization: When an innovation becomes entrenched into regular activities and loses distinct identity [3].

Institutionalization: The "staying power" or relative endurance of change in an organization [11]. The change becomes part of everyday activities or normal practices in an organization.

Reinvention: Adapting the innovation to fit with a local situation or the degree of modification by the adopters [3,12].

Spread: "The process through which new working methods developed in one setting are adopted, perhaps with appropriate modifications, in other organizational contexts" [13].

Expanded: In addition to sustaining knowledge use over time, there is a broader implementation to transcend disciplines, organizational units of care, health care sectors, and/or communities (e.g., service, academic) [14].

Scaling up: "Efforts to increase the impact of health service innovations tested in pilot or experimental projects so as to benefit more people and to foster policy and program development" [15].

health care systems to change models of care delivery; sustainability strategies for knowledge implementation must have the flexibility to respond to these shifts. There are several interrelated concepts about sustainability, and some authors use various terms interchangeably. Tables 3.7.1 and 3.7.2 provide a list and brief description of some related terms.

Why is sustainability planning rarely addressed?

Although sustainability is seen as important because many innovations are valuable only if they continue to be used [3], researchers have paid little attention to sustainability. A systematic review of the diffusion of innovations in health services organizations noted that only 2 of 1000 sources screened mentioned the term sustainability [10]. Perhaps this dearth of attention is due to the fact that many theories of planned change focus on shorter-term perspectives and clinical researchers may consider system-level change processes outside their realm of research. In addition, funding opportunities for research are typically short-term with follow-up measurement feasible for only 1 or 2 years. Thus, even for studies designed to examine change within an organization, funding windows typically only allow shorter-term change processes to be assessed. Furthermore, policy cycles are on different time scales across system levels and between sectors. Consequently, successfully producing a change at one system level does not ensure its uptake at another

Table 3.7.2 Terms related to lack of sustainability

Improvement evaporation, initiative decay, or erosion: Decreased application of the innovation over time [13].

Discontinuance: A decision to de-adopt or stop the implementation of an innovation [3].

Sticky knowledge: Knowledge is sticky and difficult to move. "Stickiness is a product of the transfer process and can be predicted by examining a number of conditions related to the knowledge, its source, the context of the transfer, and the characteristics of the recipient" [16].

Relapse: Reverting to previous ways of operating [17].

system level. Finally, a common view is that sustainability should be done toward the end of a project/program rather than at the outset. Thus, sustainability may be threatened if project leaders change or become disengaged.

Addressing sustainability requires planning for "scaling up" knowledge use. Conditions critical for scaling up include adequate human capacity and supportive financial, organizational, governance, and regulatory structures [18,19]. Some authors advocate the use of computer models to help provide better estimates of what will be required to scale up interventions [20]. Such models could be used to aid the design of research and pilot interventions to avoid the problem of testing "boutique interventions" [21]; those that require costs and human resources that are beyond the absorptive capacity of a social or health care system. Without systematic ways to address the scalability of interventions when research is planned, we may end up with "proven" interventions that hold little or no potential for system sustainability due to their inherent scaling-up limitations. For example, antiretrovirals for the treatment of HIV and AIDS have demonstrated efficacy and effectiveness, but scaling up these regimens at a national level in lower-income countries has been challenging due, in part, to human resource capacity issues within the health care system.

Facilitators and barriers to consider in developing a sustainability action plan

A paradox has been described in which the same factors can both facilitate and inhibit sustainability [22] in the same program or in other settings. Thus, we have identified eight factors, based on the literature and our experience, to consider in the development of a sustainability action plan [4,9,13,14,23,24,25].

1 Relevance of the topic: Is there a well-defined need and priority for the knowledge that is being implemented? Is there consensus about what knowledge needs to be sustained and what is needed to create conditions for sustainability? How does the new knowledge fit with current priorities?

2 Benefits: What are the anticipated outcomes of knowledge implementation from a biological, economic, psychological, organizational, social, political, or other perspective? How meaningful are these benefits to the various stakeholders?

3 Attitudes: What are the attitudes (i.e., potential resistance) of the patient/client, their family, the public, health care providers, and relevant decision-makers toward the innovation?

4 Networks: What teams or groups can be engaged to facilitate the sustainability of knowledge use? Are there people who can be engaged to cross disciplines, settings, or sectors of the health care system (e.g., interprofessional collaborative practice, academic programs, health care organizations, community-based care)?

5 Leadership: What actions might leaders and managers at all levels of involvement take to support the sustainability of knowledge use? Are there champions for the change? Who is responsible for continued implementation of the innovation and making modifications as new knowledge is brought forward? Who will be responsible for ensuring that relevant outcomes are met?

6 Policy articulation and integration: How will the fit between new knowledge and existing policies be assessed? How might the knowledge be integrated in relevant policies, procedures, regulatory and documentation systems (e.g., electronic clinical decision support systems)?

7 Financial: What funding is required to implement, sustain, and scale up knowledge? What flexibility in funding is necessary and available for reimbursement? Can cost-effective strategies be used?

8 Political: Who are the stakeholders and what power or support might be leveraged? Who will initiate scaling up processes?

Adaptation and why sustainability is difficult to predict

The complex adaptive systems theory helps us "understand why sustainability is difficult to predict" and also "tells us that sustainability ultimately comes down to the ability to adapt" [25]. This theory explains how dynamic and ongoing changes at one level of the system may eventually influence changes at another system level [26]. Simply put, adaptation theory tells us that there are continuous dynamic change processes at work within each level of the system. Thus, even when an innovation is introduced at one system level, it invariably has the potential to impact or be influenced by factors at the same and other system levels. For example, introducing evidence-informed best practice guidelines for asthma management by nurses has implications for care provision by other members of the health care team. Changes that the other health care team members make to support or thwart this shift in practice will influence whether these changes in nursing practice are sustained.

Over time, change processes at one system level may lead to change processes at the next system level. Continuing with our asthma example, changes at other system levels may include a shift in policies and procedures for asthma management, inclusion of new practices in orientation sessions for new nursing staff, and changes in patient referral and follow-up procedures. However, if these kinds of structures at the next level do not fundamentally change to accommodate the innovation, practitioners will have a tendency to revert to the former ways of doing things. Many intersystem factors may support these changes. Notably, vertical social connections (e.g., nurses being formal members of organizational decision-making committees) facilitate synergistic and multilevel adaptation processes. There are also factors that tend to maintain the status quo. These include power hierarchies among professional groups, institutionalized routines, and established governance structures that yield unequal benefits or burdens for one social group relative to another [26, 27].

Monitoring sustainability

Monitoring systems and data feedback mechanisms are needed to determine relevant process and outcome factors to assess sustainability. Whereas some relapse is to be expected, a decision will be necessary to determine how much relapse is acceptable to claim that sustainability is achieved [17]. Sustainability assessment is not an all-or-nothing phenomenon. One Canadian research team describes four degrees of sustainability from absent, precarious, weak to the ultimate sustainability level involving routinization [28]. A 53-item Program Sustainability Index (PSI) has been proposed along with suggested modifications for further testing [29].

Future research

There remains much to be learned about sustainability in the knowledge-to-action process. Sustainability is a complex construct; thus, mixed methods and participatory research designs will be required to advance our understanding of sustainability. For example, qualitative studies about process factors and quantitative studies about outcomes following knowledge implementation over time are necessary. There is a strong need for research programs and not just isolated single knowledge-to-action projects. Intriguing research questions have been proposed, such as whether to embed knowledge use in one area before use spreads to another area or whether it is better to spread new knowledge or an innovation as widely and quickly as possible so that saturation contributes to sustainability [13]. Although several scales to measure sustainability are available, further development of measurement tools is necessary [17].

Summary

Sustaining knowledge use is essential to the knowledge-to-action process. The knowledge-to-action framework depicts the sustainability phase after the evaluate outcomes step. However, many authors advocate planning for sustainability as early as possible, such as when the interventions for knowledge use are being selected and tailored. Sustainability and adaptation models are available to help with planning. Numerous potentially relevant factors have been documented in the literature, and aspects such as leadership, assessment of attitudes, and determining the financial implications are vital for thoughtful planning to continuously strive for a better health care system.

References

1 Canadian Health Services Research Foundation. URL http://www.chsrf.ca/about/do_statement_purpose_e.php [accessed 2008].

2 Canadian Institutes of Health Research. URL http://www.cihr-irsc.gc.ca/e/30240 html#slide1_e [accessed 2008].

3 Rogers EM, *Diffusion of Innovations.* 5th ed. New York: Free Press; 2005;429.

4 Maher L, Gustafson D, Evans A. *Sustainability model and guide. NHS Institute for Innovation and Improvement*; 2007. URL www.institute.nhs.uk/sustainability.

5 Mendel P, Meredith LS, Schoenbaum M, Sherbourne CD, Wells KB. Interventions in organizational and community context: a framework for building evidence on dissemination and implementation in health services research. *Adm Policy Ment Health* 2008;35[1–2]:21–37.

6 Graham ID, Tetroe J, and the KT Theories Research Group. Some theoretical underpinnings of knowledge translation. *Acad Emerg Med* 2007;14[11]:936–41.

7 NHS Institute for Innovation and Improvement. *Improvement Leader's Guide to Sustainability and Its Relationship with Spread and Adoption.* 2007. URL www.institute.nhs.uk/sustainability.

8 Bodenheimer T. *The science of spread: how innovations in care become the norm.* California HealthCare Foundation; 2007. URL http://www.chcf.org/topics/chronicdisease/index.cfm?itemID=133461.

9 Lomas J. *Formalised informality: an action plan to spread proven health innovations.* Wellington: Ministry of Health, New Zealand. URL http://www.moh.govt.nz/moh.nsf/pagesmh/7365/.

10 Greenhalgh T, Robert G, Bate P, MacFarlane F, Kyriakidou O. *Diffusion of Innovations in Health Service Organizations: A Systematic Literature Review.* Boston: Blackwell Publishing; 2005.

11 Goodman RM, Steckler A. A model for the institutionalization of health promotion programs. *Family and Community Health* 1989;11[4]:63–78.

12 Ray-Couquard T, Philip M, Lehman B, Fervers F, Farsi F, Chauvin F. Impact of a clinical guidelines program for breast and colon cancer in a French cancer center. *JAMA* 1997;278[19]:1591–5.

13 Buchanan DA, Fitzgerald L, Ketley D. *The Sustainability and Spread of Organizational Change.* New York: Routledge; 2007: xxiii.

14 Davies B, Edwards N, Ploeg J, Virani T, Skelly J, Dobbins M. *Determinants of the sustained use of research evidence in nursing: final report.* Canadian Health Services Research Foundation & Canadian Institutes for Health Research. Ottawa, Ontario, Canada; 2006. URL http://www.chsrf.ca/final_research/ogc/pdf/davies_final_e.pdf.

15 ExpandNet. URL http://www.expandnet.net/PDFs/ExpandNet_Practical_Guide .pdf [accesssed 2008].

16 Elwyn G, Taubert M, Kowalczuk J. Sticky knowledge: a possible model for investigating implementation in healthcare contexts. *Implement Sci* 2007;44[2].

17 Bowman CC, Sobo EJ, Asch SM, Gifford AL. Measuring persistence of implementation: QUERI series. *Implement Sci* 2008;21[3].

18 Simmons R, Fajans P, Ghiron L. (eds.). *Scaling up health service delivery: from pilot innovations to policies and programmes.* WHO World Health Report; 2006.

19 Hanson K, Ranson MK, Oliveira-Cruz V, Mills A. Expanding access to priority health interventions: a framework for understanding the constraints to scaling up. *Journal of Knowledge Management* 2003;15[1]:1–14.

20 Riegelman R, Verme D, Rochon J, El-Mohandes A. Interaction and intervention modeling: predicting and extrapolating the impact of multiple interventions. *Ann Epidemiol* 2002;12[3]:151–6.

21 African Youth Alliance. *Scaling-up.* URL http://www.ayaonline.org/Strategies/PDFs/ScalingUp.pdf [accessed 2008].

22 Wakerman J, Chalmers EM, Humphreys JS, Clarence CL, Bell AI, Larson A, et al. Sustainable chronic disease management in remote Australia. *MJA* 2005;183[10]:S64–S68.

23 Nolan K, Schall MW, Erb F, Nolan T. Using a framework for spread: the case of patient access in the veterans health administration. *Jt Comm J Qual Patient Saf* 2005;31[6]:339–47.

24 Shediac-Rizkallah MC, Bone LR. Planning for the sustainability of community-based health programs: conceptual frameworks and future directions for research, practice and policy. *Health Educ Res* 1998;3[1]:87–108.

25 Sibthorpe BM, Glasgow NJ, Wells RW. Emergent themes in the sustainability of primary health care innovation. *MJA* 2005;183[10 Suppl]:S77–S80, page S79.

26 Gunderson LH, Holling CS. *Panarchy: Understanding Transformations in Human and Natural Systems.* Washington, DC: Island Press; 2002.

27 Denis JL, Langley A. The dynamics of collective leadership and strategic change in pluralistic organizations. *Acad Manage J* 2001;44:809–37.

28 Pluye P, Potvin L, Denis JL, Pelletier J. Program sustainability: focus on organizational routines. *Health Promot Int* 2004;19[4]:489–500.

29 Mancini JA, Marek L. Sustaining community-based programs for families: conceptualization and measurement. *Family Relations* 2004;53[4]:339–47.

3.8 Case examples

Sumit R. Majumdar

Department of Medicine, University of Alberta, Edmonton, AB, Canada

---

KEY LEARNING POINTS

- Like any drug or device, a knowledge translation (KT) intervention should be tested in a rigorous controlled fashion and compared with usual care *before* widespread adoption and implementation.

- Most KT interventions either do not improve quality of care or do so only to a modest degree; therefore, better attention needs to be paid to reproducibility and persistence of effects, and health economics needs to be considered more often.

- During the design, implementation, and outcomes evaluation phases, mixed (quantitative and qualitative) methods need to be more often employed to better understand how or why some KT interventions work and some do not.

- Rigorously conducted studies of KT can (and should) be funded by peer review agencies and published in mainstream peer review scientific journals.

Previous chapters in this book have examined aspects of knowledge translation (KT) in detail, including various theoretical frameworks, types of interventions, implementation methods, issues related to measurement and evaluation of processes and care outcomes, and strengths and limitations of various study designs. This chapter draws upon what has come before and presents case examples of rigorous and successful knowledge-to-action studies. Although each study has its own strengths and limitations, the three examples chosen share the following features: they address a common and clinically important problem; evaluate well-designed interventions; have adequate sample sizes; use reasonable and robust analytic plans without any unit-of-analysis errors; deliver valid results; and were published in high-impact mainstream general medical journals. Each case example consists of a summary of the main features and results of the trial, a brief discussion of the main strengths and limitations of the work, some take-home messages, and

---

Knowledge Translation in Health Care: Moving from Evidence to Practice. Edited by S. Straus, J. Tetroe, and I. Graham. © 2009 Blackwell Publishing, ISBN: 978-1-4051-8106-8.

a Web link to the original article for interested readers. The chapter ends by synthesizing observations from the three case examples.

Case example #1. Using physician-specific performance feedback and achievable benchmarks to improve quality of primary care [1]

Background: Patients receive about half the recommended evidence-based primary care for which they are eligible. Physicians currently receive a great deal of audit and feedback about how they are doing, but whether such efforts are warranted is poorly understood.

Question: Over and above traditional quality improvement interventions that included physician-specific feedback, would provision of "achievable benchmark" data lead to better patient outcomes?

Intervention: Most benchmark data are provided as either the mean or median performance achieved or as an attainable value determined by consensus. In contrast, achievable benchmarks (derived from the same types of data) represent the average performance for the top 10% of physicians being evaluated within the same local context.

Study Design: Cluster randomized controlled trial with blinded ascertainment of outcomes comparing standard quality improvement efforts plus traditional audit and feedback (48 physicians, 965 patients) versus receipt of achievable benchmark data (49 physicians, 966 patients) in one state in the United States.

Outcomes: Changes in the process of care before and after the intervention among eligible patients with diabetes; specifically, changes in influenza vaccination, foot examination, and laboratory measurements of A1c, cholesterol, and triglycerides.

Results: Achievable benchmarks were 82% for influenza vaccination, 86% for foot examination, 97% for A1c, 99% for cholesterol, and 98% for triglycerides. Compared with controls, achievable benchmark data led to an additional 12% increase in influenza vaccination ($p < 0.001$), an additional 2% increase in foot examination ($p = 0.02$), and a 4% additional increase in A1c measurement ($p = 0.02$). There were no improvements in the two lipid measurements.

Discussion: As a proof of concept, this rigorous trial of KT was able to demonstrate that providing individual physicians with their own data and a comparison with what other top performers in the same environment are able to achieve can lead to improvements in the quality of primary care. A major strength of this study was that it examined multiple processes of care. That said, it should be acknowledged that improvements in two measures were small (2–4%) and that two measures did not improve at all. There are two important limitations to this work. First, improvements were only related to processes-of-care—whether clinical outcomes improved or whether there were unintended (unmeasured) consequences of this intervention are not known. Second, investigators did not (a priori) define a clinically important or clinically worthwhile improvement. Although a 12% increase in influenza vaccination may be clinically worthwhile, is a 2% increase in foot examination also worthwhile?

Take-home messages: Achievable benchmarks may be an important addition to standard audit and feedback. Replication studies and a deeper understanding of why this was not more (and not more uniformly) effective are warranted.

Link: http://jama.ama-assn.org/cgi/content/abstract/285/22/2871.

Case example #2. Using clinical decision support with electronic prompts to increase thromboprophylaxis and decrease venous thromboembolism in hospitalized patients [2]

Background: Despite the fact that deep venous thrombosis and pulmonary embolism (DVT/PE) are a common but largely preventable complication of hospitalization, inexpensive and evidence-based thromboprophylactic measures are universally underused. Many attempts to increase rates of DVT/PE prophylaxis have been made.

Question: Will an automated clinical decision support system with physician prompts improve quality of care and reduce rates of DVT/PE?

Intervention: A computerized decision support system using various predefined algorithms to identify high-risk patients based on clinical risk factors determined whether they received some form of thromboprophylaxis and prompted providers in real time to order thromboprophylaxis if it was not ordered. The prompts were not "passive"—they were delivered to the physician order entry screen and acknowledged, and then explicit orders to continue withholding prophylaxis or to deliver some form of prophylaxis had to be entered, that is, a forcing function was present.

Study design: Quasi-randomized (allocation based on even or odd patient medical record numbers) controlled trial comparing usual care controls (1251 patients) versus computerized decision support with real-time prompts (1255 patients) at a single U.S. hospital.

Outcomes: Rates of DVT/PE prophylaxis among potentially eligible patients and rates of clinically diagnosed DVT/PE within 90 days of hospitalization; the latter was the primary study endpoint.

Results: Baseline rates of prophylaxis were about 85%. Of all the patients deemed eligible for DVT/PE prophylaxis who were not receiving it, 15% of controls versus 34% of intervention patients were appropriately treated (19% improvement, $p < 0.001$). Overall, 8% of control patients versus 5% of intervention patients had clinically diagnosed DVT or PE within 90 days of hospitalization (3% reduction in clinical events, $p < 0.001$). As a measure of safety, rates of death, rehospitalization, and bleeding were similar between study groups.

Discussion: Unlike most studies in the field, this study was designed to detect differences in clinically important outcomes rather than restricting examination to processes-of-care. Indeed, for this particular clinical area, this is the first study to demonstrate that improvements in processes-of-care are tightly linked with outcomes, suggesting (for future studies) that the former are a reasonable surrogate measure of quality. Although the investigators defined all patients in the study as at sufficient risk to warrant prophylaxis, two-thirds of intervention patients (and 85% of controls) still did not receive guideline-concordant care. This result implies that either there is much greater uncertainty in the thromboprophylaxis literature than acknowledged by the investigators or that the decision support tool itself needs more refinement. This latter point is one of the major limitations of the study—the algorithm and scoring system to define "high-risk" had not been previously validated and was not commonly used. There are two other major limitations. First, contrary to the authors' statements, this was not a randomized trial—it was a quasi-randomized study, and it is possible that outcomes assessors could have broken the allocation code and been influenced in their ascertainment. Second, only one prompt was studied. In isolation, this particular reminder worked, but at what point will providers start to experience "reminder-fatigue" as numerous well-intended pop-ups prevent them from quickly and efficiently caring for their patients?

Take-home messages: This is one of the few clear demonstrations that a knowledge translation intervention can improve both process ("surrogate") measures of care and lead to important changes in clinical events that directly reflect how patients feel, function, or survive. Replication studies, with different and multiple concurrent reminders, are warranted. In addition, a better explication for why this particular intervention (conducted at what is considered one of four U.S. benchmark institutions for the implementation and study of health information technology) was not far more effective than observed is needed.

Link: http://content.nejm.org/cgi/content/abstract/352/10/969.

Case example #3. Using a multifaceted intervention directed at patients and physicians to decrease antibiotic use for acute bronchitis [3]

Background: Almost all cases of acute bronchitis treated on an outpatient basis are caused by viruses. Despite the widespread dissemination of evidence-based guidelines, the majority of patients still receive antibiotics leading to adverse events, increased antibiotic resistance in the community, and excess costs. Antibiotic use in this setting needs to be safely curtailed, but most attempts have not been able to change practice.

Question: Will interventions directed at patients and/or their physicians reduce the rate of antibiotic use in patients with viral illness such as acute bronchitis?

Interventions: High-intensity (household and office-based educational materials for patients and education, audit and feedback, and academic detailing for physicians) versus low-intensity (office-based educational materials only) interventions versus usual care in a group-model health maintenance organization.

Study design: Nonrandomized before-after study with concurrent controls. Specifically, high-intensity site (34,978 patients and 28 providers) versus low-intensity site (36,404 patients and 31 providers) versus two usual care sites (46,767 patients and 34 providers).

Outcomes: Rate of antibiotic prescriptions for acute bronchitis. Rates of antibiotic prescription for control conditions (other upper respiratory tract infections and acute sinusitis) and unintended consequences (use of nonantibiotic treatments and return visits) were secondary endpoints.

Results: Before the interventions, rates of antibiotic prescription for acute bronchitis were about 80%. Over and above changes in practice at the usual care control sites, the high-intensity intervention led to a 24% absolute reduction in antibiotic use ($p = 0.003$) while the low-intensity intervention led to a 3% reduction ($p = 0.68$). Rates of antibiotic use for control conditions, use of nonantibiotic treatments, and visit rates were similar across all three arms, suggesting that the interventions were safe and did not lead to unintended consequences.

Discussion: Acknowledging that the study design is valid albeit nonrandomized, the effect size reported is among the largest ever documented for antibiotic reduction in primary care. Most important, the investigators clearly demonstrated that all study sites were comparable before intervention and that there were no unintended consequences. For example, if providers were "aware" of the study and its intentions, a simple way to game the system and reduce antibiotic use for acute bronchitis is to diagnose patients with "upper respiratory tract infection" or "pneumonia" and give them antibiotics. This finding was not observed, and there did not appear to be any difference in downstream health resource consumption across sites. Other than the fact that the study was nonrandomized, there are two major limitations to this work. First, although two intensities of intervention were tested, this was not a factorial trial. The high-intensity intervention was effective, but whether it was the physician component, the patient education component, or their combination that mediated study effect is not known. This limitation has resource implications with respect to continuing the intervention or using similar interventions for other conditions where antibiotics may be overused. Second, this was a one-off intervention. Whether patients, providers, and the system "learn" and continue to improve or simply lapse back to usual patterns of practice after the study is complete is an important question that cannot be answered from this study.

Take-home messages: Multifaceted interventions directed at patients and their physicians can decrease the unnecessary use of antibiotics, and the methods can probably be extended to other conditions associated with overuse that are sensitive to patient demands. More important than replication in this case, studies that examine the relative importance (and cost-effectiveness) of the components of the intervention are warranted.

Link: http://jama.ama-assn.org/cgi/content/abstract/281/16/1512.

Future research

These case examples illuminate three common problems in KT research that need to be better addressed. First, investigators often test multifaceted (or multiple component) interventions. If such an intervention is found to work, those wanting to apply the work in their own settings must apply *all* components of the intervention as described. KT researchers need to start conducting more three-to-four-armed trials or formal factorial trials to better determine what works and what does not. Importantly, given how many interventions do not work and how often secular improvements in quality occur, some form of "usual care" should be considered the most appropriate control group for most trials. Only in this way will we get a better idea of which components are "mandatory" and which might be "optional." Quantitative data (e.g., end-user surveys) and qualitative studies can help better understand how elements of the intervention package work.

Second, investigators rarely provide enough information for others to replicate their work. Replicability is an important facet of science, especially the science of KT. Often, details are absent or missing because of journal word count limits and the like. For example, in an overview of systematic reviews published in *ACP Journal Club* and *Evidence-Based Medicine Journal* (journals of secondary publication), Glasziou and Shepperd found that less than 15% of reports have sufficient information about the intervention itself to allow clinicians or policymakers to implement it [4]. Open-access publication of detailed methods papers in journals like *Implementation Science* is now easier than ever, and many journals permit Web links and unfettered electronic appendices with their articles. Hopefully, this will make it much easier for those trying to apply results or for those undertaking systematic reviews.

Third, investigators rarely describe what would be considered a clinically worthwhile difference to adopt the intervention if it were found to work. In particular, as studies get larger, it will become easier to detect small and clinically unimportant but statistically significant improvements in quality of care. But at some point, preferably before the study starts, it is important to define how much of an improvement is worthwhile versus how much of an effect is statistically detectable. The former is more important than the latter; perhaps a way to begin reconciling these two measures is to define how much a practice or organization would be willing to pay for a certain amount of improvement. Regardless, formal health–economic analyses are rarely undertaken alongside most KT interventions, and this too seems unfortunate.

Summary

These three case examples in successful KT are each important contributions to the literature. They each demonstrate how disparate various clinical problems may be, how complex interventions may need to be, and how difficult implementation and evaluation will be. Nevertheless, collectively, these investigators overcame many problems endemic to the field. These cases are state-of-the-art examples of rigorous KT research. They illustrate how far the field has come over the last 2 decades (acknowledging that even the oldest study described is <10 years old) and also demonstrate how much more work needs to be done in this relatively young scientific field.

References

1 Kiefe CI, Allison JJ, Williams OD, et al. Improving quality improvement using achievable benchmarks for physician feedback: a randomized controlled trial. *JAMA* 2001;285:2871–9.

2 Kucher N, Koo S, Quiroz R, et al. Electronic alerts to prevent venous thromboembolism among hospitalized patients. *N Engl J Med* 2005;352:969–77.

3 Gonzales R, Steiner JF, Lum A, Barrett PH. Decreasing antibiotic use in ambulatory practice: impact of a multidimensional intervention on the treatment of uncomplicated acute bronchitis in adults. *JAMA* 1999;281:1512–19.

4 Glasziou P, Shepperd S. Ability to apply evidence from systematic reviews. Abstract presented, Society for Academic Primary Care, July 5, 2007, UK.

Section 4
Theories and Models of Knowledge to Action

4.1 Planned action theories

Ian D. Graham[1], Jacqueline Tetroe[2], and KT Theories Group

[1]Knowledge Translation Portfolio, Canadian Institutes of Health, and School of Nursing, University of Ottawa, Ottawa, ON, Canada
[2]Knowledge Translation Portfolio, Canadian Institutes of Health, Ottawa, ON, Canada

---

KEY LEARNING POINTS

- Data on the validity and transferability of planned action theories are limited.
- A planned action theory can focus implementation efforts and provide all stakeholders with a common script or understanding of the action plan.

There has been a growing focus on moving research into practice in recent years and, alongside, interest in theories of knowledge implementationhas been increasingincreased. For example, the idea of using conceptual models to help nurses implement research evidence gained strength in the 1970s and 1980s when a number of models were tried [1–3]. Conceptual models of implementing knowledge are essentially models or theories of change. Change theories fall into two basic kinds: classical and planned [4]. Classical theories of change (sometimes referred to as descriptive or normative theories) are passive; they explain or describe how change occurs. An example of a classical theory of change is Rogers' diffusion theory [5,6] or Kuhn's [7] conceptualization of scientific revolutions. These theories describe change but were not specifically designed to cause or guide change in practice. Other implementation theories within this category are the models that are proposed as ways of thinking about or researching knowledge translation (KT), such as Lomas's Coordinated Implementation Model [8,9]. Although classical theories of change can be informative and helpful for identifying the determinants of change, researchers, policymakers, and change agents tend to be more interested in planned change theories that are specifically intended to be used to guide or cause change [4].

A planned change theory is a set of logically interrelated concepts that explain, in a systematic way, the means by which planned change occurs, that predict how various forces in an environment will react in specified

---

Knowledge Translation in Health Care: Moving from Evidence to Practice. Edited by S. Straus, J. Tetroe, and I. Graham. © 2009 Blackwell Publishing, ISBN: 978-1-4051-8106-8.

change situations, and that help planners or change agents control variables that increase or decrease the likelihood of the occurrence of change [10,11]. Planned change, in this context, refers to deliberately engineering change that occurs in groups that vary in size and setting. Planned change theories are also referred to as prescriptive theories [4]. Those who use planned change theories may work with individuals, but their objective is to alter ways of doing things in social systems. This chapter describes our review and analysis of planned action models.

We undertook a focused search of the social science, education, management, and health sciences literature that has been documented elsewhere [12]. We restricted all searches to literature published in English or French. The literature search yielded 78 articles that were subject to data abstraction by two reviewers. This involved abstracting the key or core concepts of each model/theory, determining the action phases, and deciding whether each fit the inclusion/exclusion criteria around being planned action theory/model/framework.

Thirty-one planned action theories (see Box 4.1.1) were identified and subjected to a "theory analysis," which is a useful process for determining the strengths and limitations of theories and to determine similarities and differences. The steps in a theory analysis [13] are to (1) determine the origins of the theory (i.e., Who developed it? Where are they from? What prompted the originator to develop it? Is it inductive or deductive in form? Is there evidence to support or refute the development of the theory?), (2) examine the meaning of the theory (What are the concepts and how do they relate to each other?), (3) analyze the logical consistency of the theory (Are there any logical fallacies?), (4) define the degree of generalizability and parsimony of the theory, (5) determine the testability of the theory, and (6) determine the usefulness of the theory. The complete categorization and synthesis of the theories is available at http://www.iceberg-grebeci.ohri.ca/research/kt_theories_db.html.

The 31 theories identified in our search were published between 1983 and 2006. Of these, 16 were interdisciplinary, 6 were from nursing, 2 were from medicine, 2 were from social work, and 1 each were from HIV/AIDS prevention occupational therapy, family planning, health education, and health informatics literature. The intended foci for these theories were health care, social work, and management. The theories were most commonly derived from the literature, followed by research or the experience of the originators. Most (21/31) of the identified theories have not yet been tested empirically. The model by Graham and Logan [14] has demonstrated face and content validity in unpublished studies and implementation projects, as has Green's model [15], which was used to conduct systematic baseline-diagnostic interviews with asthma patients treated in the emergency room or as outpatients [16].

Box 4.1.1 List of planned action theories in the database

Ashford J, Eccles M, Bond S, Hall LA, Bond J. Improving health care through professional behaviour change: introducing a framework for identifying behaviour change strategies. *British Journal of Clinical Governance* 1999;4[1]:14–23.

How: Information was sought from books, articles, and "grey literature." Prominent current researchers in different areas relating to change were also approached for their advice regarding relevant texts, reviews, and articles. Searches were made in several disciplinary databases including social science, psychology, and education. Articles were included if their context was pertinent to change in health care.

Bartholomew LK, Parcel GS, Kok G, Gottlieb NH. *Intervention Mapping: Designing Theory and Evidence-Based Health Promotion Programs.* Mountain View, CA: Mayfield Publishing Company; 2001.

How: N/A

Benefield LE. Implementing evidence-based practice in home care. *Home Healthc Nurse* 2003;21[12]:804–9.

How: N/A

Craik J, Rappolt S. Theory of research utilization enhancement: a model for occupational therapy. *Can J Occup Ther* 2003;70[5]:266–75.

How: The conceptual foundation of this study builds on the theoretical stages of research utilization presented by Knott and Wildavsky (1980). The model of research utilization in occupational therapy builds upon the existing theoretical concepts and stages of clinical decision making as outlined in the Occupational Performance Process Model (Fearing et al., 1997) and the stages of research utilization by Knott and Wildavsky (1980).

Dearing J. Improving the state of health programming by using diffusion theory. *J Health Commun* 2004;9:21–36.

How: Draws on diffusion of innovations (Rogers), especially concepts of attributes, opinion leadership, and clustering, to create steps for planned diffusion.

DiCenso A, Virani T, Bajnok I, Borycki E, Davies B, Graham I, et al. A toolkit to facilitate the implementation of clinical practice guidelines in healthcare settings. *Hosp Q* 2002;5[3]:55–60.

How: Over 8-month period, panel reviewed, and critiqued research on dissemination, transfer, and uptake of clinical practice guidelines.

Dixon DR. The behavioral side of information technology. *Int J Med Inform* 1999;56[1–3]:117–23.

How: N/A

Doyle DM, Dauterive R, Chuang KH, Ellrodt AG. Translating evidence into practice: pursuing perfection in pneumococcal vaccination in a rural community. *Respir Care* 2001;46[11]:1258–72.

How: References a British survey on GP's perceptions of the route to EBP, which influenced the authors' perception of the need for behavioral methods to overcome real/ perceived barriers.

Tracy S, Dufault M. Testing a collaborative research utilization model to translate best practices in pain management. *Worldviews Evid Based Nurs* 2004;1[S1]:S26–S32.

How: Based on Rogers' Diffusion of Innovation Theory (1983) and Havelock and Havelock (1973).

Feifer C, Ornstein SM. Strategies for increasing adherence to clinical guidelines and improving patient outcomes in small primary care practices. *Jt Comm J Qual Patient Saf* 2004;30[8]:432–41.

How: During the PPRNet-TRIP study, practices experimented with new approaches to practice operations and care delivery and documented the activities and structures that emerged in each practice as part of the trial's process evaluation. One aim of this evaluation was to develop a model of improvement strategies that might serve as an example for others. Used grounded theory—an analysis style that yields categories and theories grounded in a given social situation—to develop the PPRNet-TRIP Improvement Model from qualitative data gathered in 10 intervention groups.

Fooks C, Cooper J, Bhatia V. *Making Research Transfer Work: Summary Report from the 1st National Workshop on Research Transfer Issues, Methods and Experiences.* Toronto: ICES, IWH, CHEPA; 1997.

How: In fall 1996, a staff at three Ontario-based research organizations felt that a workshop to address the issues and experiences of research transfer in Canada may be of some benefit to those in the field. "We had three questions in mind—what is research transfer, who is doing it, and, if so, how?"

Graham ID, Logan J. Innovations in knowledge transfer and continuity of care. *Can J Nurs Res* 2004;36[2]:89–103.

How: Adaptation of model published in Science Communication, 1998, 20[2]: 227–246: "Toward a Comprehensive Interdisciplinary Model of Health Care Research Use." Elements are primarily drawn from literature related to research utilization, the diffusion of innovations, physician behavior change, and development and implementation of practice guidelines (1998). TheOMRU was refined through discussions with participants in workshops we conducted for the Ontario Health Care Evaluation Network, conference presentations, and clinical education rounds (1998). Derived from theories of change, from the literature, and from a process of reflection. Captures characteristics and important social factors related to Donabedian's (1988) germinal work, but not explicitly linked (2004).

Green LW, Kreuter MW. Health Promotion Planning: An Educational and Ecological Approach. 3rd ed. Mountain View, CA: Mayfield Publishing Company; 1999.

How: Built on Andersen's model of family use of health services and original work on use of family-planning services, hypertension, and asthma self-management. Later work in community health promotion grants and health services.

Grol R, Grimshaw J. Evidence-based implementation of evidence-based medicine. *Jt Comm J Qual Improv* 1999;25[10]:135–40.

How: In this article, propose a general framework for changing practice based on theoretical approaches for translating evidence into clinical practice and on empirical evidence about the effectiveness of different implementation strategies (1999). Reviews theoretical approaches to change and integrates these into a framework for changing clinical practice.

Grol R, Wensing M. What drives change? Barriers to and incentives for achieving evidence-based practice. *Med J Aust* 2004;180[6 Suppl]:S57–S60.

How: Integrating various stages of change theories, we have compiled a 10-step model for inducing change in professional behavior.

Herie M, Martin GW. Knowledge diffusion in social work: a new approach to bridging the gap. *Soc Work* 2002;47[1]:85–95.

How: The project integrated theory and research in knowledge diffusion and social marketing to develop a dissemination model for moving these clinical tools and techniques into the direct practice arena.

Hickey M. The role of the clinical nurse specialist in the research utilization process. *Clin Nurse Spec* 1990;4[2]:93–6.

How: N/A

Hyde PS, Falls K, Morris JA, Schoenwald SK. *Turning Knowledge into Practice.* Boston: The Technical Assistance Collaborative Inc.; 2003.

How: There are substantial bodies of knowledge underlying this manual: the clinical interventions or practices themselves, the process and structure of change management, and the increasingly complex issues of financing services and supports for people with disabilities. To develop practical help to clinicians and administrators in provider organizations.

Kraft JM, Mezoff JS, Sogolow ED, Neumann MS, Thomas PA. A technology transfer model for effective HIV/AIDS interventions: science and practice. *AIDS Educ Prev* 2000;12[5 Suppl]:7–20.

How: Starting with a review of diffusion of innovations and technology transfer literature, we offer a technology transfer model for HIV interventions. We identify participants and activities directed toward the use of effective interventions by prevention service providers (e.g., health departments and community-based organizations) in each phase of technology transfer. To identify potential elements for the model, we reviewed the literature, developed a draft model, and sought feedback from prevention services providers and researchers.

Lavis JN, Robertson D, Woodside JM, McLeod CB, Abelson J. How can research organizations more effectively transfer research knowledge to decision makers? *Milbank Q* 2003;81[2]:221–2.

How: We conducted a qualitative review of both systematic reviews and original studies across the five questions, four target audiences, and full range of disciplinary perspectives and methodological approaches. Surveyed directors of applied health and economic/social research organizations regarding how their organizations transfer research knowledge to decision-makers.

Lundquist G. A rich vision of technology transfer: technology value management. *J Technol Transf* 2003;28:265–84.

How: By addressing seven distinct lines of description/questions: Why? Who? Where? When? What? At what cost? And how? (Lundquist comments: The seven sections simplify content for readers. The real key is that the authors start with the core definitions, then put those concepts into context of a multifaceted view of technology transfer.)

Motwani J, Sower VE, Brashier LW. Implementing TQM in the health care sector. *Health Care Manage Rev* 1996;21[1]:73–82.

How: N/A

Moulding NT, Silagy CA, Weller DP. A framework for effective management of change in clinical practice: dissemination and implementation of clinical practice guidelines. *Qual Health Care* 1999;8:177–83.

How: Draws on social and behavior theory, diffusion of innovation theory, transtheoretical model of behavior change, health education theory, social influence theory, social ecology theory.

National Health and Medical Research Council. *How to Put the Evidence into Practice: Implementation and Dissemination Strategies.* Canberra: Commonwealth of Australia, National Health and Medical Research Council; 2000.

How: Developed by a multidisciplinary committee and approved by the NHMRC.

Pape TM. Evidence-based nursing practice: to infinity and beyond. *J Contin Educ Nurs* 2003;34[4]:154–61.

How: N/A

Proctor EK. Leverage points for the implementation of evidence-based practice. *Brief Treatment and Crisis Intervention* 2004 4[3]227–42.

How: Drawing on literature on knowledge diffusion, innovation, and quality improvement, this article proposes a conceptual framework for the multiple tasks, participants, and leverage points required for the adoption of EBP.

Roberts-Gray C, Gray T. Implementing innovations: a model to bridge the gap between diffusion and utilization. *Knowledge: Creation, Diffusion, Utilization* 1983;5[2]:213–32.

How: Assembled around five essential elements of programmed implementation. Parts based on Lewin's theory of social change (1947).

Rosswurm MA, Larrabee JH. A model for change to evidence-based practice. *Image J Nurs Sch* 1999;31[4]:317–22.

How: The model is based on theoretical and research literature related to evidence-based practice, research utilization, standardized language, and change theory. The authors developed and tested the usefulness of the model as they mentored nurses in defining and integrating evidence-based practice protocols at a regional medical center.

Simmons R, Brown J, Diaz M. Facilitating large-scale transitions to quality of care: an idea whose time has come. *Stud Fam Plann* 2002;33[1]:61–75.

How: Review of literature (social science, family planning, political science, reproductive health, policy and organizational sciences) 61–62, 66.

Stetler C. Updating the Stetler Model of research use to facilitate evidence-based practice. *Nurs Outlook* 2003;[49]:272–9.

How: First developed in 1976 with Marram as a pragmatic tool to fill a void re: how to go from a traditional research critique to application. The model was refined in 1994 with conceptual underpinnings and a set of assumptions, plus additional detail related to critical thinking based on current science re: knowledge and research utilization plus review of and experience of CNSs with the model. Then in 2001, the model was further refined on the basis of a related utilization-focused integrative review methodology, targeted evidence concepts, and continuing experience through use of the model with primarily, but not exclusively, clinical nurse specialists. Its evolution is further described in the 2001.

Titler MG, Kleiber C, Steelman V, Goode C, Rakel B, Barry-Walker J, et al. Infusing research into practice to promote quality care. *Nurs Res* 1994;43[5]:307–13.

How: Outgrowth of the quality assurance model using research.

We examined all of the components in each of the theories to determine commonalities and to develop a framework to compare the focus of each. This exercise resulted in 10 action steps with some steps having subactions (Table 4.1.1). Each theory was analyzed for whether it addressed each action category. Planned action theories generally outline the following steps to deliberately engineer change ($n =$ the number of models that include that particular step):

1 Identify a problem that needs addressing ($n = 19$)

   - Identify the need for change ($n = 22$)
   - Identify change agents (i.e., necessary participants to bring about the change) ($n = 15$)
   - Identify target audience ($n = 13$)
   - Link to appropriate individuals or groups with vested interests in the project ($n = 15$)

2 Review the evidence or literature ($n = 21$)
3 Adapt the evidence and/or develop the innovation ($n = 11$)
4 Assess barriers to using the knowledge ($n = 18$)
5 Select and tailor interventions to promote the use of the knowledge ($n = 26$)
6 Implement the innovation ($n = 22$)
7 Develop a plan to evaluate use of the knowledge ($n = 14$)

   - Pilot test ($n = 11$)
   - Evaluate the process to determine whether and how the innovation is used ($n = 19$)

8 Evaluate the outcomes or impact of the innovation ($n = 20$)
9 Maintain change. Sustain ongoing knowledge use ($n = 11$)
10 Disseminate results of the implementation process ($n = 7$)

None of the theories included all of the action steps and no action step was included in all of the theories. Some theories focused more on evaluation, whereas others focused on identification of the problem and their barriers to implementation. In choosing a planned action theory to guide implementation efforts, we advise careful review of the component elements and how they have been coded into action categories and determine which theory is the best fit for the context and culture in which individuals are working. Regardless of the selected theory (or whether we choose to use the list of action categories as a kind of "metatheory") documenting experiences with the model will advance understanding of its use and provide information to others who are attempting a similar project.

Table 4.1.1 Comparison of planned action theories

	Ashford	Bartholomew	Benefield	Craik	Dearing	DiCenso/RNAO	Dixon	Dufault	Doyle	Feifer	Fooks	Graham/Logan	Green	Grol/Grimshaw	Grol/Wensing	Herie	Hickey	Hyde	Kraft	Lavis 2003	Lundquist	Motwani	Moulding	NHMRC	Pape	Proctor	Rosswurm	Simmons	Stetler	Titler	Total /30
Identify problem	x	x	x	x	x	x		x	x		x	x	x				x	x	x		x			x	x		x		x	x	19
Identify need for change	x	x	x	x	x	x			x	x	x	x	x			x	x	x	x		x	x	x	x			x	x	x	x	22
Identify change agents			x			x	x		x	x	x	x					x	x	x		x			x				x		x	15
Identify target audience			x	x	x	x	x	x		x	x	x		x	x		x	x	x		x			x		x	x	x		x	13
Link(age)	x	x		x	x	x		x	x	x	x					x		x	x		x			x	x	x	x	x		x	15
Review evidence/literature	x		x	x	x	x		x	x		x	x	x	x	x		x	x	x	x	x			x	x	x			x	x	21
Adapt/	x		x					x						x		x				x				x		x			x	x	11
Assess barriers			x			x	x	x	x	x	x	x	x	x	x	x	x	x	x	x	x		x	x	x	x		x	x	x	18
Tailor/develop intervention	x	x	x	x	x	x	x	x	x	x	x	x	x	x	x	x	x	x	x	x		x	x	x	x	x		x	x	x	26
Implement	x	x	x	x	x	x	x	x	x	x	x	x	x	x	x	x	x	x		x	x	x		x	x	x	x	x	x	x	22
Develop evaluation plan	x					x			x					x	x	x	x	x				x		x	x		x		x	x	14
Pilot test	x					x	x	x			x						x			x				x			x		x	x	11
Evaluate the process	x		x	x	x	x	x	x	x	x	x	x	x	x			x	x	x	x	x	x		x	x	x	x	x	x	x	19
Evaluate outcomes	x		x	x	x	x		x	x		x	x	x	x	x		x	x	x	x	x	x		x	x	x	x	x	x	x	20
Maintain change		x					x							x		x		x					x	x			x			x	11
Disseminate			x				x	x								x	x							x			x	x	x	x	7
Total # Elements/16	7	5	10	5	9	12	3	10	9	7	11	11	6	8	7	8	11	12	11	8	10	7	4	14	9	7	10	9	12	12	

Future research

An important area for research in the coming years will be the empirically testing of planned action theories. More research is also needed to determine if there are advantages in using one theory over another.

Summary

We believe that theory-driven implementation will further the study of KT by providing a framework in which we can understand the change process and see which implementation components were successful and which were not. At each action category of the knowledge-to-action cycle, there may be a host of theories from multiple disciplines to draw from when planning to move knowledge into action.

Acknowledgment

Members of the KT Theories group include Doug Angus, University of Ottawa; Melissa Brouwers, McMaster University; Barbara Davies, University of Ottawa; Michelle Driedger, University of Manitoba; Martin Eccles, Newcastle upon Tyne; Gaston Godin, University of Laval; Ian D. Graham, seconded from University of Ottawa to the Canadian Institutes of Health Research; Jeremy Grimshaw, University of Ottawa; Karen Harlos, McGill University; Margaret Harrison, Queen's University; Sylvie Lauzon, University of Ottawa; France Légaré, University of Laval; Louise Lemyre, University of Ottawa; Jo Logan, University of Ottawa; Jessie McGowan, University of Ottawa; Marie Pascal Pomey, University of Montreal; Nicole Robinson, Ottawa Health Research Institute, Dawn Stacey, University of Ottawa; Jacqueline Tetroe, the Canadian Institutes of Health Research; Michel Wensing, University of Nijmegen.

References

1 Krueger JC, Nelson AH, Wolanin MO. Nursing Research: Development, Collaboration and Utilization. Germantown, MD: Aspen Systems; 1978.
2 Horsley J, Crane J, Bingle JD. Research utilization as an organizational process. *J Nurs Admin* 1978;8[7]:4–6.
3 Stetler CB, Marram G. Evaluation of research findings for applicability in practice. *Nurs Outlook* 1976;24[9]:559–63.
4 Rimmer Tiffany C, Johnson Lutjens L. *Planned Change Theories for Nursing. Review, Analysis and Implications.* Thousand Oaks, CA: Sage; 1998.

5 Logan J, Graham ID. Toward a comprehensive interdisciplinary model of health care research use. *Sci Commun* 1998;20[2]:227–46.

6 Rogers EM. *Diffusion of Innovations.* 4th ed. New York: The Free Press; 1995.

7 Kuhn T. *The structure of Scientific Revolutions.* 2nd ed. Chicago: University of Chicago Press; 1970.

8 Lomas J. Retailing research: increasing the role of evidence in clinical services for childbirth. *Milbank Q* 1993;71[3], 439–75.

9 Lomas J. Teaching old (and not so old) docs new tricks: effective ways to implement research findings. In EV Dunn, PG Norton, M Stewart, F Tudiver, MJ Bass (Eds.), *Disseminating Research/Changing Practice.* 1st ed. Thousand Oaks, CA: Sage; 1994:1–18.

10 Tiffany C. Analysis of planned change theories. *Nurs Manage* 1994;25[2]:60–2.

11 Tiffany C, Cheatham A, Doornbos D, Loudermelt L, Momadi G. Planned change theory: survey of nursing periodical literature. *Nurs Manage* 1994;25[2]:54–9.

12 Graham ID, Tetroe J. Some theoretical underpinnings of knowledge translation. *Acad Emerg Med* 2007;14[11]:936–41.

13 Walker L, Avant K. Strategies for Theory Construction in Nursing. 4th ed. Upper Saddle River, NJ: Prentice Hall; 2005.

14 Graham ID, Logan J. Innovations in knowledge transfer and continuity of care. *Can J Nurs Res* 2004;36[2]:89–103.

15 Green LW, Kreuter MW. *Health Promotion Planning: an Educational and Ecological Approach.* 3rd ed. Mountain View, CA: Mayfield Publishing Company; 1999.

16 Levine DM, Green LW, Deeds SG, Chwalow J, Russell RP, Finlay J. Health education for hypertensive patients. *JAMA* 1979;241[16]:1700–3.

4.2 Cognitive psychology theories of change

Alison Hutchinson and Carole A. Estabrooks

Faculty of Nursing, University of Alberta, Edmonton, AB, Canada

---

KEY LEARNING POINTS

- Cognitive psychology theories related to motivation, action, stages of change, and decision making have been influential in the field of knowledge translation (KT).
- These theories provide a framework for examining, measuring, and understanding research use behavior.
- According to cognitive psychology theories, interventions designed to influence individual cognitive characteristics can be used to mediate/moderate individual behavior.
- A limited but growing body of empirical evidence exists to validate the theoretical assumptions of cognitive psychology theories.

Cognitive psychology theories have predominantly been used to examine and understand the determinants of health-related behavior of the *individual*, and in particular the role of cognitive factors in predicting behaviors such as smoking, exercise, eating habits, and vaccination adoption. These theories have the potential to aid understanding of the use of research. As such, some knowledge translation (KT) scholars have applied these theories to inform research design and to guide intervention development to influence adoption of research evidence in practice. Like health-related behaviors, health professionals' research-use behavior is considered to be, in part, within the individual's control. Furthermore, social cognitive factors, including beliefs, attitudes, and knowledge, are considered to be more amenable to change than factors such as personality. These features underlie the premise that interventions designed to influence individual cognitive characteristics can be used to mediate/moderate individual behavior [1].

Theories related to *motivation,* such as social cognitive theory [2] and the theory of planned behavior [3]; theories related to *action,* such as

---

Knowledge Translation in Health Care: Moving from Evidence to Practice. Edited by S. Straus, J. Tetroe, and I. Graham. © 2009 Blackwell Publishing, ISBN: 978-1-4051-8106-8.

implementation intentions [4] and the theory of operant conditioning [5]; theories related to *stages of change,* such as the transtheoretical model of change [6]; and theories related to *decision making,* such as the cognitive continuum theory [7], have been influential in the field of KT. Such theories offer frameworks for examining and understanding determinants of behavior and potential mechanisms to promote behavior change. Most of these theories assume that individuals make rational decisions based upon systematic analysis of the information available to them [1]. Failure to consider external factors and the social construction of knowledge are potential limitations of these theories. A brief description of the aforementioned theories and their application to KT follows.

Theories related to motivation

According to motivational theories, behavior is determined and, therefore, predicted by motivation. Two theories in this area are examined. First, social cognitive theory [2,8] assumes that behavior is determined by incentives and expectations related to situation-outcomes (beliefs about anticipated consequences if the individual abstains from the respective behavior); action-outcomes (beliefs about the likelihood of certain outcomes occurring as a result of the behavior); and perceived self-efficacy (beliefs about the extent to which the behavior is within the individual's control). Bandura [2,8] hypothesizes that four sources of information influence self-efficacy and expectations: performance accomplishments, vicarious experience, verbal persuasion, and physiological feedback. Performance accomplishment is the most influential information source and results from personal or professional experience, for example, acquisition of the necessary skills to conduct a physical examination. Vicarious experience arises from observing the behavior of and outcomes achieved by others, such as mentors, role models, or opinion leaders. Verbal persuasion includes nurturing individuals' self-confidence in their ability to accomplish a specific behavior and persuading them of the benefits of that behavior. This could be achieved through academic detailing (see Chapter 3.5.4) and continuing education (see Chapter 3.5.2). Physiological feedback resulting from a particular behavior is the least relevant of Bandura's sources of information for health professionals interested in translating knowledge into practice.

Second, according to the theory of planned behavior [3], the determinants and, therefore, potential predictors of behavior are the *intention to engage in* and *perceived control over* the behavior. Intention is a function of *attitudes* toward the behavior, *subjective norms* (beliefs about the opinions of others with respect to the behavior) and *behavioral control* (perceived ease of engagement in the behavior). Attitudes are determined by perceptions of the consequences of the behavior. Subjective norms are based on normative beliefs, that is, perceptions of the preferences of others for the individual to adopt the specific behavior. The consideration of normative beliefs is balanced against the individual's desire to comply with the perceived expectations of the group. An individual's behavior may be influenced by patients, managers, and other members of the multidisciplinary team, including those who are persuasive, respected, or in positions of power. Behavioral control, a construct derived from the notion of self-efficacy in social cognitive theory, is influenced by perceived access to resources and opportunities to engage in the behavior, balanced by the capacity of each of these to enable or impede the behavior. Behavioral control includes factors such as time, the existence of necessary equipment or staff, or patient preferences, which may influence the course of action pursued by a health professional.

The theory of planned behavior has been employed in a number of studies to predict health professionals' behavior with respect to the uptake of specific research evidence [9,10]. The demonstrated predictive power of the constructs—attitudes, subjective norms, and behavioral control, offers some evidence for their value in informing the development of interventions to influence behavior [9,11]. In general populations, intention to act has been identified as one of the most important determinants of behavior [12–14]. In the case of clinical practice guideline implementation, for example, an education intervention may be designed to address negative attitudes toward the guidelines. In the case of limited perceived behavioral control, academic detailing might be implemented to enhance confidence in skills, and/or constraints identified within the environment may be removed to promote the guideline uptake. The theory of planned behavior and social cognitive theory have been successfully used to guide development of interventions to influence primary care physicians' antibiotic prescribing behavior for patients presenting with sore throats [15,16].

Theories related to action

Theories of action focus on predictors of behavior in individuals who are motivated to change. The theory of implementation intentions [4] proposes that intentions to engage in behavior are distinct from the intention of achieving a certain goal. Specifically, implementation intentions relate to the logistics surrounding when, where, and how the behavior will be carried out to achieve a goal. Hence, when certain conditions are met the individual is mentally committed to specific behavior to accomplish particular intentions. The process of planning for a change is premised to increase the likelihood of an individual actually adopting the behavior [17]. According to this approach, interventions designed to facilitate planning and preparation may help promote the adoption of specific behavior.

The operant conditioning theory [5] proposes that positive feedback, such as a reward or incentive in response to certain behavior, is likely to encourage behavior repetition. Such repetition over time may result in the behavior becoming part of routine practice. On the other hand, negative feedback, such as a reprimand or financial disincentive, is likely to discourage the behavior. Interventions may be targeted to either encourage or discourage certain behavior. An expanding body of evidence suggests that the theory of operant conditioning helps in understanding and predicting health professionals' behavior [10,18].

Theories related to stages of change

The transtheoretical model of change is one stage of change theory. It includes five stages through which an individual progresses over time: precontemplation, contemplation, preparation, action, and maintenance [6]. In the *precontemplation* stage the individual does not plan to adopt the behavior in the foreseeable future. When individuals intend to adopt the behavior within the next 6 months they have advanced to the *contemplation* stage. The *preparation* stage is reached when the individual intends to adopt the behavior within the ensuing month. The *action* stage is reached when the individual has been using the behavior for the previous 6 months. The *maintenance* stage involves actively working to maintain the change. Finally, the *termination* stage is attained when the behavior is firmly entrenched; individuals are not tempted to abandon the behavior and are entirely confident of their self-efficacy in carrying out the behavior. One of the assumptions of the transtheoretical model of change is that interventions targeted to specific stages on the change continuum will facilitate transition along the continuum [6].

Progression from precontemplation to the contemplation stage involves changes in knowledge or attitudes and is sensitive to strategies designed to enhance awareness and re-evaluate values. Such strategies may include continuing education, educational outreach, exposure to consensus statements, and performance feedback [19], which are described in Chapters 3.5.2 and 3.5.3. Movement from the contemplation stage to preparation and action stages involves changes in the way individuals think about the particular behavior and their beliefs about their capacity and ability (self-efficacy) to make the change. Strategies useful in promoting *action* include the provision of appropriate resources and support. Reminder systems and prompts (which are described in Chapter 3.5.5) and the provision of appropriate equipment can be used to facilitate progression and promote adherence to the *action*. To progress from preparation and action to maintenance involves change in the environment and may include the provision of social support, incentive schemes, and audit and feedback [19]. There is limited evidence in support of stages of change theories. Stage of change was not a predictor of behavior when applied in the study of health professionals' use of clinical practice guidelines [18]. However, in the general population stages of change were useful for detecting barriers to certain behavior, matching interventions, and predicting outcomes [20].

Theories related to decision making

According to the cognitive continuum theory [7,21], the mode of cognition used in decision making exists on a continuum, with analysis and intuition at opposite poles. Analytic thought involves slow, conscious thought that is consistent and mostly accurate, while intuition involves rapid, unconscious thought that lacks consistency and is characterized by moderate accuracy [22]. The point on the continuum adopted by an individual in the process of decision making is a function of the characteristics of the decision task at hand [7]. The decision task structure also ranges on a continuum from ill-structured to well-structured. The greater the task structure, the higher the level of analysis incorporated in the decision-making process. Task characteristics are determined by the complexity of the available information, the degree of uncertainty associated with the content area, and the presentation of the information, including the time available for making the decision, the format of the information, and capacity for the decision to be divided into subcomponents. Hamm [22] identifies six modes of health care decision making on the cognition and task characteristics continua (Figure 4.2.1). Each mode involves a different combination of analytic and intuitive reasoning strategies, with the most analytical strategies employed in mode 1, scientific experiment, and intuition-dominating decision making in mode 6.

The cognitive continuum theory may be applied in the field of KT to help health professionals improve their clinical decision making in situations of uncertainty, for instance, when scientific evidence is equivocal or a patient presents with atypical signs and symptoms. It enables health professionals to understand and predict modes of cognition appropriate for certain decisions depending on the form and availability of information. Cognitive continuum theory can help explain and justify health professionals' decisions [23]. Additionally, adoption of appropriate modes of cognition will help health professionals maximize decision-making accuracy [22]. Research to

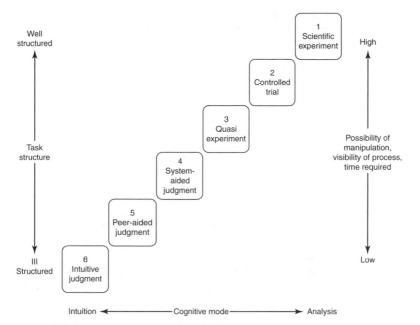

Figure 4.2.1 Cognition modes on the cognitive continuum. (From [22]. Reprinted with permission.)

substantiate the cognitive continuum theory is scant. However, some research has demonstrated health professionals' use of analytical and intuitive modes of decision making [24]. Research in other professional groups has also lent support to the theory [25].

Constructs common to psychological theories

There is considerable overlap or commonality of constructs contained in psychological theories. To promote the success of KT research in explaining as well as predicting behavior change, Michie and colleagues [26] identified key theoretical constructs embedded in psychological theories. Through a process of brainstorming and prioritizing they identified 12 theoretical domains to explain behavior change (Table 4.2.1). Following validation, a series of domain-specific interview questions were generated to assess behavior change. In addition, the researchers developed an instrument to map each theoretical domain to techniques that can be employed to promote behavior change within the respective domain [27]. This framework is designed to help researchers and health professionals diagnose and explain failed attempts to

Table 4.2.1 Theoretical domains identified by Michie et al. [25]

Domains
1. Knowledge
2. Skills
3. Social/professional role and identity (self-standards)
4. Beliefs about capabilities (self-efficacy)
5. Beliefs about consequences (anticipated outcomes/attitude)
6. Motivation and goals (intention)
7. Memory, attention, and decision processes
8. Environmental context and resources (environmental constraints)
9. Social influences (norms)
10. Emotion
11. Behavioral regulation
12. Nature of the behaviors

move knowledge to action and to guide the design of interventions to promote successful KT.

Future research

Future research in this field should be undertaken using a programmatic approach to systematically and incrementally develop and test theory-based interventions and to validate their theoretical assumptions. Consistent with this approach, a process modeling method based on the U.K. Medical Research Council Framework for Trials of Complex Interventions (discussed in Chapter 3.6.2) [28], has been adopted to examine interventions underpinned by psychological theory [17,29]. According to this framework, theory should be used to guide selection of interventions to maximize the uptake of research evidence. Importantly, the use of theory will facilitate understanding of how and why the intervention worked under certain conditions [15,16]. The theory selection phase should be followed by a modeling phase comprising theory-informed identification of measurable components of the intervention and their mechanisms of action. These constructs can then be measured and used to understand and predict outcomes. Exploratory studies should then be conducted to assess the feasibility and guide refinement of the intervention. This phase precedes the conduct of definitive randomized controlled trials to test the effectiveness of the intervention, which should then be followed by replications studies in different settings. The adoption of such an approach will help strengthen the evidence base and promote understanding of how, why, and under what circumstances interventions underpinned by cognitive psychological theory work. Importantly, detailed reporting of research methodology and intervention design and refinement is necessary for the conduct of replication studies and to maximize intervention fidelity.

Summary

Cognitive psychology theories can be useful for identifying cognitions that are amenable to change and providing a theory-based rationale for and guiding development of strategies to increase the adoption of relevant research evidence by health professionals. Such theories also offer a theoretical foundation for research designed to explore, measure, and understand health professionals' research use behavior and to study the effectiveness of interventions designed to influence such behavior.

References

1 Conner M, Norman P. Predicting health behaviour: a social cognition approach. In M Conner & P Norman (Eds.), *Predicting Health Behavior*. New York: Open University Press; 2005.

2 Bandura A. Self-efficacy mechanism in human agency. *Am Psychologist* 1982;37:122–47.

3 Azjen I. The theory of planned behavior. *Organ Behav Hum Decis Process* 1991;50:179–211.

4 Gollwitzer PM. Implementation intentions: strong effects of simple plans. *Am Psychologist* 1999;54:493–503.

5 Blackman D. *Operant Conditioning: An Experimental Analysis of Behaviour*. London: Methuen; 1974.

6 Prochaska JO, Velicer WF. The transtheoretical model of health behavior change. *Am J Health Prom* 1997;12[1]:38–48.

7 Hammond KR. *Principles of Organization in Intuitive and Analytical Cognition* (Report 231). Boulder, CO: University of Colorado, Center for Research on Judgement and Policy; 1981. Report No.: 231.

8 Bandura A. Self-efficacy: towards a unifying theory of behaviour change. *Psycholog Review* 1977;84:191–215.

9 Perkins MB, Jensen PS, Jaccard J, Gollwitzer P, Oettingen G, Pappadopulos E, et al. Applying theory-driven approaches to understanding and modifying clinicians' behavior: What do we know? *Psych Serv* 2007;58[3]:342–8.

10 Eccles MP, Grimshaw JM, Johnston M, Steen N, Pitts NB, Thomas R, et al. Applying psychological theories to evidence-based clinical practice: identifying factors predictive of managing upper respiratory tract infections without antibiotics. *Impl Sci* 2007;2[26]. URL http://www.implementationscience.com/content/2/1/26 [accessed February 7, 2008].

11 Eccles MP, Johnston M, Hrisos S, Francis J, Grimshaw J, Steen N, et al. Translating clinicians' beliefs into implementation interventions (TRACII): a protocol for an intervention modeling experiment to change clinicians' intentions to implement evidence-based practice. *Impl Sci* 2007;2[27]. URL http://www.implementationscience.com/content/2/1/27 [accessed February 7, 2008].

12 Godin G, Conner M, Sheeran P, Belanger-Gravel A, Germain M. Determinants of repeated blood donation among new and experienced blood donors. *Transfusion* 2007;47:1607–15.

13 Giles M, McClenahan C, Cairns E, Mallet J. An application of the theory of planned behaviour to blood donation: the importance of self-efficacy. *Health Educ Res* 2004;19[4]:380–91.

14 Armitage CJ, Conner M. Efficacy of the theory of planned behaviour: a meta-analytic review. *Br J Soc Psychol* 2001;40:471–99.

15 Hrisos S, Eccles M, Johnston M, Francis J, Kaner EFS, Steen N, et al. Developing the content of two behavioural interventions: using theory-based interventions to promote GP management of upper respiratory tract infection without prescribing antibiotics #1. *BMC Health Serv Res* 2008;8[11]. URL http://www.biomedcentral.com/1472-6963/8/11 [accessed February 10, 2008].

16 Hrisos S, Eccles M, Johnston M, Francis J, Kaner EFS, Steen N, et al. An intervention modelling experiment to change GPs' intentions to implement evidence-based practice: using theory-based interventions to promote GP management of upper respiratory tract infection without prescribing antibiotics #2. *BMC Health Serv Res* 2008;8[10]. URL http://www.biomedcentral.com/1472-6963/8/10 [accessed February 10, 2008].

17 Walker A, Grimshaw J, Johnston M, Pitts N, Steen N, Eccles M. PRIME - PRocess modeling in ImpleMEntation research: selecting a theoretical basis for interventions to change clinical practice. *BMC Health Serv Res* 2003;3[22]. URL http://www.biomedcentral.com/1472-6963/3/22 [accessed January 31, 2005].

18 Bonetti D, Pitts NB, Eccles M, Grimshaw J, Johnston M, Steen N, et al. Applying psychological theory to evidence-based clinical practice: identifying factors predictive of taking intra-oral radiographs. *Soc Sci Med* 2006;63:1889–99.

19 Cohen SJ, Halvorson HW, Gosselink CA. Changing physician behavior to improve disease prevention. *Prev Med* 1994;23:284–91.

20 Weinstein ND, Lyon JE, Sandman PM, Cuite CL. Experimental evidence for stages of health behavior change: the Precaution Adoption Process Model applied to home radon testing. *Health Psychol* 1998;17[5]:445–53.

21 Hammond KR. *The Integration of Research in Judgment and Decision theory* (Report 226). Boulder, CO: University of Colorado, Center for Research on Judgment and Policy; 1980.

22 Hamm RM. Clinical intuition and clinical analysis: expertise and the cognitive continuum. In J Dowie & A Elstein (Eds.), *Professional Judgment: A Reader in Clinical Decision Making.* Cambridge, UK: Cambridge University Press; 1988.

23 Cader R, Campbell S, Watson D. Cognitive Continuum Theory in nursing decision-making. *J Adv Nurs* 2005;49[4]:397–405.

24 Lauri S, Salantera S, Chalmers K, Ekman S-L, Kim HS, Kappeli S, et al. An exploratory study of clinical decision-making in five countries. *J Nurs Scholarship* 2001;33[1]:83–90.

25 Hamm RM. Moment-by-moment variation in experts' analytic and intuitive cognitive activity. *IEEE Trans Syst Man Cybern B Cybern* 1989;18[5]:757–76.

26 Michie S, Johnston M, Abraham C, Lawton R, Parker D, Walker AE. Making psychological theory useful for implementing evidence based practice: a consensus approach. *Qual Safe Health Care* 2005;14[1]:26–33.

27 Francis J, Michie S, Johnston M, Hardeman W, Eccles MP. How do behaviour change techniques map on to psychological constructs? Results of a consensus process. *PsycholHealth* 2005;20[Suppl 1]:83–4.

28 Medical Research Council. *A Framework for Development and Evaluation of RCTs for Complex Interventions to Improve Health.* London, UK; 2000.

29 Walker AE, Grimshaw JM, Armstrong EM. Salient beliefs and intentions to prescribe antibiotics for patients with a sore throat. *Br J Health Psychol* 2001;6:347–60.

4.3 **Educational theories**

Alison Hutchinson and Carole A. Estabrooks

Faculty of Nursing, University of Alberta, Edmonton, Alberta, Canada

---

KEY LEARNING POINTS

- Cognitive, affective, and psychomotor domains as well as individual learning styles should be considered when designing an educational intervention.
- Behaviorist, cognitivist, constructionist, humanist, and social learning perspectives can inform choice of educational interventions.
- Baseline assessment of learning needs, facilitation of social interaction between learners, provision of opportunities to practice newly acquired skills, and the inclusion of a series of multifaceted educational interventions have been shown to improve performance.
- Despite strong theoretical foundations, there is a limited evidence base for educational theories.

In Chapter 3.5.2, it was suggested that where there are knowledge deficits around specific and relevant research evidence, educational interventions can be used to enhance practitioners' learning, understanding, and ability to apply the evidence. Educational theories are useful for explaining the effectiveness of educational interventions and for developing frameworks to design and test new educational interventions [1]. There are a number of education theories and principles to guide the development of educational interventions [1–3]. In this chapter we will discuss educational theories targeted at the individual level and how they can be used to inform the development of interventions to move knowledge to action.

Learning domains

Educational theorists identify three broad areas of learning, the *cognitive*, *affective*, and *psychomotor* domains [2,4]. The *cognitive* domain involves the

---

Knowledge Translation in Health Care: Moving from Evidence to Practice. Edited by S. Straus, J. Tetroe, and I. Graham. © 2009 Blackwell Publishing, ISBN: 978-1-4051-8106-8.

acquisition of academic knowledge and reflects teaching methods directed toward the delivery of information, which are traditionally used in the education of health professionals. Educational interventions that are typically used to promote this form of learning include didactic lectures, academic detailing, and computer-based modules [2]. The *affective* domain of learning involves adoption of attitudes, values, and beliefs, which are important precursors to behavior change. Educational interventions such as group interaction, self-evaluation, role play, use of case studies, and simulation are recommended to advance this form of learning [2]. Finally, the *psychomotor* domain refers to psychomotor skill acquisition and development, and interventions such as demonstration followed by supervised skill performance and practice can be used to develop skill mastery [2]. All three domains are fundamental to health professionals' knowledge, skill development, and ability to deliver high-quality health care and should be taken into consideration when designing an educational intervention.

Learning styles

A range of learning styles among health professionals, including *activist, reflective, theoretical,* and *pragmatic* styles, have been described [5,6]. The *activist* prefers to learn through experience, enjoys group work and discussion, readily adopts an innovation but has a tendency to become bored with the process of implementation, and therefore quickly rejects the innovation. The *reflective* learner is systematic in collecting information on all available options before acting but can be indecisive, resulting in delayed innovation adoption. The *theoretical* learner prefers to analyze and consider the information and develop models of cause and effect before deciding to act. The *pragmatic* learner is more inclined to base his or her behavior on practical experience with an innovation. To engage the learner and maximize learning outcomes, the individual learning styles of health professionals should be considered when designing educational interventions. Inclusion of a range of teaching techniques can be used to satisfy the styles of all learners [7].

Motivation to learn

An understanding of motivators for behavior change is important when designing interventions to promote learning. Sources of motivation are considered intrinsic or extrinsic [8]. Intrinsic motivation comes from within individuals and relates, for example, to their personal interest in acquiring new knowledge or to their desire to advance or contribute service to the community. Extrinsic sources of motivation for learning include conditions such as employment requirements, career advancement requirements, or a directive from a higher authority. Intrinsic sources of motivation, such as the desire for professional competence, are considered to provide a more powerful impetus for behavior change than external sources [8].

Learning theories

Five perspectives from which we can understand learning have been described: behaviorist, cognitivist, constructionist, humanist, and social learning [9]. These theoretical approaches to learning and how they inform choice of educational interventions are discussed in turn.

Behaviorist approaches

According to behavior theorists, the context in which individuals work influences their behavior. Behavior theorists are interested in observable and measurable behavioral responses to certain stimuli [9]. The notion of behavior reinforcement is seen as an important aspect of learning. Hence, individual feedback is perceived to be important to the success of education interventions [3]. The instructor's role is to create an environment that encourages desirable behavior and discourages undesirable behavior [9]. Behavior theory can be used to design interventions including regular performance appraisal, the setting of behavioral learning objectives and plans, peer review, the use of competencies and standards against which to measure performance, and computer-based learning modules.

Cognitivist approaches

Cognitive theorists study the processes used to acquire, interpret, store, and use information to formulate awareness, understanding, and meaning [9]. Modeling behavior based on the observation of others' behavior is one mechanism through which cognitive theorists believe learning occurs. Cognitive theory has helped describe the process of problem solving and how skills acquired to solve one problem can be applied to new situations [3]. The use of mentorship or preceptor programs and role models to support training of novice learners is an example of cognitive theory use. Problem-based learning approaches have also emerged as a method for teaching health professionals. This approach typically involves the use of small groups, self-directed learning, tutorial instruction, examination of a relevant and realistic problem, and skill development. This approach has been recommended because knowledge acquisition as a result of problem solving is thought to result in sustained and readily accessible knowledge [2]. A recent systematic review indicates that problem-based learning approaches in medical school positively affect the social and cognitive aspects of physician competence [10].

Constructivist approaches

Constructivist theorists believe that learning is based on experience, from which meaning and understanding are constructed [9]. Constructivism draws on the notion of reflection on practice and the potential for learning through reflection and evaluation of past experience. Schon [11] was influential in highlighting the importance of reflection to professional practice, and Mezirow's [12] theory of transformative learning focuses on the concepts of experience and critical reflection. According to Mezirow, change in beliefs, attitudes, and behavior requires critical reflection on experiences to transform an individual's perspective. Schon [11] also advocated for coaching by senior professionals to facilitate learning in novice professionals. Benner [13] argues that clinical practice experience is essential to the development of critical thinking skills and reflective practice. Promotion of opportunities for reflective practice, reflective journaling, evaluation of information such as quality reports, and critical incident debriefing reflect the use of constructivist theory. Further, preceptorship programs can be employed to coach learners and stimulate reflective practice.

Humanist approaches

According to humanist theorists, learning is a function of growth; humans have control over their future, will actively work toward improvement, and have unlimited learning potential [9]. Humanism focuses on learning through experience and stresses the importance of autonomy and individual responsibility to achieve betterment [9]. Benner's work [13] is situated in the intuitive–humanistic paradigm [14] and draws on the Dreyfus model of skill acquisition to understand how nurses learn. According to this model the learner progresses through five stages of proficiency: novice, advanced beginner, competent, proficient, and expert. Benner [13] contends that practitioners reach the expert level as a result of a combination of gaining, over time, a sound knowledge base and extensive practical experience.

Adult learning theory is a dominant perspective among humanist theories. Knowles [15,16] introduced the term *androgogy* to describe adult learning and proposed a number of oft-cited principles of adult learning (Table 4.3.1). These principles can be used to guide planning for educational interventions directed at adults and have had considerable influence on delivery of education for health professionals [8,17]. Adult learning theory is based on the assumptions that adults have already acquired a range of life experiences and knowledge, are more motivated to learn something that is immediately

Table 4.3.1 Principles of adult learning theory

Adults are self-directed. They need to decide what they want to learn.

Adults have acquired a range of experiences and knowledge. Learning can be more meaningful when prior knowledge can be integrated with new knowledge.

Adults are goal-directed. Encountering situations that require certain knowledge stimulates readiness to learn.

Adults are relevancy-oriented. They require new knowledge to be relevant.

Adults focus on acquiring practical knowledge. They need to know that new knowledge is applicable and beneficial.

Adults want to be treated with respect.

Adapted from Leib (1991) [25].

relevant to their needs, and are self-directed in their learning style. This approach differs from the pedagogical approach, in which education involves instruction, most commonly using traditional teacher-centered methods, and learning is perceived as a passive process with the learner being the recipient of instruction [9].

According to Knowles [15,16], adults are goal-oriented and they want to know how an educational session is going to help them achieve their objectives. To address this need the teacher should provide clear objectives at the beginning of any educational session so the learner is informed and has realistic expectations of the session [7,16]. Adults are motivated by realistic practical problems or issues in preference to abstract or conceptual issues [8]. In addition, adult learners want to integrate new knowledge with existing knowledge. Learning activities should, therefore, allow for different knowledge levels and provide opportunities for the learner to integrate prior learning with new knowledge. Furthermore, adult learners want the new knowledge to be relevant and readily transferable to their practice. Based on the premise that adult learners are self-directed, they should be allowed to discover new knowledge with the guidance of a facilitator. The learning atmosphere should foster interaction and challenge learners to consider new ideas [2]. Timely, regular, constructive, and sensitively delivered feedback is important to successful learning and skill acquisition [7].

The principles of adult learning theory can be used to inform the design of education interventions to maximize knowledge translation (KT) in health care. Specifically, the intervention should include an assessment of the health professional's learning needs, acknowledgment of their existing knowledge in relation to the subject [7], the provision of clear objectives that are relevant and meaningful to the health professional's practice, and the use of creative interventions or activities to engage them in the learning process. The interventions may involve approaches such as self-directed learning, small group work and discussion forums, problem solving, use of case studies, practice sessions, computer-based modules and simulation, academic detailing, and educational outreach visits as discussed in Chapter 3.5.2. Formal feedback sessions should be factored into the intervention design. Opportunities to provide informal feedback should also be used when appropriate.

Social learning approaches

Social learning theorists concentrate on understanding how learning occurs through social and environmental interaction [9]. Learning, according to this theory, can result from observation of others' behavior and the consequences of their actions [18]. Drawing on elements of behaviorist, cognitivist, and humanist theory, social learning theory views experience, motivation, self-direction, setting of objectives, and observation as important aspects of learning [3]. Role modeling appropriate behavior has been identified by social learning theorists as an important mechanism to facilitate learning [3]. Further, mentorship models to promote learning through social interaction are strongly grounded in social learning theory [9].

Evidence for educational theories and interventions

Although educational theories have strong theoretical foundations, the evidential base for these theories is somewhat limited [2]. Research efforts to validate the theoretical assumptions underlying these theories have been hampered by methodological limitations, practical, and ethical issues [2]. Acknowledging these limitations, scholars continue to argue for the use of theory to guide the design of educational interventions and to make recommendations for continued research to test the theoretical assumptions of educational theories [2].

Considerable research has been undertaken to study the effectiveness of educational interventions in influencing knowledge use [19,20]. Research in the field of continuing education has demonstrated that traditional passive, noninteractive teaching methods have had minimal effect on the behavior of health professionals and have had no discernable effect on clinical outcomes [2,21]. However, as outlined in Chapter 3.5.2, evidence in support of the effectiveness of educational interventions, including interactive education sessions [22], academic detailing [23], and educational outreach visits [19,22–24] on the behavior of health professionals and on patient outcomes does exist. From research examining the effectiveness of continuing education efforts, some factors have consistently shown to be effective in improving physician performance [21]. These factors include baseline assessment of learning needs, facilitation of social interaction between learners, provision of opportunities to practice newly acquired skills, and the inclusion of a series of multifaceted educational interventions. Although the evidence suggests that educational interventions have the potential to influence the uptake of knowledge, it appears such interventions alone are unlikely to be sufficient.

Future research

Future research to test the effectiveness of educational interventions should promote generalizability, be underpinned by educational theory, and be carefully designed and conducted with rigor to avoid methodological limitations, such as unit of analysis error. Such research is required to test and validate the assumptions of educational theories as well as determine the effectiveness of the intervention. Reporting should include a careful and detailed description of the intervention as well as a detailed description of the education, if any, received by the control group in the event that a control is employed. In addition, rich description of context in which the research is conducted will help in the assessment of the generalizability of the findings. Finally, detailed economic evaluation will enable decision-makers to make informed decisions about the suitability and feasibility of the intervention.

Summary

Theory-informed educational interventions can be used to facilitate research use when they are tailored to individual learning styles and needs, matched to the skills of the learner, relevant to practice, problem- and goal-oriented, and when they enable the integration of new knowledge with existing knowledge and experience. They should be delivered in a cooperative and respectful atmosphere, using teaching approaches designed to accomplish learning objectives, to allow active involvement and self-directed learning, and to address key learning domains. Research to validate the assumptions of educational theories has been constrained by methodological limitations. However, evidence in favor of the effectiveness of some educational interventions in facilitating knowledge-to-action is promising and can be used to guide the design, implementation, and evaluation of such interventions.

References

1 Laidley TL, Braddock III CH. Role of adult learning theory in evaluating and designing strategies for teaching residents in ambulatory settings. *Adv Health Sci Educ* 2000;5:43–54.

2 Stuart GW, Tondora J, Hoge MA. Evidence-based teaching practice: implications for behavioral health. *Admin Pol Mental Health* 2004;32[2]:107–30.

3 Mann KV. The role of educational theory in continuing medical education: has it helped us? *J Cont EducHealth Prof* 2004;24:S22–S30.

4 Krathwohl DR, Bloom BS, Masia BB. *Taxonomy of Educational Objectives: The Classification of Educational Goals. Handbook II: Affective Domain.* New York: David McKay; 1969.

5 Grol RPTM, Bosch MC, Hulscher MEJL, Eccles MP, Wensing M. Planning and studying improvement in patient care: the use of theoretical perspectives. *Milbank Q* 2007;85[1]:93–138.

6 Lewis AP, Bolden KJ. General practitioners and their learning styles. *J R Coll Gen Pract* 1989;39:187–99.

7 Collins J. Education techniques for lifelong learning. *RadioGraphics* 2004;24: 1483–9.

8 Grol R, Wensing M, Hulscher M, Eccles MP. Theories on implementation of change in healthcare. In R Grol, M Wensing, & MP Eccles (Eds.), *Improving Patient Care. The Implementation of Change in Clinical Practice.* London: Elsevier; 2005.

9 Merriam SB, Caffarella RS. *Learning in Adulthood.* 2nd ed. San Francisco: Jossey-Bass; 1999.

10 Koh GC-H, Khoo HE, Wong ML, Koh D. The effects of problem-based learning during medical school on physician competency: a systematic review. *CMAJ* 2008;178[1]:34–41.

11 Schon D. *The Reflective Practitioner. How Professionals Think in Action.* London: Temple Smith; 1983.

12 Mezirow J. *Transformative Dimensions of Adult Learning.* San Francisco, CA: Jossey-Bass; 1991.

13 Benner P. *From Novice to Expert.* Menlo Park, CA: Addison-Wesley Publishing; 1984.

14 Thompson C. A conceptual treadmill: the need for 'middle ground' in clinical decision making theory in nursing. *J Adv Nurs* 1999;30[5]:1222–9.

15 Knowles MS. *The Modern Practice of Adult Education: Andragogy versus Pedagogy.* New York: Association Press; 1970.

16 Knowles MS. *The Modern Practice of Adult Education.* Revised ed. Chicago: Association Press/Follett; 1980.

17 Fox RD, Bennett NL. Learning and change: implications for continuing medical education. *Br Med J* 1998;316[7129]:466–8.

18 Bandura A. *Social Learning Theory.* New York: General Learning Press; 1977.

19 Grimshaw JM, Thomas RE, MacLennan G, Fraser C, Ramsay CR, Vale L, et al. Effectiveness and efficiency of guideline dissemination and implementation strategies. *Health Technol Assess* 2004;8[6].

20 Gilbody S, Whitty P, Grimshaw J, Thomas R. Educational and organizational interventions to improve the management of depression in primary care. A systematic review. *JAMA* 2003;289:3145–51.

21 Mazmanian PE, Davis DA. Continuing medical education and the physician as a learner. Guide to the evidence. *JAMA* 2002;288[9]:1057–60.

22 O'Brien MA, Freemantle N, Oxman AD, Wolf F, Davis DA, Herrin J. Continuing education meetings and workshops: Effects of professional practice and health care outcomes. *Cochrane Database of Systematic Reviews* 2001 [Issue 1].

23 O'Brien MA, Rogers S, Jamtvedt G, Oxman AD, Odgaard-Jensen J, Kristoffersen DT, et al. Educational outreach visits: effects on professional practice and health care outcomes. *Cochrane Database of Systematic Reviews* 2007 [Issue 4].

24 NHS Centre for Reviews and Dissemination. Effective health care. Getting evidence into practice. In *Bulletin on the Effectiveness of Health Service Interventions for Decision Makers* 1999;5[1]:1–16.

25 Leib S. *Principles of adult learning.* Vision 1991. URL http://honolulu.hawaii.edu/intranet/committees/FacDevCom/guidebk/teachtip/adults-2.htm [accessed February 12, 2008].

4.4 Organizational theory

Jean-Louis Denis, Pascale Lehoux

Department of Health Administration, University of Montreal, Montreal, QC, Canada

---

KEY LEARNING POINTS

- An organizational perspective on knowledge use focuses on the enrichment of organizational context.
- Three concepts form the core of an organizational perspective on knowledge use: capabilities, process, and codification.
- Specific knowledge use strategies can be derived from each of these three concepts.
- Knowledge management in organizations can be based on the integration of these three views of knowledge.

Our main objective in this chapter is to present an organizational perspective on knowledge use in health care organizations and systems. Taking an organizational perspective means we scrutinize the intellectual and system capabilities that organizations develop and nurture to improve their use of knowledge and, consequently, their performance, adaptation, and innovation [1,2]. Broadly speaking, an organizational perspective addresses the concept of receptive capacity, which includes learning by organizational participants and their involvement in the creation and coproduction of knowledge [3]. Organizations are resources capable of increasing the development and use of knowledge.

The idea that organizations can develop strategies to increase knowledge use is based on extensive scholarly work on learning organizations [1,4,5] and evidence-informed management [6–11]. Whereas the abilities to capture knowledge, put knowledge into action, and learn from experience is based on the behaviors, talents, and intellectual capacities of individuals, an organizational perspective on knowledge use emphasizes the steps organizations can take to stimulate closer connections among their decisions, operations, and emerging knowledge. Overall, we suggest that the net impact of strategies

---

Knowledge Translation in Health Care: Moving from Evidence to Practice. Edited by S. Straus, J. Tetroe, and I. Graham. © 2009 Blackwell Publishing, ISBN: 978-1-4051-8106-8.

designed to increase the use of research-based evidence in health care organizations and systems highly depends on the enrichment of organizational contexts.

The problem of knowledge use in health care organizations and systems

Health care organizations are traditionally defined as professional bureaucracies [12] in which work processes are in the hands of highly qualified experts and where managers and support services are at the service of those experts. Through the autonomy delegated to experts within the operating core of these organizations, the mobilization of up-to-date knowledge is ensured. Also through the interactions of well-trained professionals within and around the clinical core, should complex problems be resolved. However, the practices of autonomous and highly qualified professionals and organizations guarantee neither the quality and safety of care [13–15] nor the adaptation or updating of practices to cutting-edge knowledge and technologies. If such things were guaranteed, concerns about how to generate more evidence-informed health care systems, organizations, and practices would not be an issue.

That expert organizations may at times underperform with respect to knowledge use is intriguing from an organizational perspective. This perspective posits three interrelated principles:

- Experts and knowledge cannot be dissociated; indeed, each empowers the other.
- Knowledge is a process phenomenon where internal and external knowledge consolidates organizations by circulating through them.
- Codified knowledge plays a key role in sustainable organizational change.

We draw on these principles to discuss three key concepts that shed light on the potential of an organizational perspective to implement knowledge. The first concept emphasizes organizational and system features that foster knowledge use. The second focuses on organizational processes involved in knowledge application. And, the third examines the use of codified knowledge to improve performance. These three concepts reflect a constant tension between the search for conformity between research-based evidence and organizational practices and the need for *in-situ* learning and adaptation to bring about quality and performance improvement.

Key concepts of knowledge use

Knowledge as capabilities

Understanding *knowledge as capabilities* requires awareness of the tangible and intangible assets that can increase the incorporation of knowledge in an organization's main operations and services [1,16–18]. Capabilities are the properties that can stimulate attention to and use of knowledge. When knowledge is endogenous, the challenge is to ensure its diffusion to other organizational units. For example, if leaders of a given clinical program develop ways to improve the functioning of multidisciplinary teams, processes should be in place to ensure knowledge-sharing with other appropriate units. When knowledge is exogenous, the challenge is to capture it rapidly and to translate it into innovative practices and/or services within the organization. A classic example of this challenge is an organization's ability to assimilate and adapt new practice or clinical guidelines. In reality, both endogenous and exogenous sources of knowledge combine in an indistinct manner.

Several studies create a solid conceptual starting point for identifying the major organizational capabilities that influence knowledge use [3,19–22]. According to these studies, competition in the form of increased performance pressures (e.g., benchmarking) and open policies regarding access to scientific knowledge (e.g., availability at nonprohibitive cost of published scientific works and vigorous dissemination policies) increase pressure on organizations to use new knowledge [19].

An organization can improve its ability to manage knowledge if its structure, strategy, and culture have certain characteristics. Structurally, organizations that leverage their organic properties such as autonomy of decision and flexibility are better prepared to capture and manage knowledge [23]. Organic properties emphasize decentralized decision making and authority in ways that foster customized solutions to emerging problems [1]. Decentralization in these types of organizations—which resemble the enabling bureaucracies described by Adler and Borys [24]—is coupled with clear strategies that value using knowledge to improve performance. In such organizations, incentive systems like group rewards foster group cohesion and performance. On the cultural front, a high level of professional autonomy is considered desirable and viable as long as an organization is in a position to monitor and stimulate commitment and performance [1,25]. Decentralization facilitates knowledge contextualization by giving a great deal of autonomy to the people in charge of resolving complex problems [3,21]. In these types of organizations some resources are provided to support innovative projects and to cover the risks of experimentation [19]. In addition to the type of organizational structure in place, research-based evidence must be accessible through various technical supports designed to increase its use in daily practices. Implementation of roles such as knowledge brokers [26] is also part of the pool of capabilities organizations may consider. Although as outlined by Eccles in Chapter 3.5, evidence to support their use is limited.

The concept of knowledge as capabilities holds that organizations will excel in knowledge management if they manage the tension between the autonomy of a decentralized structure and the need to stimulate professionals to improve their performance [1,23]. This tension will be constructive as long as professionals and other staff members have the resources to access new sources of knowledge and to develop local or customized strategies to put knowledge into action. Knowledge understood as capabilities also mandates that organizations must tolerate risk and accept that not all the initiatives deriving from the incorporation or dissemination of knowledge will be genuine innovations and will necessarily affect performance in a positive manner. Organizational mechanisms like systematic evaluation geared to identifying and selecting promising innovations or practices derived from new knowledge are key ingredients of an effective knowledge management strategy [27].

Knowledge as process

Whereas the focus on capabilities emphasizes resources, design, and norms that organizations may put in place to foster knowledge use, *knowledge as process* looks at processes that condition knowledge's acceptability and potential. Knowledge is considered an innovation from the point of view of potential users. Social processes that support the constitution and circulation of knowledge in networks of organizations are regarded as determining levels of use and application. From a process perspective, knowledge is a dynamic and ambiguous entity characterized by fluid boundaries [28]. Knowledge is used because it is transformed within networks of concerned individuals and organizations [29]. Accordingly, context is not something given to people but a social construct or phenomenon that results from day-to-day interaction [30].

The role of scientific evidence in spreading clinical–administrative innovations offers a good example of knowledge as process [31]. Using a case study approach, this study tracks the spread of innovations among clinical and organizational settings through interviews with key informants and analysis of secondary data available on the diffusion process. Although in each of the four innovations they studied the authors identified a core of hard evidence (i.e., evidence that is less subject to controversies), they also identified a soft periphery for each innovation (a soft periphery is a space in which an innovation's boundaries are more negotiable, the notion of credible scientific evidence is much less settled, and the evaluation of an innovation in terms of costs and benefits is much more controversial). For example, in their research, Denis and colleagues studied the case of assertive community treatment (ACT), a care-delivery model for patients with severe mental health problems. This innovation was subjected to various assessments by stakeholders regarding the value and credibility of scientific demonstrations of its benefits. Community health organizations looked for alternative approaches that place greater value on patient autonomy, and they were reluctant to adopt a standardized approach that would impose control over patients' daily lives. ACT required adaptations in the organization of work, scheduling, and staffing. Denis and colleagues found that evaluations of gains and losses varied across promoters, patient representatives (e.g., community groups), and staff. Dissemination of ACT appeared to depend on the type of networks that developed around the innovation and on the ability to transform opponents into adherents or promoters of this new approach. In a similar initiative, Denis and colleagues studied cholecystectomy by laparoscopic surgery. They found that the procedure rapidly diffused throughout a network of physicians and patients. For surgeons, the procedure was the only way to keep pace with an expanding market; nonadopters risked being shut out of the sector or losing significant portions of their activity. For patients, the promise of rapid recovery with fewer visible traces on their bodies transformed them into supporters despite the risks associated with the procedure's rapid diffusion and extension of the scope of its indications. The ACT and laparoscopic surgery examples reveal that a complex web of interactions and meaning systems determine what is considered knowledge and the credibility people attach to innovations. From a process view of knowledge, these examples illustrate that knowledge use is the customization of knowledge to fit situations involving organizational pluralism.

Lehoux's [32] work on the social analysis of technology in health care illuminates another aspect of knowledge as key process concept. In her study of technological diffusion, Lehoux emphasizes the role of normative assumptions in the shaping and level of acceptability of these technologies [see also 33]. Such assumptions—for example, beliefs about the kinds of innovations that are desirable for modern health care systems—are often tacit, but they determine how people and organizations regard new knowledge. Normative expectations are also embedded in a political economy of health where certain technologies, such as low-cost portable radiology equipment for primary care [34], have less chance of being diffused and adopted than others.

Knowledge is a social construct that at times transcends and, at other times, is circumscribed by professional and clinical boundaries [35]. People who engage in epistemic conversations develop various definitions of the forms that valid and useful knowledge can take. In such situations, knowledge is used when convergence arises among a plurality of people and organizations. It is important to point out that this process of accommodation cannot be totally identified with pure political considerations where concerned actors promote a certain kind of knowledge to gain power and preserve their interests. From a process perspective, knowledge is used when it contributes to increasing individuals' problem-solving capacities, when it increases their sense of self-control over their working contexts and day-to-day practices [4], and when it reflects normative preferences of what an innovation should do.

Although it comes from a disciplinary tradition that differs greatly from our own, Wenger's work [36] on communities of practice provides a basis for thinking about knowledge use within the context of networks. According to Wenger, communities of practice develop around three key components: identity, problem-sharing, and artefact development. Because of their organic and contextual nature, communities of practice link social dynamics and learning in forms that hold the potential to translate and appropriate knowledge processes within and across organizations. It must be noted, however, that learning processes in communities of practice are constrained or enabled by governance structures and normative frames embedded in organizational or social settings.

Knowledge understood as process suggests that organizations should go beyond implementing formal capabilities, such as design, incentives, and accessibility and availability of knowledge. Instead, they should devise interventions that blend social processes, learning, and knowledge use. The concept of knowledge as process suggests that use of research-based evidence is contingent on the ability of people within an organization to agree on a common set of problems and to maintain cooperation and communication despite inevitable controversies.

Knowledge as codification

Polanyi [37] made the classic distinction between tacit and explicit—or codified—forms of knowledge. *Knowledge as codification* refers to knowledge that is embedded in formal and visible codes and well-circumscribed technologies. Codified knowledge in health care organizations includes clinical practice guidelines, quality indicators, performance management systems, information systems, and electronic patient records.

Current research on clinical governance underscores the importance of codified knowledge for improving organizational and clinical performance [38,39]. In health care organizations, codified knowledge development is often associated with a search for increased accountability and the need to open the black box of resource use. When undertaken with the development of technological capacities, codified knowledge also plays a (growing) role in the governance of health care organizations and systems. The Canadian Institute for Health Information (CIHI), for instance, is dedicated to increasing codified knowledge within the regulation of Canada's health care system. Organizations in the United Kingdom such as the National Institute for Health and Clinical Excellence (NICE) and the Institute for Innovation and Improvement also promote elevated use of codified knowledge aimed at influencing the behavior of health care decision makers and professionals. In the United States, meanwhile, the pivotal role of information systems in the Veterans Administration restructuring further illustrates the potential of codified knowledge to improve performance [40].

An organizational perspective on knowledge use sees both potential for and limits to the expansion of codified knowledge for governing health care organizations. Potential resides in the possibility of inducing desirable changes by providing information about processes and outcomes that support organizations in their improvement efforts. Studies of improvements and performance in health care organizations tend to emphasize this positive (instrumental) side of codified knowledge.

An organizational perspective, however, highlights the importance of paying attention to the limits of codified knowledge. Such limits are found in the undesirable dynamics that codified knowledge systems can stimulate. Such systems are populated with indicators that can be used to perform summary evaluations of activities and performance assessments. The gaming that often develops to comply with embedded expectations is a classic example of such effects. A recent review of the benefits of public reporting of health care performance suggests that, to obtain maximum benefits from such systems, the pressures providers feel to comply with standards of care in such contexts should be addressed [41].

Another limit (or risk) is found in the potential inadequacy of such systems when they are used to assess care quality and service performance. For example, there is a difference between assessing care quality in a hospital at a discrete point in time and evaluating it across a full episode of care that goes beyond a single organization's boundaries. Quality or performance appraisal systems may provide a reductionist view of activities and responsibilities and might leave aside important segments or dimensions of activities. In addition, codified knowledge systems can take on lives of their own and thereby reduce the agency of individuals and their ability to adjust or to take more desirable courses of action. A recent study [42] reported on this phenomenon in an empirical exploration of the use of indicators to restructure health care systems and to close facilities. The researchers found that decision makers used a limited set of indicators to target hospital closures. Whereas in most cases the system of indicators seemed to support sound decision making, in the case of one hospital it was much less clear, considering the role played by this organization and its dynamism. Despite that shortcoming, decision makers were unable to adjust their decisions, thereby becoming trapped by a system of indicators. Publicly recognizing the system's limits would have compromised the indicators' legitimacy and, ultimately, the legitimacy of the entire decision-making process involved in the restructuring project.

By using this example of contestable decision making, we do not want to devalue the potential of codified knowledge systems. Rather, we suggest that the use of such systems will be more beneficial if one pays attention to the organizational dynamics that develop around the implementation of such tools. Although accountability issues are important and probably inevitable, studies of governance [e.g., 43] suggest that accountability relations between various individuals and organizations can be developed in an argumentative framework in which people debate the quality and appropriateness of their behavior and achievements. In such a process, codified knowledge couples with systems and actions that favor argumentation and deliberation, with a focus on continuous improvements instead of an overemphasis on control. This position is also in line with recent studies of care safety that promote the need for a culture of learning instead of a culture of blaming [44].

Future research

From an organizational perspective, future research on knowledge use should look at the specific attributes and dynamics that transform codified knowledge into learning opportunities and improvements. There is a pressing need to better understand the interplay between formalized knowledge systems and more organic processes, as well as the ways both contribute to increased performance in health care organizations. We also must be more specific about certain organizational assets (e.g., technology, new organizational roles such as knowledge broker) that may contribute to learning and improvements. And, finally, there is still much to be discovered about how new organizational forms such as networks can assist knowledge exchange and about how to stimulate network development across various organizational forms and health care systems to increase mutual learning.

Summary

Organizational perspective is useful for understanding the factors and processes that can impede or facilitate the use of research-based evidence to enhance decisions and practices. This perspective builds on three key knowledge concepts: capability, process, and codification. Each of these concepts embodies different strategies for promoting the use of knowledge or research-based evidence in health care organizations and systems.

Knowledge as capability underlines the potential of organizational structures and resources to support people in their attempts to use knowledge. *Knowledge as process*, meanwhile, emphasizes flexibility in knowledge use and the need to contextualize knowledge to adapt to local settings and dynamics. Experimentation and trialability are, therefore, key to success. *Knowledge as codification* focuses on the potential of sophisticated information systems to govern health care organizations, an approach that is most beneficial when people confront their views on information that can be extracted from such tools. Ideally, the search for increased accountability should not be conducted at the expense of learning.

References

1 Quinn JB, Anderson P, Finkelstein S. Managing professional intellect: making the most of the best. *Harv Bus Rev* 1996;74[2]:71–80.

2 Quinn JB. *Intelligent Enterprise: A Knowledge and Service Based Paradigm for Industry.* New York: Free Press; 1992.

3 Greenhalgh T, Robert G, Bate P, Kyriakidou O, Macfarlane F, Peacock R. *How to spread good ideas: asystematic review of the literature on diffusion, dissemination and sustainability of innovations in health service delivery and organisation.* Report for the National Co-ordinating Centre for NHS Service Delivery and Organisation. London: NCCSDO; 2004.

4 Schön DA. *The Reflective Practitioner: How Professionals Think in Action.* New York: Basic Books; 1983.

5 Nonaka I. A dynamic theory of organizational knowledge creation. *Organization Science* 1994;5[1]:14–37.

6 Rousseau DM. Is there such a thing as "evidence-based management"? *Acad Manage Rev* 2006;31[2]:256–69.

7 Rousseau DM, McCarthy S. Educating managers from an evidence-based perspective. *AMLE* 2007;61[1]:84–101.

8 Pfeffer J, Sutton RI. *The Knowing-Doing Gap: How Smart Companies Turn Knowledge into Action.* Cambridge, MA: Harvard Business School Press; 1999.

9 Walshe K, Rundall T. Evidence-based management: from theory to practice in health care. *Milbank Q* 2001;79[3]:429–57, iv–v.

10 Kovner AR, Rundall TG. Evidence-based management reconsidered. *Front Health Serv Manage* 2006;22[3]:3–22.

11 Denis JL, Lomas J, Stipich N. Creating receptor capacity for research in the health system: the Executive Training for Research Application (EXTRA) program in Canada. *J Health Serv Res Policy* 2008;13[Suppl 1]:1–7.

12 Mintzberg H. *The Structure of Organizations.* Englewood Cliffs, NJ: Prentice Hall; 1979.

13 Baker R, Norton P. *La sécurité des patients et les erreurs médicales dans le système de santé canadien: Un examen et une analyse systématiques des principales initiatives*

prises dans le monde. Ottawa: Health Canada. URL http://www.hc-sc.gc.ca/hcs-sss/pubs/care-soins/2002-patient-securit-rev-exam/index_f.html [accessed 2002].

14 Institute of Medicine, Committee on Quality of Health Care in America. *Crossing the Quality Chasm: A New System for the 21st Century.* Washington, DC: National Academy Press; 2001.

15 McGlynn EA, Asch SM, Adams J, Keesey J, Hicks J, DeCristofaro A, et al. The quality of health care delivered to adults in the United States. *NEJM* 2003;348[26]:2635–45.

16 Cohen WM, Levinthal DA. Absorptive capacity: a new perspective on learning and innovation. *Adm Sci Q* 1990;35[1]:128–52.

17 Zahra SA, George G. Absorptive capacity: a review, reconceptualization, and extension. *Acad Manage Rev* 2002;27[2]:185–203.

18 Barney J. Firm resources and sustained competitive advantage. *J Manage* 1991; 17[1]:99–120.

19 Cummings J. *Knowledge Sharing: A Review of the Literature.* Washington, DC: World Bank Operations Evaluation Department; 2003.

20 Lane PJ, Lubatkin M. Relative absorptive capacity and interorganizational learning. *Strategic Management Journal* 1998;19[5]:461–77.

21 Champagne F, Lemieux-Charles L, McGuire W. Introduction: towards a broader understanding of the use of knowledge and evidence. In L Lemieux-Charles & F Champagne (Eds.), *Using Knowledge and Evidence in Health Care* (p. 3–17). Toronto: University of Toronto Press; 2004.

22 Mitton C, Adair CE, McKenzie E, Patten SB, Waye Perry B. Knowledge transfer and exchange: review and synthesis of the literature. *Milbank Q* 2007;85[4]:729–68.

23 Burns T, Stalker GM. *The Management of Innovation.* London: Tavistock; 1961.

24 Adler PS, Borys B. Two types of bureaucracy: enabling and coercitive. *Adm Sci Q* 1996;41[1]:61–89.

25 Brunsson N, Sahlin-Andersson K. Constructing organizations: the example of public sector reform. *Organization Studies* 2000;21[4]:721–46.

26 CHSRF. 2008. URL http://www.chsrf.ca/brokering.

27 Langley A. Innovativeness in large public systems. *Optimum* 1997;27[2]:21–31.

28 Waddell C, Lavis J, Abelson J, Lomas J, Sheperd C, Bird-Gayson T, et al. Research use in children's mental health policy in Canada: maintaining vigilance amid ambiguity. *Soc Science Med* 2005;61[8]:1649–57.

29 Latour B. *La science en action: introduction à la sociologie des sciences.* Paris: Gallimard; 1989.

30 Dopson S. A view from organization studies. *Nurs Res* 2007;56[4, Suppl 1]:S72–7.

31 Denis JL, Hébert Y, Langley A, Trottier LH, Lozeau D. Explaining diffusion patterns for complex health care innovations. *Health Care Manage Rev* 2002;27[3]:60–73.

32 Lehoux P. *The Problem of Health Technology: Policy Implications for Modern Health Care Systems.* New York: Routledge; 2006.

33 Campbell JL. Ideas, politics, and public policy. *Annual Rev Soc* 2002;28:21–38.

34 Christensen CM, Bohmer R, Kenagy J. Will disruptive innovations cure health care? *Harv Bus Rev* 2000;78[5]:102–12.

35 Lehoux P, Daudelin G, Denis JL, Miller F. Scientists and policymakers at work: listening to epistemic conversations in a genetics science network. *Science and Public Policy* 2008;35[3]:207–20.

36 Wenger E. *Communities of Practice: Learning, Meaning and Identity.* New York: Cambridge University Press; 1999.

37 Polanyi M. *The Tacit Dimension.* London: Routledge & Kegan Paul; 1966.

38 Starey N. What is clinical governance? *Evidence-Based Medicine* 2003;1[12].

39 Scally G, Donaldson LJ. Clinical governance and the drive for quality improvement in the NHS in England. *BMJ* 1998;317[7150]:61–5.

40 Perlin JB, Kolodner RM, Roswell RH. The Veterans Health Administration: quality, value, accountability, and information as transforming strategies for patient-centered care, *Healthcare Papers* 2005;5[4]:10–24.

41 Marshall M, Shekelle PG, Davies HTO, Smith PC. Public reporting on quality in the United States and the United Kingdom. *Health Affairs* 2003;22[3]:134–48.

42 Denis JL, Langley A, Rouleau L. The power of numbers in strategizing. *Strategic Organization* 2006;4[4]:349–77.

43 Denis JL, Champagne F, Pomey MP, Preval J, Tré G. *An analytical framework for governance of health care organizations.* Report submitted to the Canadian Council on Health Services Accreditation. Ottawa, Ontario, Canada; 2005.

44 Leape LL, Berwick DM. Safe health care: are we up to it? *BMJ* 2000;320[7237]: 725–6.

4.5 **Quality improvement**

Anne Sales

Faculty of Nursing, University of Alberta, Edmonton, AB, Canada

---

KEY LEARNING POINTS

- Quality improvement (QI) and knowledge translation (KT) have similarities, but they are not identical.
- QI is by nature more local and less generalizable than KT.
- There are conceptual frameworks for QI that have strong overlap with conceptual frameworks for KT, but there may not be a strong theory base for QI.
- There is much published literature on QI, including methods for doing QI and reports of the processes and outcomes of QI.

Defining quality improvement

The Institute of Medicine in the United States defines quality of care as "[t]he degree to which health services for individuals and populations increase the likelihood of desired health outcomes and are consistent with current professional knowledge" [1]. Although there are other definitions of quality of care, most are consistent with this definition. It follows that quality improvement (QI) is the effort to increase or improve the degree to which health services increase the likelihood of desired health outcomes and are consistent with current professional knowledge.

Relating quality improvement to knowledge translation research

The overlap between QI and knowledge translation (KT) is embedded in the desire to increase the degree to which health services are consistent with "current professional knowledge." However, despite this overlap, much of the work done as part of QI may not be related to this goal but is related instead to

---

Knowledge Translation in Health Care: Moving from Evidence to Practice. Edited by S. Straus, J. Tetroe, and I. Graham. © 2009 Blackwell Publishing, ISBN: 978-1-4051-8106-8.

efforts to address problems or issues that are perceived as affecting the degree to which health services "increase the likelihood of desired health outcomes" or are perceived as inefficient, harmful, or violating other precepts of high-quality care, including safety, effectiveness, patient-centeredness, timeliness, efficiency, and equity [1]. All of these may be part of "desired health outcomes" but may not relate to whether professional knowledge and practice are current and effective. QI and KT may not share the same specific goals, but both are intended to improve care.

Frameworks for QI

Avedis Donabedian traces the history of QI models and proposals to the early part of the twentieth century [2]. His proposed framework for understanding factors influencing quality of care, and in particular outcomes of health services, is widely adopted in the literature on health care QI. He proposed that *structure* of health services, which include the physical facilities in which health services are delivered, the types of services available (e.g., level of intensive care, availability of surgery or specialty services), and factors such as staffing levels or per capita ratios of key inputs to health services (e.g., physicians per 1000 population), influence the *process* of care. Care processes include specific interventions such as surgery, prescribing medications, and monitoring processes of care [3], including monitoring vital signs during a hospital admission. These factors, in Donabedian's framework, influence *outcomes*, which can be at several different levels, although his framework focuses on patient-level outcomes of care. These outcomes include whether a patient survives a care episode delivered during an acute event, such as hospitalization following myocardial infarction, the quality of life someone has after receiving health services for a health condition or problem (e.g., chemotherapy or radiation therapy for cancer care), and other sequelae of the health condition and of health services received. These sequelae may include iatrogenic or adverse events resulting from health care services. It should be noted that although Donabedian is best known for the *structure–process–outcome* framework, he elaborated several additional principles to guide improvement of quality in health care, many of which are similar to the six core principles outlined by the Institute of Medicine [4]. In addition to patient-level outcomes, he also focused on system-level outcomes, such as cost and efficiency [5–10].

Negative outcomes—iatrogenic or adverse events resulting from health services delivered—have received a considerable amount of attention in recent years. In response, additional frameworks for conceptualizing health care quality improvement have been proposed. This strategy comes originally from manufacturing industries and is credited to Joseph Juran and W. Edwards Deming, separately, both of whom were engaged in quality improvement and the development of *total quality management* and *continuous quality improvement* processes and techniques [11]. The translation of these approaches to health care can largely be credited to Donald Berwick. His work has resulted in the adoption of quality improvement principles in the hospital and health care organization accreditation procedures of the Joint Commission in the United States as well as in other jurisdictions. Through the Institute for Healthcare Improvement (IHI), Berwick has had considerable influence in many different countries. The core framework for continuous quality improvement includes several tenets, which include the use of data and statistical analysis to identify processes and control of processes; the use of benchmarking for comparison with relevant groups; the use of teams to identify problems, processes, and solutions; and the use of some form of improvement process, usually described as a cycle: *plan, do, study* (or *check*), *act*. Following action, the cycle repeats with further planning, doing, studying or checking results, and further action [12]. These tenets have been developed by IHI into processes called *Collaboratives*, in which several health care organizations come together over a period of 12–18 months and engage in activities designed to address specific problems such as surgical wound infections [13–15].

Assessments of quality improvement as a means of knowledge translation

Over the last several years, there have been several systematic reviews addressing the degree to which QI processes and techniques achieve their intended goals of improving quality of care [16–18]. Some of these reviews have attempted to assess the global impact of QI initiatives, while others have focused on specific aspects of the way QI is done. In a series of reports for the Agency for Healthcare Research and Quality, a group at Stanford University and the University of California at San Francisco evaluated effects of QI activities on care for a series of chronic health conditions, including hypertension [16] and type 2 diabetes [17]. They found that QI initiatives spanned a wide variety of activities and that, overall, the results of QI methods are mixed in terms of effectiveness. In a related article, Shojania and Grimshaw reviewed the evidence base for QI techniques and found it problematic because many of the methods used for QI have little basis in evidence, produce mixed and inconsistent findings at best, and demonstrate a scattered approach [18]. Similarly, Øvretveit and colleagues found relatively little evidence for sustainability of QI initiatives over time, suggesting that many QI initiatives are limited in effect duration, even when they demonstrate effectiveness in short-term projects [15,19–21].

These reviews point out substantive differences between some QI and KT or implementation science efforts. QI initiatives tend to be local in nature. Problems are identified at a local level and often do not generalize, particularly in their specificity, to other settings or organizations. In addition, QI efforts are geared toward dealing with immediate problems and toward attempting to address concerns with how care is delivered in real time to specific patients. KT research often attempts to derive generalizable knowledge through the systematic application of research methods and principles and to apply lessons learned from one specific setting to another or across a relatively large number of settings or organizations.

Issues and concerns in quality improvement as a means of knowledge translation

Issues have been raised about the role of ethical or human subjects review and protections for both patients and health care providers in QI activities. In research activities, there is no question about the need for ethical or human subjects protection review, but this is rarely considered an issue in QI, even when similar activities and interventions are used [22,23]. Concerns have been raised about whether some forms of KT, particularly attempts to implement evidence-based medicine or evidence-based care, might conflict with attempts to engage in meaningful QI activities [24,25]. These concerns are echoed in terms of concern about the lack of an evidence base of QI activities on one hand [18,26] and concerns about standards used for evidence on the other [27]. Additional concerns include how quality of care issues are identified, the role of professional and individual lenses in identifying issues initially [28], and how different health care professionals may rate the seriousness of quality issues [29]. The highly localized nature of QI may make these issues more of a concern than they might be for KT research, with its broader scope and greater emphasis on generalizability.

Despite these concerns and caveats, QI remains a mainstay of efforts to improve patient experiences when they receive health care services. There is an increasing merger between the perspectives of QI and KT research, evidenced by large, multisite QI initiatives, including approaches using collaboratives similar to those pioneered by IHI as well as other approaches [30–32]. In many of these, attempts are being made to provide evidence for Donabedian's *structure–process–outcome* framework, bolstering the theory base for QI activities [19,33]. Overall, there is an increasing convergence in viewpoint between proponents of evidence-based practice, KT, and QI, which will lead to improvements in the care patients and consumers receive from health care organizations and systems [34].

Future research

Given the nature and intent of QI, it is not clear whether there is a need for a science of QI, although there have been calls for developing such a science [34]. There are, however, areas for improving the reliability and effectiveness of QI interventions that depend on developing reliable and effective methods for improving quality of care. These methods are shared with implementation or KT science, and research related to QI and QI efforts can contribute to building generalizable knowledge and reliable, effective interventions. One important approach that has been neglected to date is the synthesizing of the vast literature reporting the processes and outcomes of QI efforts; this alone will constitute a long-term research agenda and will contribute substantively to our knowledge about methods for improving care.

References

1 Institute of Medicine. Committee on Quality of Health Care in America. *Crossing the Quality Chasm: A New Health System for the 21st Century.* Washington, DC: National Academy Press; 2001.
2 Donabedian A. 20 years of research on the quality of medical care, 1964–1984. *Salud Publica Mex* 1988;30[2]:202–15.
3 Donabedian A. Monitoring: the eyes and ears of healthcare. *Health Prog* 1988; 69[9]:38–43.
4 Donabedian A. The seven pillars of quality. *Arch Pathol Lab Med* 1990;114[11]: 1115–8.
5 Donabedian A. Quality and cost: choices and responsibilities. *J Occup Med* 1990; 32[12]:1167–72.
6 Donabedian A. The price of quality and the perplexities of care. *HMO Pract* 1991; 5[1]:24–8.
7 Frenk J, Ruelas E, Donabedian A. Staffing and training aspects of hospital management: some issues for research. *Med Care Rev* 1989;46[2]:189–220.
8 Donabedian A. Quality, cost, and cost containment. *Nurs Outlook* 1984;32[3]: 142–5.
9 Donabedian A. Quality, cost, and clinical decisions. *Ann Am Acad Pol Soc Sci* 1983; [468]:196–204.
10 Donabedian A, Wheeler JR, Wyszewianski L. Quality, cost, and health: an integrative model. *Med Care* 1982;20[10]:975–92.
11 Berwick DM. Harvesting knowledge from improvement. *JAMA* 1996;275[11]: 877–8.

12 McLaughlin CP, Kaluzny AD. *Continuous Quality Improvement in Health Care: Theory, Implementation, and Applications.* 2nd ed. Sudbury, MA; Boston; London: Jones and Bartlett; 2004.

13 Marsteller JA, Shortell SM, Lin M, Mendel P, Dell E, Wang S, et al. Teamwork and communication: how do teams in quality improvement collaboratives interact? *Jt Comm J Qual Patient Saf* 2007;33[5]:267–76.

14 Cretin S, Shortell SM, Keeler EB. An evaluation of collaborative interventions to improve chronic illness care framework and study design. *Eval Rev* 2004;28[1]: 28–51.

15 Øvretveit J, Bate P, Cleary P, Cretin S, Gustafson D, McInnes K, et al. Quality collaboratives: lessons from research. *Qual Saf Health Care* 2002;11[4]:345–51.

16 Walsh JME, McDonald KM, Shojania KG, Sundaram V, Nayak S, Lewis R, et al. Quality improvement strategies for hypertension management: a systematic review. *Med Care* 2006;44[7]:646–57.

17 Shojania KG, Ranji SR, McDonald KM, Grimshaw JM, Sundaram V, Rushakoff RJ, et al. Effects of quality improvement strategies for type 2 diabetes on glycemic control: a meta-regression analysis. *JAMA* 2006;296[4]:427–40.

18 Shojania KG, Grimshaw JM. Evidence-based quality improvement: the state of the science. *Health Aff (Millwood)* 2005;24[1]:138–50.

19 Ovretveit J. The convergence of evidence-based health care and quality improvement. *Healthcare Review Online* 1998;2[9].

20 Øvretveit J, Gustafson D. Evaluation of quality improvement programmes. *Qual Saf Health Care* 2002;11[3]:270–5.

21 Buchanan D, Fitzgerald L, Ketley D, Gollop R, Jones JL, Lamont SS, et al. No going back: a review of the literature on sustaining organizational change. *Int J Manage Rev* 2005;7[3]:189–205.

22 Cretin S, Keeler EB, Lynn J, Batalden PB, Berwick DM, Bisognano M. Should patients in quality-improvement activities have the same protections as participants in research studies? *JAMA* 2000;284[14]:1786; author reply 1787–8.

23 Casarett D, Karlawish JHT, Sugarman J. Determining when quality improvement initiatives should be considered research: proposed criteria and potential implications. *JAMA* 2000;283[17]:2275–80.

24 Harvey G, Wensing M. Methods for evaluation of small scale quality improvement projects. *Qual Saf Health Care* 2003;12[3]:210–4.

25 Harvey G. Quality improvement and evidence-based practice: as one or at odds in the effort to promote better health care? *Worldviews Evid Based Nurs* 2005;2[2]: 52–4.

26 Auerbach AD, Landefeld CS, Shojania KG. The tension between needing to improve care and knowing how to do it. *N Engl J Med* 2007;357[6]:608–13.

27 Berwick DM. Broadening the view of evidence-based medicine. *Qual Saf Health Care* 2005;14[5]:315–6.

28 Sales A, Lurie N, Moscovice I, Goes J. Is quality in the eye of the beholder? *Jt Comm J Qual Improv* 1995;21[5]:219–25.

29 Sales A, Moscovice I, Lurie N. Measuring seriousness of hospital quality of care issues. *Jt Comm J Qual Improv* 1996;22[12]:811–6.

30 Berwick DM, Calkins DR, Joseph McCannon C, Hackbarth AD. The 100 000 lives campaign: setting a goal and a deadline for improving health care quality. *JAMA* 2006;295[3]:324–7.

31 Jain M, Miller L, Belt D, King D, Berwick DM. Decline in ICU adverse events, nosocomial infections and cost through a quality improvement initiative focusing on teamwork and culture change. *Qual Saf Health Care* 2006;15[4]:235–9.

32 Alexander KP, Roe MT, Chen AY, Lytle BL, Pollack CV, Jr, Foody JM, et al. Evolution in cardiovascular care for elderly patients with non-ST-segment elevation acute coronary syndromes: results from the CRUSADE National Quality Improvement Initiative. *J Am Coll Cardiol* 2005;46[8]:1479–87.

33 Peterson ED, Roe MT, Mulgund J, DeLong ER, Lytle BL, Brindis RG, et al. Association between hospital process performance and outcomes among patients with acute coronary syndromes. *JAMA* 2006;295[16]:1912–20.

34 Berwick DM. The science of improvement. *JAMA* 2008;299[10]:1182–4.

Section 5
Knowledge Exchange

5.1 Knowledge dissemination and exchange of knowledge

Michelle Gagnon

Knowledge Synthesis and Exchange Branch, Canadian Institutes of Health Research, Ottawa, ON, Canada

---

KEY LEARNING POINTS

- Dissemination targets research findings to specific audiences.
- Dissemination activities should be considered and outlined in a dissemination plan that focuses on the needs of the audience that will use the knowledge.
- Researchers should engage knowledge users to craft messages and help disseminate research findings.
- Knowledge brokers, networks, and practice communities hold promise as innovative ways to disseminate and facilitate the application of knowledge.
- Knowledge exchange, or integrated KT, involves active collaboration and exchange between researchers and knowledge users throughout the research process.

The dissemination and exchange of knowledge are critical components of the knowledge translation (KT) process and are frequently thought to occur between the generation and synthesis of knowledge and its application or use. Researchers are often asked to consider their knowledge dissemination or translation strategy when preparing grant applications. Dissemination and exchange of knowledge are not necessarily isolated activities that take place at the end of a research project. Depending on the intent of the research endeavor, these activities can be woven into the research process itself. Traditional end-of-grant or project KT typically involves publication in peer-reviewed journals or presentation of results at appropriate meetings. Whereas in some circumstances, end-of-grant KT is highly appropriate [1], in others, integrating knowledge exchange and mutual learning into the research process through an interactive process that involves both researchers and knowledge users may be a more effective way to minimize the knowledge-to-action gap [1,2].

Knowledge Translation in Health Care: Moving from Evidence to Practice. Edited by S. Straus, J. Tetroe, and I. Graham. © 2009 Blackwell Publishing, ISBN: 978-1-4051-8106-8.

Knowledge dissemination

What is knowledge dissemination?

Lomas (1993) provides a useful taxonomy of KT activities that groups them into three conceptually distinct types: diffusion, dissemination, and implementation. He defines *diffusion* as passive and largely unplanned efforts, uncontrolled and primarily horizontal or mediated by peers [3,4]. Publishing in peer-reviewed journals or presenting research results to peers at an academic conference are examples of this type of dissemination. In this category of KT activities, the onus is on the potential adopter to seek out the information.

Dissemination of knowledge, also known as knowledge transfer or end-of-grant KT [1,5], focuses primarily on communicating research results by targeting and tailoring the findings and the message to a particular target audience [2]. As we move along the continuum and want to reach audiences other than academics and researchers, more active dissemination approaches include tailoring the message and medium to the specific audience; linking researchers and knowledge users through linkage and exchange mechanisms, such as small workshops focused on the dissemination of a synthesized body of knowledge or those focused on developing a user-driven dissemination strategy; media engagement; the use of knowledge brokers; and the creation of networks or communities of practice involving both researchers and knowledge users focused on ongoing monitoring, dissemination, and uptake of research evidence to improve health and/or the health system [1,3,4, 6–15].

Whether passive or active dissemination activities are called for, researchers (and their knowledge user partners, where relevant) are encouraged, and increasingly required, to develop dissemination plans as part of their grant proposals. Such plans should describe the plan for disseminating the outcomes of the project and consider what knowledge should be transferred, to whom, how, and with what effect [16–18].

Finally, the last category in Lomas' taxonomy, *implementation or application*, is an even more active process than dissemination and involves systematic efforts to encourage adoption of the research findings by identifying and overcoming barriers, discussed further in Chapter 3.4.

Fundamentals of dissemination

Regardless of the type of dissemination activity and who is involved in the process, based on the literature review undertaken for this chapter, a number of fundamental guidelines appear to underpin knowledge dissemination:

- Where available, the design of dissemination processes and approaches should be informed by high-quality evidence that considers the contextual or locally applicable factors that are critical to successful KT [19]. In the health services and clinical realms, such evidence might include systematic reviews that examine the effectiveness and efficiency of dissemination strategies targeted at health professionals [20,21]. In the public policy-making arena, dissemination plans could be informed by systematic reviews of studies focusing on factors that influence evidence use in policy making [19,22].
- Messages should be clear, simple, action-oriented, and tailored for each audience based on knowledge user need [23].
- Messengers or message sources should be individuals or organizations that are influential and credible with each target audience [23].
- Dissemination approaches should be knowledge user-driven or tailored to how and when knowledge users want to receive the information. Possibilities include face-to-face meetings, written reports, or presentations [23].
- A dissemination strategy should include a plan to evaluate the impact of the chosen approach, including ways to measure success [19].

Reardon, Lavis, and Gibson's [24] knowledge transfer planning guide summarizes these points in five questions to consider when undertaking knowledge dissemination: (1) What is the message? (2) Who is the audience? (3) Who is the messenger? (4) What is the transfer method? (5) What is the expected outcome [24–28]?

Approaches to disseminating knowledge

Knowledge brokers
As mentioned in Chapter 3.5.1, knowledge brokers are a potential strategy for moving knowledge to action, although evidence in support of their use is not yet available [4,7,13,29,30]. The rationale for knowledge brokers is the need to provide an intermediary who can facilitate collaborations between researchers and research users and find research evidence to shape decisions, assess this evidence, interpret and adapt it to circumstances, and identify emerging management and policy issues that research can help solve [29]. Knowledge of marketing and communication and the capacity to span boundaries and understand potentially disparate worlds that researchers and knowledge users live in is also needed. Based on this skill set, individuals with diverse experience in research and decision or policy-making worlds or organizations whose mandate is to span these worlds would be ideal knowledge brokers. From this description, we can conclude that knowledge brokering is certainly not

new. Relationship brokers exist in most organizations and sectors. What is new, however, are growing calls to recognize and formalize this role in the KT process not only to evaluate its effectiveness but to capitalize on the benefits it brings to the process while also learning more about its potential drawbacks [7,29–31].

Networks

Networks, including communities of practice, knowledge networks, and soft networks, are potentially effective mechanisms for knowledge dissemination and application because their principal purpose is to connect people who might not otherwise have an opportunity to interact, enable dialogue, stimulate learning, and capture and diffuse knowledge [11,12,32]. A community of practice is a group of people who share a common concern, a set of problems, or interest in a topic and who come together to fulfill both individual and group goals usually focused on improving professional practice [32]. Although communities of practice tend to be relatively informal, a knowledge network is a more formal community consisting of groups of experts from different fields who come together around a common goal or issue [33]. Finally, a soft network is a large referral system where members sign onto a listserv primarily to make connections [33]. Each type of network plays a role in the dissemination of knowledge. Network examples are provided in the boxes below.

> The Canadian Neonatal Network is a KT initiative aimed at improving the health and quality of health care for newborn babies. The network, made up of researchers, clinicians, and administrators from neonatal intensive care units and universities across Canada, conducts evidence-based collaborative research with an emphasis on implementation of practice and policy changes. The network contributes to the development of policies related to the allocation of neonatal resources in British Columbia, Canada [34].

> The Australian National Institute of Clinical Studies has established a community of practice for clinicians, health managers, and health care professionals involved in the delivery of emergency care so that they can share their knowledge and expertise to help close evidence–practice gaps and improve patient care. Objectives of the program include assisting the uptake of evidence-based practice in emergency care, providing access to evidence-based research information, and developing processes for making the best use of good quality clinical care data.

> The community of practice also gathers and disseminates "stories of improvement" on its Web site about the impact of KT projects and activities related to emergency health care systems and practices. (http://www.nhmrc.gov.au/nics/asp/index.asp?cid=5263&gid=207&page=programs/programs_article.)

Another taxonomy for KT activities

Push, pull, and exchange are concepts that provide another way to categorize and understand the KT process [19,24]. Push efforts occur when producers of research knowledge plan and implement approaches to push (disseminate) knowledge toward audiences who they believe need to receive it [24]. A workshop organized by researchers focused on sharing and discussing research results with knowledge users is one example of a push strategy [19]. Pull efforts occur when knowledge users plan and implement strategies to pull knowledge from sources they identify as producing knowledge useful to their own decision making [24]. Commissioning a systematic review on a relevant topic to inform decision making is one example of a pull strategy. Finally, in contrast to push and pull, exchange efforts aim to bring the researcher and knowledge user communities together through an interactive process [6,19]. Such exchange can take place throughout the research process using an integrated KT approach that will be described more fully in the next section of this chapter. Knowledge exchange can also focus on end-of-grant KT. In this context, exchange refers to the collaborative process taking place at the end of a grant once research findings are available [35]. Researchers and knowledge users work together to develop and implement a dissemination strategy that is appropriate for the knowledge user audience(s). This collaborative process that builds relationships between researchers and knowledge users may significantly enhance dissemination efforts. Whatever approach is taken—push, pull, or exchange, there is significant evidence to support the premise that the dissemination of results is most effective when researchers and knowledge users already have existing relationships built on ongoing exchange of information and ideas [24,35].

What is knowledge exchange?

As noted earlier, knowledge exchange or integrated knowledge translation (IKT), also known as collaborative research, action research, participatory research, community-based participatory research, coproduction of knowledge, or Mode 2 research, involves active collaboration and exchange between researchers and knowledge users throughout the research process, from identifying and shaping the research questions to collecting data and interpreting findings and disseminating and applying results [1,36]. This methodology is most appropriately used to understand and address complex, relevant, and timely "real-life" health or health system issues that require the engagement of multiple stakeholders in both the research and change processes. Therefore, it may not be an effective or necessary approach when conducting basic discovery research.

Depending on the intent of the research project and potential actions, knowledge users engaged in the IKT process could include other researchers, clinicians, policy makers, or the public. An integrated approach is potentially more time-consuming, demanding, and resource intensive than other strategies because it requires both researchers and knowledge users to develop new skills, knowledge, and perspectives. However, involving knowledge users as partners in the research process is a strong predictor that research findings will be used and that the research endeavor will achieve a greater impact [6,36–41]. Over the last several years, health research funding agencies have designed and implemented research initiatives that aim to support and promote integrated KT approaches [42,43].

What makes the integrated KT process work effectively?

Significant evidence exists about the collaborative research process, including barriers, facilitators, and conditions for success from which several key success factors about this process can be drawn [34,36,44–50]. The following key success factors can be applied to any type of collaborative research endeavor that brings together researchers and knowledge users to generate, exchange, and apply knowledge to understand and address a health or health system issue. Such factors include:

- A process to develop a shared perspective, common language, and common understanding about the health problem/issue that the team will focus on
- A plan for collaboration with explicit description of roles and responsibilities and a commitment to regularly assess its effectiveness
- A plan for the inclusion of team members who are collaborative
- A strategy for ensuring that trusting relationships among team members are maintained and conflicts are resolved appropriately when they arise

Institutional support, including incentives in both academic and knowledge user environments, can facilitate this process. For example academic institutions could recognize the importance and significance of engaging in the applied research exemplified by IKT in their tenure and promotion policies [51,52]. Knowledge user organizations could similarly "credit" such activities in their performance evaluation frameworks and provide release time for their staff to engage in research activities.

An interdisciplinary team of health services researchers was asked by a regional Home Care authority to work on improving best practice for venous leg ulcers. Working collaboratively with the Home Care authority and a community nursing agency, the team undertook research to determine the extent of the research-practice gap, identified existing best practice, and adapted existing international guidelines for local use, redesigned the delivery of services to leg ulcer clients by establishing a dedicated leg ulcer services, implemented an evidence-based approach to leg ulcer care, and evaluated it. The evidence-based approach increased healing rates from 23% to 56%, reduced nursing visits from 3 to 2.1 per week, and decreased the median cost per case from $1923 to $406. In this case, implementation of best practice was not only more effective but less costly than usual care [34,53].

Safe Kids Canada's strong relationships with Canadian health researchers led to a collaboration aimed at reducing scald burns among children based on compelling evidence of the effectiveness of an intervention to reduce hot tap water temperature. This collaborative knowledge translation (KT) process led to a change in policy on setting of hot water heaters through changes to the Ontario Plumbing Code and provides lessons for those entering into integrated knowledge translation (IKT) partnerships. For example, through this process, it became apparent that researchers, nongovernmental organizations, policymakers, and industry interpreted and weighed the same body of evidence differently. Context and expert advice as well as research evidence played a role in decision making. As well, the IKT team concluded that a successful collaboration requires active listening, mutual respect as equal partners, and early discussion of timelines and outputs of meaning to all participants [54].

Future research

Several gaps need to be addressed in future research, including identifying optimal strategies for performing knowledge dissemination. In particular, studies are needed to evaluate the impact of knowledge brokers and networks.

Summary

Regardless of whether an integrated or end-of-grant KT approach is used, collaborative relationships built on trust and frequent interaction between researchers and knowledge users are key determinants of successful exchange and dissemination efforts. As innovative approaches to exchange and dissemination grow and evolve, increasing focus must be placed on developing indicators to evaluate these processes and on rigorously evaluating their effectiveness on relevant short, medium, and long-term outcomes.

References

1 Graham ID, Tetroe J. CIHR research: how to translate health research knowledge into effective healthcare action. *Healthcare Quarterly* 2007;10[3]:20–2.

2 Graham ID, Logan J, Harrison MB, Straus SE, Tetroe J, Caswell W, et al. Lost in knowledge translation: time for a map? *J Contin Educ Health Prof* 2006;26:13–24.

3 Greenhalgh T, Robert G, Macfarlane F, Bate P, Kyriakidou O. Diffusion of innovations in service organizations: systematic review and recommendations. *Milbank Q* 2004;82[4]:581–629.

4 Lomas J. Diffusion, dissemination, and implementation: who should do what? *Ann NY Acad Sci* 1993;703[1]:226–37.

5 Tetroe J. *Knowledge translation at the Canadian Institutes of Health Research: a primer.* National Center for the Dissemination of Disability Research Focus 2007. Technical Brief No. 18:1–11.

6 Lomas J. Using 'linkage and exchange' to move research into policy at a Canadian foundation. *Health Aff* 2000;19[3]:236–40.

7 Lomas J. The in-between world of knowledge brokering. *BMJ* 2007;334[7585]: 129–32.

8 Crosswaite C, Curtice L. Disseminating research results-the challenge of bridging the gap between health research and health action. *Health Promot Int* 1994;9[4]:289–96.

9 Nutley S, Walter I, Davies HTO. From knowing to doing: a framework for understanding the evidence-into-practice agenda. *Evaluation* 2003;9[2]:125–48.

10 Pfeffer J, Sutton RI. *The Knowing-Doing Gap: How Smart Companies Turn Knowledge into Action.* Boston: Harvard Business School Press; 2000.

11 Wenger E, McDermott R, Snyder WM. *Cultivating Communities of Practice.* Boston: Harvard Business School Press; 2002.

12 Birdsell J, Matthias S. *Networks and their role in enhancing research impact in Alberta;* 2003. Workshop Report.

13 Lawrence R. Research dissemination: actively bringing the research and policy worlds together. *Evidence & Policy: A Journal of Research, Debate and Practice.* 2006 Aug;2:373–84.

14 Rogers EM. *Diffusion of Innovations.* 5th ed. New York: Free Press; 2003.

15 Mitton C, Adair CE, McKenzie E, Patten SB, Perry BW. Knowledge transfer and exchange: review and synthesis of the literature. *Milbank Q* 2007;85[4]:729–68.

16 Canadian Institutes of Health Research. *2007–2008 CIHR Grants and Awards Guide;* 2007.

17 Canadian Institutes of Health Research. *Knowledge to Action 2008–2009;* 2008.

18 Canadian Institutes of Health Research. *Knowledge Synthesis Grant 2008-2009;* 2008.

19 Lavis JN. Research, public policymaking, and knowledge-translation processes: Canadian efforts to build bridges. *J Contin Educ Health Prof* 2006;26[1]:37–45.

20 Dobbins M, Ciliska D, DiCenso A. Dissemination and use of research evidence for policy and practice: a framework for developing, implementing and evaluating strategies. *NLM Gateway: a Service of the U.S. National Institutes of Health;* 1998. URL http://gateway.nlm.nih.gov/MeetingAbstracts/ma?f=102237186.html [accessed March 21, 2008].

21 Grimshaw J, Thomas RE, MacLennan G, Fraser C, Ramsay CR, Vale L, et al. Effectiveness and efficiency of guideline dissemination and implementation strategies. *Health Technology Assessment* 2004;8[6].

22 Lavis J, Davies H, Oxman A, Denis SL, Golden-Biddle K, Ferlie E. Towards reviews that inform health care management and policy-making. *J Health Serv Res Policy* 2005;10[Suppl 1]:35–47.

23 Canadian Health Services Research Foundation. *Disseminating Research. Tools to Help Organizations Create, Share and Use Research;* 2008. URL http://www.chsrf.ca/keys/use_disseminating_e.php.

24 Reardon R, Lavis J, Gibson J. *From Research to Practice: A Knowledge Transfer Planning Guide;* 2006.

25 Canadian Institutes of Health Research. *The Research-Media Partnership;* 2008.

26 Lavis J, Robertson D, Woodside JM, McLeod CB, Abelson J. Knowledge Ttransfer Study Group. How can research organizations more effectively transfer research knowledge to decision makers? *Milbank Q* 2003;81[2]:221–47.

27 Health Council of New Zealand. *Implementing Research—A Guideline for Health Researchers;* 2007.

28 Landry R, Lyons R, Amara N, Warner G, Ziam S, Halilem N, et al. *Knowledge Translation Planning Tools for Stroke Researchers;* 2006.

29 Canadian Health Services Research Foundation. *The Theory and Practice of Knowledge Brokering in Canada's Health System;* 2003.

30 Lyons R, Warner G, Langille L, Phillips SJ. *Piloting knowledge brokers to promote integrated stroke care in Atlantic Canada. Evidence in Action, Acting on Evidence: a Casebook of Health Services and Policy Research Knowledge Translation Stories.* Ottawa, Ontario, Canada: Canadian Institutes of Health Research; 2006.

31 Canadian Health Services Research Foundation. *Knowledge Brokering Evaluation Program;* 2004. URL http://www.chsrf.ca/brokering/evaluation_program_e.php.

32 Cambridge D, Suter V. *Community of practice design guide: a step-by-step guide for designing & cultivating communities of practice in higher education.* Educause CONNECT Transforming Education through Information Technologies; 2005. URL www.educause.edu/ir/library/pdf/NLI0531.pdf.

33 Canadian Health Services Research Foundation. *Network Notes I: what's all this talk about networks?* CHSRF; 2005. URL www.chsrf.ca.

34 Canadian Institutes of Health Research. Evidence in action, acting on evidence; 2006.

35 Canadian Health Services Research Foundation. Summary of the article: From research to practice: a knowledge transfer planning guide. *Insight and Action* 2007:1.

36 Denis J-L, Lomas J. Convergent evolution: the academic and policy roots of collaborative research. *J Health Serv Res Policy* 2003;2[8]:1–6.

37 Lomas J. CHSRF knowledge transfer: decision support: a new approach to making the best healthcare management and policy choices. *Healthc Q* 2007;10[3]:16–18.

38 Lomas J. *Improving research dissemination and uptake in the health sector: beyond the sound of one hand clapping.* McMaster University Centre for Health Economics and Policy Analysis Policy Commentary; 1997. Report No.: C97-1.

39 Ross S, Lavis J, Rodriguez C, Woodside J, Denis J-L. Partnership experiences: involving decision-makers in the research process. *J Health Serv Res Policy* 2003;2[8]: 26–34.

40 Kothari A, Birch S, Charles C. "Interaction" and research utilisation in health policies and programs: does it work? *Health Policy* 2005;71[1]:117–25.

41 Minkler M. Community-based research partnerships: challenges and opportunities. *J Urban Health* 2005;82[Suppl 2]:ii3–ii12.

42 Canadian Institutes of Health Research. *Partnerships for Health System Improvement; 2008.* URL http://www.cihr-irsc.gc.ca/e/34347.html.

43 Canadian Health Services Research Foundation. *Research, Exchange and Impact for System Support (REISS);* 2008. URL http://www.chsrf.ca/funding_opportunities/reiss/index_e.php.

44 Ducharme F. Partnership in research: a tandem of opportunities and constraints. *Nursing Leadership* 2003;16[1]:61–74.

45 Ross S, Lavis J, Rodriguez C, Woodside J, Denis J-L. Partnership experiences: involving decision-makers in the research process. *J Health Serv Res Policy* 2003 Oct 2;8:26–34.

46 Canadian Institutes of Health Research. *Moving Population and Public Health Knowledge into Action:* A *Casebook of Knowledge Translation Stories;* 2006.

47 Walter I, Davies H, Nutley S. Increasing research impact through partnerships: evidence from outside health care. *J Health Serv Res Policy* 2003 Oct 2;8:58–61.

48 Golden-Biddle K, Reay T, Petz S, Witt C, Casebeer A, Pablo A, et al. Toward a communicative perspective of collaborating in research: the case of the researcher-decision-maker partnership. *J Health Serv Res Policy* 2003 Oct 2;8:20–5.

49 Denis J-L, Lehoux P, Hivon M, Champagne F. Creating a new articulation between research and practice through policy? The views and experiences of researchers and practitioners. *J Health Serv Res Policy* 2003 Oct 2;8:44–50.

50 Roussos ST, Fawcett SB. A review of collaborative partnerships as a strategy for improving community health. *Annu Rev Public Health* 2000;21[1]:369–402.

51 Jacobson N, Butterill D, Goering P. Organizational factors that influence university-based researchers' engagement in knowledge transfer activities. *Science Communication* 2004;25[3]:246–59.

52 Canadian Health Services Research Foundation. The creative professional activity-how one university department weighs knowledge transfer and exchange activities in its promotion decisions. *Recognition* 2006;[1].

53 Harrison MB, Graham ID, Lorimer K, Friedberg E, Pierscianowski T, Brandys T. Leg-ulcer care in the community, before and after implementation of an evidence-based service. *CMAJ* 2005;172[11]:1447–52.

54 Hewitt A, MacArthur C, Raina PS. The role of evidence in public health policy: an example of linkage and exchange in the prevention of scald burns. *Healthcare Policy/Politiques de Sant θ* 2007;3[2]:59–66.

Section 6
Evaluation of Knowledge to Action

6.1 Methodologies to evaluate effectiveness of knowledge translation interventions

Onil Bhattacharyya[1] and Merrick Zwarenstein[2]

[1]Li Ka Shing Knowledge Institute, St. Michael's Hospital, and Department of Family and Community Medicine, University of Toronto, Toronto, OR, Canada

[2]Sunnybrook Research Institute, Sunnybrook Health Sciences Center; Department of Health Policy Management and Evaluation, University of Toronto; and Institute for Clinical Evaluation Sciences, Toronto, OR, Canada

---

KEY LEARNING POINTS

- The evidence base for interventions to change clinical practice is modest but growing.
- Given the cost of implementing knowledge translation (KT) interventions and their variable impact on practice, they should be rigorously evaluated.
- Evaluation studies should address internal validity, the degree to which an observed outcome can be attributed to an intervention.
- Randomized controlled trials provide the highest degree of internal validity, followed by interrupted time series, controlled before–after studies, and uncontrolled before–after studies.
- The degree to which results from a particular study apply to a regular practice setting is called external validity.
- Evaluations should be selected based on available resources, the need for rigor, and the interest in producing results that will be locally or generally applicable.

Evidence based medicine should be complemented by evidence based implementation.   Richard Grol

Knowledge translation (KT) promotes the uptake of evidence-based practices, but the methods used to promote these practices are often not evidence-based [1,2]. On one hand, there is pressure to improve quality of care using sensible approaches [3]. On the other hand, there is a dearth of information on which interventions actually work [4] and under what circumstances. The complexity of implementation research is daunting. It requires taking into account multiple levels: patients nested within a provider's practice nested within a multidisciplinary team nested within a health facility nested in local and national health care systems. The conceptual and methodological

---

Knowledge Translation in Health Care: Moving from Evidence to Practice. Edited by S. Straus, J. Tetroe, and I. Graham. © 2009 Blackwell Publishing, ISBN: 978-1-4051-8106-8.

challenges are significant. These challenges are likely why the average impact of implementation interventions has so far been modest [5]. Furthermore, the conclusions one draws about the most effective approaches and how they should be applied in a given setting are also limited [6]. The Cochrane Collaboration has registered over 350,000 randomized controlled trials in clinical medicine [1] but only 2400 experimental and quasi-experimental trials of interventions to improve health care delivery [7]. The complexity of changing the behavior of organizations and service providers and the potential benefits of doing so warrants a shift of effort from the development of new treatments to developing approaches to consistently deliver what is already known to work [8].

Given the limited evidence base to work from, people involved in quality improvement have a responsibility to evaluate the effectiveness of their efforts [9], not only because many interventions are ineffective and may lead to a waste of resources [4], but also because evaluation creates knowledge that may benefit others. When considering how to evaluate the impact of an intervention, the first issue is whether we are interested in local or generalizable knowledge. The former is the concern of managers responsible for quality improvement in an institution, and the latter is of interest to KT researchers. Those who are interested in locally applicable knowledge (i.e., whether an intervention worked in the context in which it was implemented) should use the most rigorous evaluation feasible within this setting. These designs are subject to bias but are likely to describe what has occurred in the context under study. They include uncontrolled before–after studies, controlled before–after studies, and interrupted time series. Those who are interested in generalizable knowledge (whether an intervention is likely to work in comparable settings) should use the most rigorous evaluation design they can afford. These more rigorous designs control for bias and include interrupted time series or randomized controlled trials. This chapter will review these designs in detail and explain the benefits and disadvantages of each for managers and researchers.

Evaluation study designs

The questions of producing local or generalizable knowledge and the resources available drive most choices in KT intervention study design. The first parameter is internal validity, the degree to which an observed effect can be attributed to the intervention under study. The second parameter is external validity or generalizability, the degree to which results of one study in a given setting can be applied to similar settings [10]. If a study has poor internal validity (the relationship between intervention and impact has not been accurately measured), it cannot have external validity, because the question of whether this spurious finding represents what would happen in other settings is moot. Nevertheless, if the practice environment is carefully selected and controlled to accurately measure the relationship between intervention and observed impact, it may not represent what would happen if the intervention were implemented in a regular practice setting. We will first discuss the elements of study design that establish internal validity and then elements that establish external validity.

Establishing internal validity

There are many reasons why an intervention may appear effective when it is not. For example, a treatment for the common cold may seem to work because a person is cured a few days after taking it. The clinical improvement may be due to the treatment's effect or to the natural course of a self-limited disease that lasts a few days. Similarly, quality of care in a given department may improve after an intervention because the intervention was effective or because quality has improved consistently for several years or because a national incentive program was started around the time of the intervention. The purpose of most evaluation studies is to determine whether there has been improvement in the outcome of interest and whether this improvement is due to the intervention under study.

The two broad categories of study design are randomized, as in randomized controlled trial, and nonrandomized or quasi-experimental designs [11]. In this section, we describe various randomized trial designs and three types of nonrandomized studies: uncontrolled before and after, controlled before and after, and interrupted time series. Randomized studies are logistically more demanding but provide more reliable results, while nonrandomized studies can be implemented more easily and are appropriate when randomization is not possible. We will describe the various design considerations in each study type.

Randomized designs
Randomized controlled trials are considered the gold standard for assessing causality and for evaluating the impact of an intervention [12]. As illustrated in Figure 6.1.1, units can be randomized to an intervention or usual care. This design controls for many of the confounders that may influence the perceived impact of a treatment or other intervention. For example, intervention groups may not be comparable at baseline, so if outcomes differ at the end of the study, this might be due to intrinsic differences between groups rather than the intervention. With randomization individuals have

an equal chance of being in one group or another and thus are more likely to be similar. Those who measure outcomes may feel that the intervention is effective, which may bias their measurement in favor of the intervention. By blinding observers to the allocation of a group (intervention or control), one is able to minimize this bias. The fact that a participant receives an intervention (and special attention) may result in a benefit unrelated to the intervention itself (the placebo effect). Placebo interventions can produce a similar effect in the control group, ensuring that the only difference is that one is receiving a particular intervention. Lastly, one group may improve due to chance alone, so randomizing large numbers of participants increases the likelihood that any observed difference is due to intervention rather than chance.

Randomized controlled trials have been widely used to test drugs, but they are particularly well-suited to testing the effectiveness of different KT interventions for a number of reasons. First, as noted in Chapter 3.5.1, the effects of most interventions are on the order of 10% [2], a modest effect that requires a large sample size to measure accurately (because this difference could easily be due to chance alone). Second, there is a poor theoretical understanding of professional behavior and behavior change, so it is more important to know if something *does* work rather than why it *should* work [13]. Third, there is limited understanding of likely confounders (e.g., age of providers, gender, organization of care), so it is hard to know if groups are actually balanced at baseline. Randomization increases the chance that groups have a similar distribution of known *and* unknown confounders. Lastly, quality improvement can be expensive, and there are substantial opportunity costs if ineffective or inefficient dissemination and implementation strategies are used.

Using a randomized controlled trial to evaluate an intervention opens up a series of design choices around number of comparators, unit of randomization, and sample size.

Number of comparison arms

There are multiple potential designs for randomized controlled trials, depending on how many interventions one cares to evaluate. Two-arm trials (Figure 6.1.1) are the most common and they can determine if an intervention is better than carrying on with usual care. Multiple-arm trials allow for comparisons of different interventions and assess the relative effectiveness of different approaches. If we want to know whether two interventions are synergistic, they can be tested in a factorial design, which compares either intervention individually or in combination with a control.

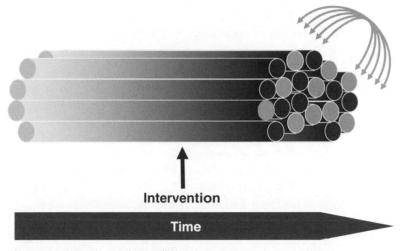

Figure 6.1.1 Randomized controlled trial.

Unit of randomization

In drug trials, patients are usually randomized to receive the study medication or a placebo (or active control). This may not be feasible in quality improvement studies. If the intervention is a change in organization of care such as introduction of an electronic medical record, then it may be difficult to include some patients and not others within the same facility. Similarly, if the intervention is an educational workshop for physicians, the physicians will not be able to apply the knowledge to some patients and not others. Contamination is another concern and can occur when participants in the control group are affected by the intervention, usually through contact with people in the intervention group. It is often easier to randomize intact units (e.g., clinics or practices), not only for administrative convenience but also to reduce contamination and because it may be the natural application level of interventions. For example, wards have been selected as the experimental unit in trials evaluating interprofessional collaboration initiatives [14]. Alternatively, clinics, communities, or physicians may be the unit of randomization. Box 6.1.1 provides an example where family physician practices are randomized.

Sample size

To minimize the likelihood of observing a change in outcome due to chance alone, randomized controlled trials must include a sufficiently large number of patients. When patients are randomized, this calculation is straightforward

Box 6.1.1 Can knowledge translation strategies be evaluated under conditions in which data on impact are difficult to obtain? CHAMP: a randomized trial to test academic outreach

Childhood asthma is common in Cape Town, a province of South Africa, but is underdiagnosed by general practitioners. Medications are often prescribed inappropriately and care is episodic. We conducted a cluster randomized trial to assess the impact of educational outreach to general practitioners on asthma symptoms of children in their practice. We randomized general practices (and their patients, who in this system are loosely affiliated) in a relatively poor dormitory suburb of Cape Town, where mostly solo general practitioners, with little practice support, operate from storefront practices. Caregiver-reported symptom data were collected for 318 eligible children (2–17 years) with moderate to severe asthma who attended 43 general practices in Mitchell's Plain. One year postintervention follow-up data were collected for 271 (85%) of these children in all 43 practices. Practices randomized to intervention [21] received two 30-minute educational outreach visits by a trained pharmacist who left materials describing key interventions to improve asthma care. Intervention and control practices received the national childhood asthma guideline. Asthma severity was measured in a parent-completed survey administered through schools using a symptom frequency and severity scale. We compared intervention and control group children on the change in score from pre- to 1-year postintervention and found that their asthma symptom scores had declined an additional 0.84 points in the intervention versus control group (on a 9-point scale, $p = 0.03$). For every 12 children with asthma exposed to a doctor allocated to the intervention, one extra child had substantially reduced symptoms. Educational outreach was accepted by general practitioners and was effective. It could be applied to other health care quality problems in this setting, and it proved feasible to conduct a rigorous evaluation of the intervention in this difficult setting [21].

and depends on the size of the effect one is trying to detect and the power of the study or the acceptable likelihood of not finding a difference if it is there.

Sample size calculation is slightly more complicated in trials where groups rather than individuals are randomized. Patients living in the same community and attending the same clinic are more likely to be similar in a trial where clinics are the unit of randomization, both because there may be community-wide similarities and because they are exposed to the same set of care providers. This means that each person is not entirely indepen-dent, which increases the required sample size because less information is contributed by each individual. The degree of similarity between subjects within a group is captured in the intracluster correlation coefficient (ICC), and the degree to which sample size is affected is called the inflation factor [15]. Generally speaking, more power is derived from adding clusters than from increasing the number of patients within each cluster, so the benefit of recruiting more than 50 patients per cluster is small [16].

Nonrandomized designs

These designs are more subject to bias than randomized trials but tend to require fewer resources and are more easily done on a small scale. Measuring quality of care at baseline and then at another point after an intervention without a control group is better than no measurement at all, and can assess whether quality has improved. However, we cannot infer whether this is due to the intervention (i.e., whether it would occur without any intervention) or whether it would work in another setting. Managers in a given facility who are more concerned with implementation than evaluation may not be interested in these issues, but it is possible to use more rigorous designs with little additional effort.

Controlled before–after studies

If we are interested in testing an intervention in a single context, identifying a control group that is comparable will double the effort in terms of data collection but also provide a much more reliable answer (Figure 6.1.2). If there are multiple wards in a given hospital service or clinics in a practice group, it may be possible to randomly select one to receive the intervention initially; the second could receive it at some specified time in the future, provided it was effective. This strategy may be done for financial and logistical reasons, in addition to the obvious scientific ones. However, with a small number of units, it may not be possible to find groups that are comparable for measurable (and, quite likely, unmeasurable) confounders. The result of this is that the secular trend in the outcome of interest may be different in the two groups such that it is not a true control [12]. Nevertheless, a well-matched control should give a sense of secular trends and sudden changes and should be attempted if a randomized trial or interrupted time series is not possible.

Interrupted time series

This design uses multiple measurements before and after an intervention to determine if it has an effect that is greater than the underlying trend

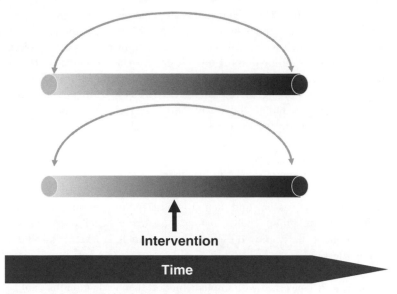

Figure 6.1.2 Controlled before and after trial.

(Figure 6.1.3) [17]. For example, in the United Kingdom, there has been a gradual improvement in quality of care that could be mistaken for the effect of an intervention if one was conducting an uncontrolled trial [18]. These studies are particularly useful when assessing an intervention where a control group cannot be identified, such as a national media campaign or a new policy that goes into effect simultaneously throughout a region. Box 6.1.2 describes one such study. An interrupted time series usually requires multiple time points before the intervention to identify the underlying trend or any cyclical phenomena and multiple points afterward to see if there is any change in the trend measured previously. From an analytic perspective, the number of time points and the time between each determines the stability of the estimate of the underlying trend. Time points that are close to each other are more likely to be similar than those that are further apart, a phenomenon known as autocorrelation [12]. Though more reliable than unbalanced controlled before–after trials, interrupted time series studies do not control for outside influence on the outcome of interest and they are difficult to do in settings where routine outcome data are not collected. This situation would require collecting data for several months or years before starting the study.

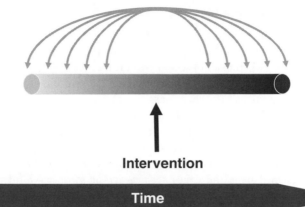

Intervention

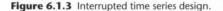

Time

Figure 6.1.3 Interrupted time series design.

Box 6.1.2 Interrupted time series of antihypertensive medications

The rates of diuretics prescription prior to and after the release of a major trial provide a natural interrupted time series experiment of media's impact on evidence-based practice. The intervention was the media attention around ALLHAT, a $120 million study with 42,000 patients recruited from 623 primary care clinics. It was a pragmatic trial intended to inform clinical and policy decision making on the best choice of antihypertensive medications. The study measured both long- and short-term trends in U.S. antihypertensive prescribing from 1990 through 2004 by extracting data from the National Disease and Therapeutic Index, a continuing survey of a national sample of US office-based physicians. Diuretics ranked among the top 3 antihypertensive drug classes throughout the entire study time span. There was an immediate but short-lived increase in the prescription of thiazide diuretics after the publication of ALLHAT in December 2002 that demonstrated the clinical equivalence of thiazides to ACE inhibitors and calcium channel blockers (CCBs). In contrast, ACE inhibitor prescriptions declined, accompanied by continuation of a pre-existing increase in the prescription of angiotensin receptor blockers (ARBs) (not studied in ALLHAT), whereas prescription of CCBs remained essentially stable after new evidence was released. The recorded long- and short-term trends indicate that evidence-based clinical recommendations had an impact on antihypertensive prescribing practices, but the magnitude of impact was smaller and of more limited duration than hoped [22].

Establishing generalizability

Pragmatic designs

The types of studies mentioned above vary in their ability to control for bias and to ascertain whether an observed effect is the result of the intervention in question. This involves having a sufficient sample size, blinding outcomes assessors and participants (where possible) to group allocation, and using a placebo when feasible. These all increase internal validity. However, even a perfectly valid study may not allow us to determine the degree to which a result is relevant to real-world conditions, that is, if a result found in one setting can be reproduced in regular practice outside of a trial [19]. Pragmatic trials are designed to maximize the relevance of results for real-world decision making, often for a broad range of settings.

Quality improvement and KT studies are often conducted by enthusiastic practitioners in supportive environments, and these conditions may have been essential to the success of the intervention. Expanding a successful pilot program to the regional or national level may not produce similar results unless efforts to maximize the generalizability of the study are taken. Pragmatic trials are the appropriate design for expansions ranging from pilot to large-scale real-world testing.

The use of broad eligibility criteria are a key feature of pragmatic designs, where a high proportion of providers or health facilities approached are recruited and analyzed. Those participants who drop out or who choose not to join studies may not be sufficiently motivated to follow through on labor-intensive interventions, so studies that only recruit enthusiastic groups may overestimate the impact in a general practice setting. Alternatively, motivated groups may have a high baseline quality, thus minimizing the impact of a quality improvement intervention because of a ceiling effect. The degree of implementation is an important factor when assessing impact, as an intervention may be ineffective because it is not feasible or acceptable in a given setting, and analyses should take these factors into account when extrapolating to other settings [10].

Summary

Given the time and resources necessary to implement KT interventions, there is a need to evaluate them rigorously. Complex strategies of this nature should be pilot-tested, and if promising, they should be evaluated in explanatory trials as outlined in Chapter 3.6.2 [20]. Randomized controlled designs are least subject to bias but require a large number of units (patients, providers, clinics), which may be logistically challenging. Controlled before–after designs and interrupted time series may be more appropriate when randomization is not feasible. Pragmatic designs also increase the confidence with which one can extrapolate to other practice settings. However, even when bias has been minimized, the wide variation in implementation of interventions and practice settings may make the results hard to interpret [4]. Limited descriptions of context and the intervention itself make it difficult to reproduce the study in another setting [5]. Ideally, qualitative studies should be run alongside the trials to assess degree of implementation and to give some insight into why an intervention was successful or not. We suggest that these methods be integrated to provide a richer knowledge base to move the field of KT forward and to increase the chance that evidence-based implementation strategies will be taken up in health systems seeking to improve quality of care.

References

1 Grol R, Grimshaw J. From best evidence to best practice: effective implementation of change in patients' care. *Lancet* 2003;362[9391]:1225–30.

2 Grimshaw JM, Eccles MP. Is evidence-based implementation of evidence-based care possible? *Med J Aust* 2004;180[6 Suppl]:S50–S51.

3 Auerbach AD, Landefeld CS, Shojania KG. The tension between needing to improve care and knowing how to do it. *N Engl J Med* 2007;357[6]:608–13.

4 Grimshaw JM, Thomas RE, Maclennan G, Fraser C, Ramsay CR, Vale L, et al. Effectiveness and efficiency of guideline dissemination and implementation strategies. *Health Technol Assess* 2004;8[6]:1–72.

5 Grimshaw J, Eccles M, Thomas R, Maclennan G, Ramsay C, Fraser C, et al. Toward evidence-based quality improvement. Evidence (and its limitations) of the effectiveness of guideline dissemination and implementation strategies 1966–1998. *J Gen Intern Med* 2006;21[Suppl. 2]:S14–S20.

6 Foy R, Eccles MP, Jamtvedt G, Young J, Grimshaw JM, Baker R. What do we know about how to do audit and feedback? Pitfalls in applying evidence from a systematic review. *BMC Health Serv Res* 2005;5[1]:50.

7 Salzwedel D. *Effective Practice and Organization of Care*. Ottawa, Ontario, Canada: Cochrane Collaboration; 2007.

8 Woolf SH, Johnson RE. The break-even point: when medical advances are less important than improving the fidelity with which they are delivered. *Ann Fam Med* 2005;3[6]:545–52.

9 Lynn J, Baily MA, Bottrell M, Jennings B, Levine RJ, Davidoff F, et al. The ethics of using quality improvement methods in health care. *Ann Intern Med* 2007;146[9]:666–73.

10 Eldridge S, Ashby D, Bennett C, Wakelin M, Feder G. Internal and external validity of cluster randomised trials: systematic review of recent trials [Miscellaneous]. *BMJ* 2008;336:876–84.

11 Campbell DT, Stanley JC. *Experimental and Quasi-Experimental Designs for Research*. Rand McNally and Co.; 1966.

12 Eccles M, Grimshaw J, Campbell M, Ramsay C. Research designs for studies evaluating the effectiveness of change and improvement strategies. *Qual Saf Health Care* 2003;12[1]:47–52.

13 Bhattacharyya O, Reeves S, Garfinkel S, Zwarenstein M. Designing theoretically-informed implementation interventions: fine in theory, but evidence of effectiveness in practice is needed. *Impl Sci* 2006;1[1]:5.

14 Zwarenstein M, Reeves S, Russell A, Kenaszchuk C, Conn LG, Miller KL, et al. Structuring communication relationships for interprofessional teamwork (SCRIPT): a cluster randomized controlled trial. *Trials* 2007;8:23.

15 Reading R, Harvey I, Mclean M. Cluster randomised trials in maternal and child health: implications for power and sample size. *Arch Dis Child* 2000;82[1]:79–83.

16 Eccles M, Grimshaw J, Campbell M, Ramsay C. Research designs for studies evaluating the effectiveness of change and improvement strategies. *Qual Saf Health Care* 2003;12[1]:47–52.

17 Cook TD, Campbell DT. *Causal inference and the language of experimentation. Quasi-Experimentation: Design and Analysis Issues for Field Settings*. Boston: Houghton Mifflin Co.; 1979.

18 Campbell S, Reeves D, Kontopantelis E, Middleton E, Sibbald B, Roland M. Quality of primary care in England with the introduction of pay for performance. *N Engl J Med* 2007;357[2]:181–90.

19 Tunis SR, Stryer DB, Clancy CM. Practical clinical trials: increasing the value of clinical research for decision making in clinical and health policy. *JAMA* 2003;290[12]:1624–32.

20 Campbell M, Fitzpatrick R, Haines A, Kinmonth AL, Sandercock P, Spiegelhalter D, et al. Framework for design and evaluation of complex interventions to improve health. *BMJ* 2000;321[7262]:694–6.

21 Zwarenstein M, Bheekie A, Lombard C, Swingler G, Ehrlich R, Eccles M, et al. Educational outreach to general practitioners reduces children's asthma symptoms: a cluster randomised controlled trial. *Impl Sci* 2007;2:30.

22 Stafford RS, Monti V, Furberg CD, Ma J. Long-term and short-term changes in antihypertensive prescribing by office-based physicians in the United States. *Hypertension* 2006;48[2]:213–8.

6.2 Economic evaluation of knowledge-to-action interventions

Deborah J. Kenny[1], Evelyn Cornelissen[2], and Craig Mitton[3]

[1] TriService Nursing Research Program, Uniformed Services, University of the Health Sciences, Bethesda, MD, USA
[2] Faculty of Health and Social Development, University of British Columbia–Okanagan, Kelowna, BC, Canada
[3] Heath Services Priority Setting, University of British Columbia–Okanagan, Kelowna, BC, Canada

---

KEY LEARNING POINTS

- Economic evaluation should be part of any knowledge translation (KT) implementation given the financial constraints in health care.
- Economic evaluation can include cost–benefit analysis, cost–utility analysis, and cost-effectiveness analysis.

Economic evaluation of clinical interventions is vital in a health care system where resources are finite and the corporate bottom line is at the forefront. Increasingly, clinical decisions and policy will be led by economic factors [1]. As the translation of knowledge to practice becomes more prevalent, so does the need to quantify improvements in care based on implementation of evidence-based clinical guidelines [2,3]. Current conventional wisdom suggests that practice guideline use can result in improved practice and patient outcomes; however, empirical evidence of improved outcomes or of cost-effectiveness has not often been provided.

Economic evaluation has been defined as the "comparative analysis of alternative courses of action in terms of both their costs and consequences" [4]. The rationale for conducting an economic evaluation generally has to do with resource scarcity: resource demand exceeds resource availability so choices must be made between competing demands for limited resources. Economic techniques help define these choices and provide an indication of value for resources spent.

Three main types of economic evaluation [5] can beconsidered in knowledge translation (KT):

Knowledge Translation in Health Care: Moving from Evidence to Practice. Edited by S. Straus, J. Tetroe, and I. Graham. © 2009 Blackwell Publishing, ISBN: 978-1-4051-8106-8.

1 If the interest is in determining how best to deliver a given service (or intervention) once a decision has been made to fund that service, the question asked is one of technical efficiency, and the appropriate type of evaluation is a *cost-effectiveness analysis*. In these studies, outcomes are generally measured in "natural units," such as life years gained or number of cases detected. The outcome depends on the anticipated effects of the intervention. For example, Mortimer et al. [6], who developed an economic evaluation protocol alongside a trial examining implementation of a low back pain clinical practice guideline, chose x-ray referrals and disability level as outcome measures.

2 If faced with determining whether to fund a given intervention or alternative resource uses that could potentially affect different client groups, the question is one of allocative efficiency, and the appropriate type of evaluation is *cost–benefit analysis*. In these studies, the decision maker attempts to discern the "worthwhileness" of a given intervention, which can only be done when explicitly considering the costs and benefits across competing demands for resources. Mekhail, Aeschbach, and Stanton-Hicks [7] performed a cost–benefit analysis of two types of neurostimulation for patients experiencing chronic pain. Their outcome measures included professional and facility fees as well as medical savings and utilization of patient health care resources for all patients.

3 The third type of economic evaluation is *cost–utility analysis*, which can be used to address questions of either technical or allocative efficiency. It is used when the intervention effect has two or more important dimensions, for example, benefit and side effect [8]. Here the unit of benefit is typically the quality adjusted life year, QALY, which considers both length and quality of life.

Quality of economic evaluations in KT

There is a clear need to understand how to quantify improvements in quality of care that might result from specific KT strategies. Cost-effectiveness data should be included in clinical practice guidelines to inform decision making regarding their use [9,10]. Starfield, Hyde, Gervas, and Heath [11] believe cost analyses estimates should be subsumed in prevention guideline recommendations. Williams, McIver, Moore, and Bryan [12] reported that practitioners hesitated to use economic information in guideline development for several reasons, including a limited ability to understand or interpret cost-effectiveness information, as well as the means to appraise cost analyses for use in clinical decision making.

Inconsistent application of appropriate methodology to determine the effectiveness of clinical guidelines is problematic in the use of economic evaluation for KT. Coyle and Graham reported that 4% of guidelines identified measurable economic outcomes [13]. Vetter [14] evaluated the chronic pain medicine literature and found some type of economic evaluation in only 142 of 1822 potentially relevant citations. His analysis found that, over time, economic analysis is becoming more prevalent, but there is a need for methodological consistency when considering economic results. Also, in a review of the literature on interventions aimed at improving physical activity, Hagberg and Lindholm [15] found methodological weaknesses in analyses of all articles they reviewed. Because of the above limitations, inaccurate assumptions are made about the positive value of certain health care interventions [16].

There have been several projects designed to help determine clinical effectiveness of guideline implementation. For example, the Agency for Healthcare Research and Quality's (AHRQ) National Guideline Clearinghouse (NGC) includes cost analysis in its clinical guidelines templates; however, we identified useful cost-effectiveness data was found in only 20% of a random selection of 100 guidelines, and when it was available it often did not provide specific cost information [17]. The NHS Economic Evaluation Database (NHS EED) was commissioned to enhance access to economic information of health interventions. Structured criteria are used to select studies for critical appraisal. To date, the database contains over 7000 abstracts containing economic evaluations [18]. However, this database contains economic data pertaining to studies and not specifically KT studies. We examined a random sample of 100 syntheses of cost and benefits in the NHS EED and found many economic evaluations of appraised studies contained flaws such as exclusion of indirect costs, failure to perform sensitivity analyses, not reporting the price year for extrapolation of future costs, and nongeneralizability of cost factors for the studies. Use of templates such as that the questions for economic examination suggested by Kernick [1] or Mason et al. [8] is needed and may help prevent the flaws we identified.

The role of economic evaluation in allocating health care resources

Once the appropriate form of economic evaluation is determined, the next step is to determine relevant "costs" and "benefits." Direct costs include resources consumed by the intervention and can be borne by the health care system, community, and/or client/family [4]. Indirect costs include time consumed (and thereby productivity losses) as a result of the intervention [4]. In KT, relevant "direct" costs include anything from intervention development to implementation that requires financial or human resources. Broader "societal" costs are also often relevant. These include costs borne by the client affected by a practice change due to a specific intervention. These costs can include lost productivity due to missed work (indirect costs) and prescriptions or alternative care not covered by provincial health insurance (direct costs). In KT, these broader costs also include those borne by participants in an intervention, for example, lost productivity (indirect costs) due to missed work to attend a workshop. These "indirect" costs are critical when assessing the total costs of a specific intervention. The perspective or viewpoint taken—for example, individual client, institutional, community, or societal—will determine costs and benefits considered in the economic analysis.

Some health economists advocate the use of incremental ratios when attempting to quantify the benefits gained in relation to resources spent. This process may entail determining costs and benefits associated with various phases of an intervention, such as development, dissemination, and implementation, and then comparing the change in costs to the change in benefits/outcomes. As an alternative to ratios, economic evaluation of the application of research results may be better suited to a "balance sheet approach" where costs and benefits are listed for the various phases of the intervention, and also for usual practice, but an actual ratio is not calculated [19].

KT can play a significant role in informing priority setting when allocating health care resources. Decision makers need to be informed of relevant and current evidence-based practices, clinical practice guidelines, and relevant economic and other evidence to make evidence-informed decisions regarding resource allocations. It is important to assess both resource use and expected benefits of various interventions. This is challenged at a system level by the multiple dimensions and multitude of effects of a particular intervention. These include the change in clinician practice and health outcome changes at the client level attributed to the change in care. In addition, interpreting the results from an economic evaluation is not always straightforward, particularly for allocative efficiency questions where the decision maker is faced with determining how much a given initiative is worth in terms of the expected return for that investment. Nevertheless, much of economics is about providing a way of thinking about, rather than a definitive solution to, a particular problem. When thought of in this way, economic evaluation can be an important methodological tool to use when developing and evaluating interventions. Alternatively, the KT process is important to consider in priority-setting activities.

Future research

Further work is needed to investigate the state of the science of economic evaluation of KT to determine parameters for evaluation, to make recommendations for appraisal of implementation studies, and to determine how best to influence the use of existing templates for economic evaluation.

Summary

There is a growing literature base on the importance of economic evaluation of health care interventions, but there are few published studies that link economic evaluation to the implementation of evidence-based guidelines. Economic evaluations, if included in study reports, often contain methodological flaws, and many health care providers are not adept at performing or understanding the many methods of evaluating the costs and/or benefits of practice interventions.

Disclaimer

The views and opinions expressed in this article are solely those of the authors and do not reflect the policy or position of the Department of the Army, the Department of Defense, or the US government.

References

1 Kernick DP. Economic evaluation in health: a thumb nail sketch. *BMJ* 1998; 316[7145]:1663–5.
2 Kennedy N, Stokes E. Discussion paper: why physiotherapy needs economics. *Physical Therapy Reviews* 2003;8:27–30.
3 Ramsey SD, Sullivan SD. Weighing the economic evidence: guidelines for critical assessment of cost-effectiveness analyses. *J Am Board Fam Pract* 1999;12[6]:477–85.
4 Drummond M, Sculpher M, Torrance G, O'Brien B, Stoddart G. *Methods for the Economic Evaluation of Health Care Programmes.* 3rd ed. Oxford: Oxford University Press; 2005.
5 Donaldson C, Currie G, Mitton C. Cost effectiveness analysis in health care: contraindications. *BMJ* 2002;325[7369]:891–4.
6 Mortimer D, French S, McKenzie J, O'Connor D, Green S. Protocol for economic evaluation alongside the IMPLEMENT cluster randomized control trial. *Implement Sci* 2008;3[1]:12.
7 Mekhail NA, Aeschbach A, Stanton-Hicks M. Cost benefit analysis of neurostimulation for chronic pain. *Clin J Pain* 2004;20[6]:462–8.

8 Greenhalgh T. *How to Read a Paper, the Basics of Evidence-Based Medicine.* 3rd ed. Boston: Blackwell Publishing; 2006.

9 Mason J, Eccles M, Freemantle N, Drummond M. A framework for incorporating cost-effectiveness in evidence-based clinical practice guidelines. *Health Policy* 1999;47[1]:37–52.

10 Helfand M. Incorporating information about cost-effectiveness into evidence-based decision making: the evidence-based practice center (EPC) model. *Med Care* 2005;43[Suppl 7]:33–43.

11 Starfield B, Hyde J, Gervas J, Heath I. The concept of prevention: a good idea gone astray? *J Epidemiol Community Health* 2008;62[7]:580–3.

12 Williams I, McIver S, Moore D, Bryan S. The use of economic evaluations in NHS decision-making: a review and empirical investigation. *Health Technol Assess* 2008;12[7]:iii, iv–v, 1–175.

13 Coyle D, Graham ID. The role of economics in Canadian clinical practice guidelines for drug therapy. *Disease Management and Health Outcomes* 2003;11:45–8.

14 Vetter TR. The application of economic evaluation methods in the chronic pain medicine literature. *Anesth Analg* 2007;105[1]:114–8.

15 Hagberg LA, Lindholm L. Cost-effectiveness of healthcare-based interventions aimed at improving physical activity. *Scand J Public Health* 2006;34[6]:641–53.

16 Niven KJ. A review of the application of health economics to health and safety in healthcare. *Health Policy* 2002;61[3]:291–304.

17 National Guideline Clearinghouse. URL http://www.guideline.gov/submit/template.aspx [accessed July 9, 2008].

18 Centre for Reviews and Evaluation. *NHS economic evaluation database.* URL http://www.york.ac.uk/inst/crd/crddatabases.htm [accessed July 2, 2008].

19 McIntosh E, Donaldson C, Ryan M. Recent advances in the methods of cost-benefit analysis in healthcare: matching the art to the science. *Pharmacoeconomics* 1999;15[4]:357–67.

Appendixes

Appendix 1 **Approaches to measurement**

Robert Parent
University of Sherbrooke, Quebec, Canada

Introduction

Linking what is known about health care to what actually gets used within the health care system to improve population health is growing in popularity, as recent articles about *linking knowledge to action* and *bridging the know–do gap* demonstrate. As Lavis [1] observed, however, although linking research to action has captured a great deal of international attention recently, statements and resolutions are easier made than acted on. This chapter provides a brief overview of some of the latest literature that attempts to shift the focus of knowledge translation (KT) toward the action or utilization component of the knowledge-to-action continuum. More specifically, we will discuss how both health care policy and practice can be informed and impacted by the best available evidence in a given context. We will also look at approaches to measure adoption of evidence and the impact it has on patient outcomes, including changes in policy decisions, clinical behavior, and patient behaviors. Finally, we will provide a KT capacity-building framework for assessing KT initiatives.

Linking knowledge to action or bridging the know–do gap

Most health care professionals agree that many more lives can be saved, and for many the quality of life can be improved, by better linking health care knowledge creation to action, including such activities as policymaking, clinical behavior, and patient behavior. Although there continues to be widespread debate within the health care community about what constitutes evidence, the issue is outside the scope of this chapter. Suffice it to say that there is a growing consensus among health care researchers and funding agencies that

Knowledge Translation in Health Care: Moving from Evidence to Practice. Edited by S. Straus, J. Tetroe, and I. Graham. © 2009 Blackwell Publishing, ISBN: 978-1-4051-8106-8.

more attention needs to be directed at how to move from the knowledge creation or generation component of the knowledge-to-action cycle to the action or utilization component of the cycle [2–12]. This does not represent a new rallying call since, back in 1993, Backer [13] defined knowledge utilization as "including a variety of interventions aimed at increasing the use of knowledge to solve human problems."

Since then, several different models or approaches for linking research to action have been proposed, ranging from early linear approaches (known as knowledge push and knowledge pull) to the latest exchange and network integration approaches. Linear approaches viewed knowledge as an object to be passed on mechanistically from the creator to a translator, who would adapt it so the information could be transmitted to the end user [14]. Within this process, the user was generally viewed as a passive actor or receptacle of knowledge, and the context within which the translation occurred was typically ignored. Numerous authors have criticized the linear model of KT for ignoring the reality of both the context in which the new knowledge was generated and the one in which it will be used. This criticism has led to a series of relatively new KT approaches, including knowledge exchange, knowledge brokers, implementation science, and knowledge mobilization. These latest approaches generally focus on the relationships required to bring change and improvements in overall health care. They imply changes within all segments of the health care system, including changes in how research is conducted, policy is made, health care is provided, and ultimately the way health care is consumed.

This modern focus on health care as a "social system" has led researchers, policymakers, funding agencies, and practitioners to look more precisely at what the system is trying to accomplish. A social system usually forms in response to a specific need by its members and is typically made up of individuals grouped in a variety of either loosely or tightly knit relationships (systems and subsystems). The purpose, problem, or need must be sufficiently complex to imply involvement of multiple stakeholders. In health care, the social system can take many forms such as a hospital, clinic, association, group of researchers, policymakers, and funding agencies. The number of social systems is infinite. To understand how knowledge gets translated within and between them, we need to understand the need that the system is attempting to address or the problem it wants to solve. For example, policymakers may look to how the country's health care system addresses problems related to constantly rising costs. To help it address vital health care issues, the academic perspective, however, may focus on the knowledge that the research community needs from the health care sector. From the health care provider's perspective, it may be addressing the question: what new knowledge does a pharmaceutical company require to meet the medication needs of the health care sector and thereby continue to compete in the global economy?

The initial identification of the system's needs is particularly important because it determines, to a large extent, the type of new knowledge to be translated. For example, saying that our society has a problem treating lung cancer leads us to generate and translate new knowledge for doing so (medical interventions). On the other hand, saying that we have a societal problem with nicotine dependence leads us to seek out and translate ways to prevent smoking (social and educational interventions as well as medical and legal means). In addition to clarifying what new knowledge the system needs, the initial needs identification also helps clarify the actors or groups that must be involved in solving the problem, as well as the current state of knowledge—both tacit and explicit—within the system. Finally, from an assessment perspective, it also provides us with measurable indicators that will ultimately allow us to assess the success or failure of a KT initiative.

Knowledge translation assessment

Assessment examines the outcomes of a health care policy, program of treatment, or project against original expectation. It ensures that lessons learned are fed back into the decision-making process. This ensures that a research activity or program, a policy decision, an approach to the provision of health care, and ultimately the consumption of health care products and services are continually refined to reflect the best ultimate health care for society. Most of the recent literature on KT assessment proposes the emergence of interesting approaches to bridging this know–do gap in health care, including Lavis' [15] model for assessing country-level efforts to link research to action; the USAID *Guide to Monitoring and Evaluating Health Information Products and Services* [16]; the World Health Organization's *Bridging the "Know-Do" Gap* [17]; the knowledge value chain proposed by Landry [18]; Lomas' [19] coordinated implementation model; and the knowledge-to-action process from Graham [20], which is the basis for this book. The overall characteristics or themes of most of these approaches can be summarized, in no particular order, in the following way:

- They focus on solving a health care problem.
- They operate from a systems perspective.
- They operate with different types of knowledge use [21]:
  1 Instrumental use
  2 Conceptual use
  3 Symbolic use
- They involve different multidirectional methods and phases.

- They operate using different levels and effectiveness categories.
- They refer to a dynamic and iterative process involving various components, aspects, and scales.
- They include not only recent research findings but also knowledge from the dynamic interaction of people who come together to solve public health problems.
- They attempt to provide core lists of both qualitative and quantitative indicators to consistently measure the impact of KT.

For a well-developed and timely introduction, readers may refer to Sudsawad's *Knowledge Translation: an Introduction to Models, Strategies and Measures* [22].

The dynamic knowledge transfer model

Clearly, evaluating the use of knowledge in health care is increasingly recognized as a complex, multidimensional process consisting of several events [23]. For Pablos-Mendez and Ramesh Shademani [24], "Translating knowledge into new or improved health policies, services and outcomes requires a clear understanding of the characteristics of this process, the ways it can be used, the conditions governing it and criteria to assess its impact." The variety of approaches to knowledge utilization considers knowledge from different perspectives or themes. Because of the complexities associated with knowledge utilization, it helps to have a comprehensive systemic framework to guide us. The dynamic knowledge transfer model (DKTC) by Parent et al. [25] suggests that understanding how social systems translate knowledge requires an understanding of the capacities associated with KT within KT systems. In this sense, KT capacities are prerequisites for effective KT, regardless of the process used.

The DKTC model advances a new systemic, generic framework to identify the components required for social systems to generate, disseminate, and use new knowledge to meet their needs. By applying a holistic, systems-thinking focus to KT, one begins to appreciate KT as linked to the relationships between and within systems—including their systems of needs, goals, and processes. This systemic perspective allows one to view KT from both how knowledge gets translated (the process) and what capacities the system possesses for KT to succeed. As all systems have limits, the model considers the boundaries within which KT typically occurs. In contrast to the more traditional KT models that describe KT as a process, the DKTC model focuses on the components or assets a social system must possess for KT to occur. As illustrated in Figure A.1.1, the model includes two pre-existing conditions (need and prior knowledge) and four capacities.

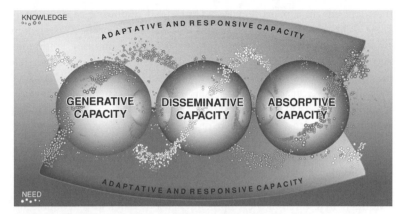

Figure A.1.1 Dynamic knowledge transfer capacity model.

The need that the system wants to address and the level of related knowledge that the system possesses constitute the model's backbone. In Figure A.1.1, tthese are illustrated with light and dark bubbles, respectively. Line porosity conveys that the four capacities are influenced by these two components at the same time they influence them. The continuous flow of the lines representing existing and required knowledge signifies that knowledge and needs are infinite. Once need and existing knowledge are identified, the social system needs to possess or acquire the four capacities for KT to be successful. By capacity, the authors mean potential for action or ability based on existing resources within or available to the social system.

Generative capacity refers to the ability to discover or improve knowledge and the processes, technologies, products, and services that derive from it. It is based on the system's intellectual and creative capital (which is present among its members), research infrastructure, and alliances. Disseminative capacity denotes the ability to contextualize, format, adapt, translate, and diffuse knowledge through a social and/or technological network and to build commitment from stakeholders. This ability is generally based on the existence of an articulated social network (social capital includes strong and weak ties), brokers, and other intermediaries, including the support of a technological and social communications infrastructure. Absorptive capacity, initially conceptualized by Cohen and Levinthal [26], is defined here as the ability to recognize the value of new external knowledge, assimilate it, and apply it to address relevant issues for a system's stakeholders. Absorptive capacity is typically found in environments that possess prior related knowledge, a readiness to change, trust between partners, flexible and adaptable work organizations, and management support. Finally, adaptive and responsive capacity refers to the ability to continuously learn and renew elements of the KT system in use for ongoing change and improvement. It is based on prior continuous learning experience, visionary and critical thinking, distributed leadership among stakeholders, multiple feedback loops, and monitoring mechanisms. All four of these capacities are necessary for a social system (e.g., network, organization, society) to translate knowledge successfully. A system wanting to translate knowledge must acquire or develop any of these capacities that it lacks.

The first three capacities—generative, disseminative, and absorptive—are central to the model. Their relative importance varies depending on the problem. In certain cases, the problem's complexity may require a significant investment in research and development, such as research for a new molecule in the pharmaceutical industry, whereas diffusion and absorption are less challenging. In other circumstances, diffusion may be problematic, typified by research findings that are published in scientific journals but never make it to the practice arena. In other circumstances, resistance to change resulting from cultural challenges may make absorption the main obstacle. An example of this would be the implementation of birth control in some countries.

The fourth capacity, called adaptive and responsive capacity, is a second-order or superior-level capacity, whose function is to reflect continuously on the appropriateness of KT activities within the system and to encourage rapid adaptations to environmental changes. For example, are knowledge brokers the best way to translate knowledge? Table A.1.1 illustrates the resources required, activities typically associated with, and results generally obtained for each capacity in the model.

Conclusion

This short chapter opens the way to a broader demonstration of the importance of striking a balance between knowledge and action in the KT cycle as a means of bridging the know–do gap. It also highlights the need for more attention to and research on KT assessment. KT is a multidimensional, nonlinear process that involves both research findings and knowledge created through the dynamic interaction of people who come together to solve health problems. Although attention should be paid to the knowledge itself, consideration also needs to be given to the purpose, people, processes, and capacities involved in the knowledge-to-action cycle. The assets or capacities required for a health care system to succeed at KT provide excellent indicators of KT success.

Table A.1.1 The Dynamic Knowledge Transfer Capacity Model

	Generative Capacity	Disseminative Capacity	Absorptive Capacity	Adaptive/ Responsive Capacity
Primary Focus	Discovery	Diffusion	Application	Renewal
Assets generally associated with each capacity	• Research & Development • Intellectual capital • Creativity & imagination • Advisory networks • Alliances	• Social capital • Social & technological infrastructure • Information technology • Knowledge brokers (translators, gatekeepers, boundary-spanners, facilitators...)	• Prior related knowledge • Readiness to change • Trust between partners • Flexible and adaptable work organization • Management support	• Prior continuous learning experience • Visionary & critical thinking • Distributed leadership among stakeholders • Multiple feedback loops • Monitoring mechanisms

Table A.1.1 (*Continued*)

| Activities generally associated with each capacity | • Matching stakeholder needs & research
• Linking researchers & practitioners
• Scanning external sources of knowledge
• Attracting creative leaders from different perspectives (discipliners, sectors, education)
• Creating "think tanks"
• Building alliances (expertise, "best practices")
• Inventing (externalizing ideas, intuitions, combining, experimenting, testing, revising) | • Networking, clustering and building commitment of stakeholders
• Brokering and negotiating knowledge transfer arrangements
• Contextualizing the new knowledge
• Adapting/translating the new knowledge to end-user reality
• Formatting knowledge (publications, activities, IT)
• Delivering transferable knowledge to different stakeholders (contamination...)
• Working with opinion leadership
• Developing iterative mechanisms to facilitate broad knowledge diffusion | • Recognizing external relevant knowledge to solve problems and/or address critical issues
• Managing stages of change
• Exploring the new knowledge
• Deciding to change (evaluation) and/or adopt the new knowledge
• Experimenting/combining/modifying practices, technologies
• Internalizing the new knowledge
• Utilizing the new knowledge | • Monitoring KT system
• Critically reflecting on KT "best practices" and mechanisms
• Exploring/comparing multiple KT systems' perspectives
• Combining/experimenting with new practices
• Upgrading or redesigning KT system |

| Outputs generally experienced | New or improved knowledge (codified or not) relevant to issues or problems:
• Concepts
• Processes/routines
• Technologies
• Products/services (patents, databases) | Knowledge adapted and shared with committed stakeholders:
• Transferable knowledge
• Adaptable/applicable knowledge
• Meaningful knowledge | Knowledge identified, assimilated, and applied by end users (other researchers, policy makers, decision makers, providers, operators, technicians) to solve problems and/or issues:
• Application of new concepts
• New integrated practices/processes/routines
• New technologies adopted
• New products/services in place | Improved knowledge transfer "best practices," mechanisms, and norms:
• KT practices continuously assessed
• Repositories of best KT practices and their specific context
• Processes and mechanisms of KT well adapted to context
• Culture of creativeness, sharing, trust, and learning |

References

1 Lavis JN. Assessing provincial or national efforts to link research to action. In *Policy Decision-Making*. Ontario, Canada: McMaster University; 2006.

2 Pablos-Méndez A, Shademani R. The role of Knowledge Translation in bridging the "know-do gap." *Global Forum Update on Research for Health* 2007;4:104–7.

3 Graham I, Tetroe J. How to translate health research knowledge into effective healthcare action. *Healthcare Quarterly* 2007;10[3]:21–3. URL http://www.longwoods.com/product.php?productid=18919&cat=492&page=1 [accessed May 15, 2008].

4 Graham I, Logan J, Harrison M, Tetroe J. KT Theories Research Group. Planned action models/theories to implement evidence-based care: a review. *Implement Sci* 2007 (under review).

5 Parent R, Roch J, Béliveau J. Learning history: spanning the great divide. *Management Research News* 2007;30[4]: 271–82.

6 Estabrooks CA. *Glossary: Knowledge Utilization Studies Program*. 2006.URL http://www.nursing.ualberta.ca/kusp/Resources_Glossary.htm [accessed May 10, 2008].

7 Lavis JN, Lomas J, Hamid M, Sewankambo NK. Assessing country-level efforts to link research to action. *Bull World Health Organ* 2006;84[8]:620–8. Available from http://www.scielosp.org.

8 *Developing a CIHR Famework to Measure to Measure the Impact of Health Research* (CIHR synthesis report). *The Canadian Institutes of Health Research*. 2005. URL http://www.cihr-irsc.gc.ca/e/30324.html [accessed September 7, 2007].

9 World Health Organization. *Report from the ministerial summit on health research*. 2004. URL http://www.who.int/rpc/summit [accessed May 7, 2008].

10 Estabrooks CA. Translating research into practice: implications for organizations and administrators. *Can J Nurs Res* 2003;35[3]:53–68.

11 Titler MG, Mentes JC, Rakel BA, Abbott L, Baumler S. From book to bedside: putting evidence to use in the care of the elderly. *Jt Comm J Qual Improv* 1999;25[10]:545–56.

12 Estabrooks CA. Will evidence-based nursing practice make practice perfect? *Can J Nurs Res* 1998;30[1]:15–36.

13 Backer TE. Information alchemy: transforming information through knowledge utilization. *J Am Soc Inf Sci* 1993;44:217–21.

14 Dissanayake W. Communication models and knowledge generation, dissemination and utilization activities: a historical survey. In GM Beal, W Dissanayake, & S Konoshima (Eds.), *Knowledge generation, exchange and utilization*. Philadelphia: Westview Press; 1986:61–76.

15 Lavis JN. *Assessing provincial or national efforts to link research to action*. Presentation made in the program in policy decision-making. Ontario, Canada: McMaster University; 2006.

16 Sullivan M, Strachan M, Timmons BK (eds.). *USAID guide to monitoring and evaluating health information products and services*. Baltimore: Center for Communication Programs, Johns Hopkins Bloomberg School of Public Health; Washington, DC: Constella Futures; Cambridge, MA: Management Sciences for Health; 2007.

17 World Health Organization. *Bridging the "know-do" gap. Meeting on knowledge translation in global health.* Oct 10-12, 2005. Geneva, Switzerland: Departments of Knowledge Management and Sharing, Research Policy and Cooperation, World Health Organization; 2006.

18 Landry R, Amara N, Pablos-Mendes A, Shademani R, Gold I. The knowledge-value chain: a conceptual framework for knowledge translation in health. *Bull World Health Organ* 2006;84[8]: 597–602.

19 Lomas J. Retailing research: increasing the role of evidence in clinical services for childbirth. *Milbank Q* 1993;71:439–75.

20 Graham ID, Logan J, Harrison MB, Straus SE, Tetroe J, Caswell W, et al. Lost in knowledge translation: time for a map? *J Contin Educ Health Prof* 2006;26:13–24.

21 Beyer JM. Research utilization: bridging the gap between communities. *Journal of Management Inquiry* 1997;6[1]:17–22.

22 Sudsawad P. *Knowledge translation: introduction to models, strategies, and measures.* Austin, TX: Southwest Educational Development Laboratory, National Center for the Dissemination of Disability Research; 2007.

23 Rich RF. Knowledge creation, diffusion, and utilization: perspectives of the founding editor of Knowledge. *Knowledge: Creation, Diffusion, Utilization* 1991;12:319–37.

24 Pablos-Méndez A, Shademani R. The role of Knowledge Translation in bridging the "know-do gap." *Global Forum Update on Research for Health* 2007;4:104–7.

25 Parent R, Roy M, St-Jacques D. A systems-based dynamic knowledge transfer capacity model. *Journal of Knowledge Management* 2007;11[6]:81–93.

26 Cohen WM, Levinthal DA. Absorptive capacity: a new perspective on learning and innovation. *Adm Sci Q* 1990;35[1]:128–53.

Appendix 2 **Knowledge management and commercialization**

Réjean Landry

Faculty of Business, Department of Management, Laval University, Quebec City, QC, Canada

Many organizations have developed programs to move knowledge into action. The primary focus of these initiatives has been on building bridges and partnerships between researchers and potential research users, and on adapting and disseminating research results to potential users in health service organizations. However, although such initiatives can improve the capability of individual health care professionals to integrate research knowledge in their practice and in the clinical services that they provide, it does not ensure that health service organizations are making the best use of existing knowledge. In this section, we focus attention on the various stages of the knowledge transformation process to shed new light on how value is created at every stage. How does knowledge transfer differ from knowledge management? Knowledge transfer is a process by which knowledge is moved from one party to another to develop or improve products, services, or practices. Knowledge management, on the other hand, involves four complementary organizational processes: recognizing or creating knowledge that carries high potential of applications, transforming this potential into actual applications (proving that the knowledge works in the real world and not just in a laboratory environment), sharing and communicating the proven value of knowledge to other units in your organization or to other organizations (this stage corresponds to knowledge transfer), and implementing or commercializing the communicated knowledge through the development of new or improved products, services, or practices.

The knowledge management approach

Knowledge management (KM) studies tend to adopt the organization as their focus of attention, thus looking at the capability of organizations to acquire, create, share, and apply knowledge to improve services and practices

---

Knowledge Translation in Health Care: Moving from Evidence to Practice. Edited by S. Straus, J. Tetroe, and I. Graham. © 2009 Blackwell Publishing, ISBN: 978-1-4051-8106-8.

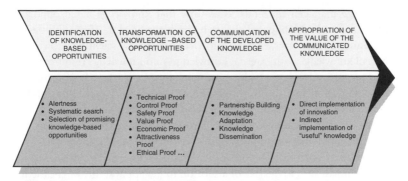

Figure A.2.1 Knowledge transfer as a value creation process.

regarding health care problems [1]. The assumption on which this section rests is that organizations that rely intensively on the use of research knowledge to develop innovation (i.e., to develop or improve policies, programs, interventions, and professional practices from research knowledge) have superior knowledge transformation processes [2]. This assumption suggests focusing on transformation processes that create value at every stage [3] and on ways to improve organizational processes that transform knowledge to add value to products, services, and practices. In this section, knowledge transformation processes refer to sets of integrated activities undertaken to transform knowledge-based opportunities into new or improved products, services, and practices. We suggest that organizations that transform knowledge to create value achieve four functions in a sequential process involving identification of knowledge-based opportunities; conversion of knowledge-based opportunities into new or improved products, services, and practices; communication of the developed knowledge to other units in an organization or to other organizations; and appropriation of the value of communicated knowledge through implementation or commercialization (Figure A.2.1). Each stage is made up of activities to convert or transform inputs into outputs. The ultimate goal of this process is to convert knowledge inputs into new or improved products, services, and practices that add value for health care customers. In turn, let us now consider different stages that make up this process.

Identification of research knowledge-based opportunities

Studies of knowledge translation (KT) tend to implicitly assume the existence of knowledge-based opportunities. By comparison, the literature on knowledge management tends to assume that knowledge-based opportunities need to be highlighted through the identification of possibilities of combining, in new ways, existing knowledge with new scientific knowledge, internal knowledge with external knowledge, and knowledge resources with other resources. However, highly promising knowledge-based opportunities may suffer from two shortcomings. First, knowledge-based opportunities tend to focus the search on highly promising research knowledge, whereas studies on the development of new products and services that show the development of such innovations usually require the mobilization of research knowledge in combination with other forms of knowledge [4]. A second shortcoming relates to the lack of attention to the applicability of knowledge (see Chapter 3.3 on adaptation), more specifically on the transformations required to convert promising knowledge to new or improved products, services, and practices.

Converting promising research opportunities into new or improved products and practices

KT and knowledge management approaches sharply differ with respect to their assumptions on the applicability of research knowledge. On the one hand, organizations promoting knowledge-to-action assume that to increase transfer, they need to forge more efficient interactions with users and to more effectively adapt and communicate research knowledge to users. On the other hand, the literature on knowledge management assumes that the KT assumption is counterproductive because research knowledge is not ready for application. Many studies confirm this second assumption. A study regarding the translation of highly promising basic research into clinical applications screened 101 articles published in top, basic science journals between 1979–1983 and found that: "Two decades later, only 5 of these promises were in licensed clinical use and only one of them had a major impact on current medical practices. Three quarters of the basic science promises had not yet been tested in a randomized trial [5]. Such an assessment suggests that promising basic science opportunities are almost never ready for application. For instance, it is not sufficient to establish an association between BRCA mutations and breast cancer (a case of discovery). There is also a need to establish the positive predictive value of BRCA mutations in at-risk women (which is about moving from health application to practice guidelines).

Research knowledge is about generic principles, but there is a gap between generic principles and their applications in the development or improvement of products, services, and practices. Filling this gap involves more than simple knowledge dissemination. It calls for the transformation of knowledge-based opportunities into viable products, services, or practices [6]. Gaining support and investment for the application of research knowledge requires proof at many complementary levels [7]:

1 *Technical proof:* demonstration that a concept (for a new good, new process, new service, new practice) is technically feasible at each stage, from theory through production and delivery to customers;

2 *Control proof:* demonstration of ownership of the intellectual property of the proven concept (for a new good, new process, new practice);

3 *Safety proof:* demonstration that the proven concept is safe and that it minimizes liabilities;

4 *Value proof:* demonstration that enough customers exist and can be served to clearly generate an economic or social value from the proven concept over time;

5 *Economic proof:* demonstration that a finished product or service based on the proven concept will deliver benefits in excess of their costs;

6 *Attractiveness proof:* demonstration that the current technology and final product, service, or practice fits the mission, goals, and strategy of the organization to which the proven concept is transferred;

7 *Ethical proof:* demonstration that the proven concept meets the organization's ethical criteria.

There is a need to judge, on a case-by-case approach, the elements of proof required to ensure that the developed knowledge moves to the next stage in the KT process. Demonstrating that promising biomedical research knowledge works in clinical practice calls for a successful translation from basic science research to humans (phase 1 and 2 clinical trials), to patients (guideline development, meta-analyses, systematic reviews), and to health care practice (implementation research). Likewise, demonstrating that promising health service research knowledge works in practice also requires a successful translation from basic science research to incubation in pilot projects, to pilot implementation, and to project implementation at a larger scale to replace existing services and practices. Chapter 3.6.2 describes a framework that can be considered for this approach in KT.

Communication of the developed knowledge to other individuals or organizations

Once the value of promising research results has been established, the next stage is to communicate it to end users. Knowledge communication is influenced by the relationship between the producers and users of knowledge [8–10]. Given the complexity of knowledge and the variability of receptor capacity of end users [11–12], knowledge managers need to answer three complementary sets of questions [13]:

1 *Partnership building*: To what extent did we interact, on a frequent and personalized basis, with end users regarding the identification of acceptable knowledge-based opportunities, technical, control, safety, value, economic, attractiveness, and ethical proof to build a strong partnership that is responsive to their needs and opportunities?

2 *Knowledge adaptation*: To what extent was knowledge proposed for transfer adapted for the recipient end user? To what extent was it presented: (1) In nontechnical language? (2) With examples or demonstrations of how to use it? (3) In documents or products that were appealing (attention to packaging, graphics, color)? (4) In reports on specific topics? (5) During discussions about the implications of the knowledge for use in the development or improvement of products and processes?

3 *Knowledge dissemination*: How did we disseminate the knowledge proposed for transfer? Did we: (1) Identify what (what part of) knowledge we want to disseminate (products)? (2) Identify individuals or organizations that could benefit by applying the knowledge proposed for transfer (end users)? (3) Identify individuals, organizations, or networks through whom we can reach end users of the knowledge proposed for transfer (dissemination partners)? (4) Identify specific communication channels for the dissemination of the knowledge proposed for transfer (e.g., newsletters, Web sites) (communication channels)? This stage also relies on knowledge of what strategies have been found to be effective. For example, as outlined in Chapter 3.5.1, printed materials alone are not effective in achieving change. (5) Dedicate time and resources to disseminate the knowledge proposed for transfer (resources and work plan)?

Appropriation of the value of the communicated knowledge through implementation or commercialization

Choosing knowledge-based opportunities is easy. Proving that knowledge implementation works is hard. Effectively communicating the increased value embodied in new products, services, or practices is very hard. Making effective value appropriation by end users is even harder. The fourth stage of the KT process involves the possibility of appropriating at least part of the created value. There appears to be at least two major mechanisms that we can rely on to appropriate value from knowledge-based opportunities: direct implementation of knowledge into innovations and indirect implementation of "useful" knowledge.

In direct implementation knowledge-based opportunities are turned into tangible routine applications. This stage is subdivided into three phases: trial, acceptance, and expansion:

1 Trial: the new product, service, or practice is adopted for trial evaluation. The adopters develop product demonstrators, prototypes, and pilot projects, undertake pilot production tests or pilot implementation. The product, service, or practice is adjusted to the particular requirements and competences of the receptor organization.

2 Acceptance: the new product, service, or practice is accepted and full-scale production and implementation are launched. The product, service, or practice is taken to the market for commercialization or implementation.

3 Expansion: the production and implementation of the new product, service, or practice are expanded and improved before replacement by another new product, service, or practice that creates more value.

In indirect implementation (meaning indirect or conceptual use of research?) of "useful" knowledge, transferred knowledge contributes to improve access to knowledge-based opportunities that are exploited or implemented below their potential value. The knowledge transferred through indirect implementation provides new ideas and hypotheses that contribute to improved access to knowledge, influencing future decisions regarding the development or improvement of existing products, services, and practices, but not to actual uptake of knowledge.

The knowledge and technology transfer literature has made a clear distinction between the creation and the appropriation of value. Organizations that create and transfer value through direct implementation into tangible applications are in a better position to retain the value they have helped create by relying on protection mechanisms such as patents, copyrights, trademarks, and confidentiality agreements. However, in the case of knowledge transfer through indirect implementation of "useful" knowledge, the organization that has created the value will lose a more or less large fraction of the value created because of value slippage. Lepak and colleagues [14] define it as follows: "Value slippage—that is, when the party creating the value does not retain all the new value that is created—occurs when use value is high while exchange value is low. Slippage obviously provides little incentive for a source to continue creating value in the long run." It is important to point out that value slippage may be socially desirable in cases involving public goods. For instance, value slippage related to improved use of research knowledge in medical practice may be desirable because it may create or increase value for patients, hospital organizations, and society.

Knowledge translation and knowledge management strategies

Organizations involved in KT appear to vary greatly on two dimensions: first, the strength of their capabilities to achieve activities involved in the identification, transformation, communication, and appropriation of value developed from promising knowledge-based opportunities, and second, the mechanisms and targets of KT. Every organization has some kind of KT strategy, although such strategies may not always be explicitly articulated [15]. Sheehen and Stabell [16] suggest that KT and KM strategies can be developed in three sequential steps:

1 *Positioning:* How is the organization positioned with respect to the identification, transformation, communication, and appropriation of knowledge, and how is the organization positioned with respect to mechanisms and targets of KT?

2 *Comparing:* How are other organizations using these positioning characteristics?

3 *Assessing:* Based on the strengths and weaknesses of other organizations, how can we improve the organization's KT performance by altering or reinforcing one or more positioning characteristics.

When considering how knowledge managers position their organizations with respect to KT mechanisms and to KT targets, we suggest differentiating two translation mechanisms [9]: the people-to-document mechanism that involves significant investments in information technologies and focuses on developing information systems that codify, store, disseminate, and allow multiple reuse of knowledge (as described in Chapter 3.5.5), and the person-to-person mechanism that involves moderate investments in information technologies but focuses on developing networks to link people to complement the dissemination of codified knowledge with the sharing of tacit knowledge.

Knowledge managers can decide to target either individuals or organizations. We suggest that when individuals are the targets of KT, the attention of managers is focused on individual attributes such as the level of training, motivation, and networks (interactions with people located in their environment) in relation to the development, improvement, and diffusion of new or improved professional practices. When such a positioning is used, the value created from transferred knowledge is predicted from individual attributes and the interactions between individuals and their professional environment. However, we hypothesize that when organizations are the targets of KT, the organizational attributes, the development and improvement of products or services, and the capabilities of organizations to manage knowledge from

Table A.2.1 Four KT strategies

	TARGETS	
Mechanisms	Individual targets	Organizational targets
People-to-document	Evidence-based professional practice strategy	Technology transfer or dissemination strategy
People-to-people	Community of practice strategy	Knowledge management strategy

the identification of knowledge opportunities to its appropriation into product, process, or practice innovations, become the managers' dominant focus of attention. This strategy may be more useful for large rather than small organizations.

Applying these positioning characteristics to organizations involved in knowledge transfer allows us to derive four emblematic KT interventions: an evidence-based professional practice strategy; a community of practice strategy; a technology transfer or dissemination strategy; and a KM strategy (Table A.2.1). Managers may use these positioning characteristics to assess their strengths and weaknesses in comparison with other organizations. Some of these distinctive positioning characteristics illustrate how various types of organizations and KT interventions share similarities and differences (Table A.2.2). These illustrations suggest that there may be significant strengths and weaknesses differentiating the four strategies portrayed in Table A.2.1. A more comprehensive diagnosis relies on a systematic benchmarking of all the strengths and weaknesses of an organization in comparison with other organizations for all the tasks involved in each of the four stages of the KT process. The results of benchmarking exercises help managers collect information on the specific strengths and weaknesses of their own organizations and improve the organization's knowledge transfer performance of their strategy by altering or reinforcing one or more positioning characteristics. Interviews would show that most organizations rely on a combination of these four strategies. However, we hypothesize that health care organizations that are effective in KT predominantly rely on one strategy and use a second or third one to support the first.

Summary

Looking at KT in organizations as a process made up of many positioning characteristics invites knowledge managers and policymakers to invest

Table A.2.2 Distinctive characteristics of four KT strategies

	People-to-document / individuals	People-to-document / organizations	Person-to-person / individuals	Person-to-person / organizations
Dominant knowledge value activity	Strong on knowledge creation and weak on communication	Strong on identification of opportunities and communication	Strong on knowledge creation	Strong on identification and communication
Dominant strategy	Evidence-based professional practice strategy	Technology transfer or dissemination strategy	Community of practice strategy	Knowledge management strategy
Exemplary cases	Institutes of Clinical Evaluation	University Technology Transfer offices National Center for the Dissemination of Disability Research	Cochrane Collaboration	World Health Organization World Bank

resources in the improvement of these positioning characteristics where their organizations are strong and in these positioning characteristics that constitute their weakest links in the process. Failure to improve the weakest activities may compromise overall KT capabilities and organizational performance. For knowledge managers, projects involving the identification, transformation, communication, and appropriation of value created through knowledge-based opportunities can be assimilated to experiments in which some projects succeed whereas others fail to deliver value. Failures, however, might provide opportunities for learning. A KM framework may help point to weaknesses in the translation process that will lead to strengthening weak links that, in turn, would improve the likelihood of success in other translation projects.

Studies on KT and technology transfer rarely focus on activities related to the transformation of promising research opportunities into new or improved products, services, or practices that work in the real world. Few organizations significantly invest in programs and projects aiming to prove that promising research knowledge works in the real world. Until now, most organizations have tended to invest in the creation of knowledge and its communication (adaptation and dissemination). Investing more significantly in proof-of-principle programs and projects will likely receive more attention in the future.

The KM framework developed in this section provides a systematic and customized approach to help managers assess the KT performance of their organization and identify the strengths of other organizations that would attenuate their weaknesses if remedial interventions were implemented. However, conceptual frameworks always focus on a limited number of issues at the expense of the complexity of the real world. The framework developed in this section should, therefore, be considered a simplification of reality that calls for further development.

Acknowledgment

The author acknowledges the financial assistance provided for this project by the Canadian Health Services Research Foundation and the Social Sciences and Humanities Research Council of Canada.

References

1 Landry R, Amara N, Pablos-Mendes A, Shademani R, Gold I. The knowledge-value chain: a conceptual framework for knowledge translation in health. *Bull World Health Organ* 2006;84[8]:597–602.

2 English MJ, Baker Jr. WH. *Winning the Knowledge Transfer Race*. New York: McGraw-Hill; 2006.

3 Landry R. *Knowledge Transfer as a Value Creation Process*. IAMOT2008 proceedings; 2008.

4 Amara N, Landry R. Sources of information as determinants of novelty of innovation in manufacturing firms: evidence from the 1999 Statistics Canada Innovation Survey. *Technovation* 2005;25:245–59.

5 Ioannidis J PA. Materializing research promises: opportunities, priorities and conflicts in translational medicine. *J Transl Med* 2004;2[5]:1–6.

6 Fontes M. The process of transformation of scientific and technological knowledge into economic value conducted by biotechnology spin-offs. *Technovation* 2003;25:339–47.

7 Lundquist G. A rich vision of technology transfer: technology value management. *J Technol Transf* 2003;28:265–84.

8 Rogers EM. *Diffusion of Innovations*. New York: The Free Press; 1995.

9 Hansen MT, Nohria N, Tierney T. What's your strategy for managing knowledge. *Harvard Business Review* 1999;March–April:106–16.

10 Argote L, Ophir R. Learning within organizations: factors affecting the creation, retention and transfer of knowledge. In J Baum (Ed.), *Blackwell Companion to Organizations*. Oxford: Blackwell; 2000.

11 Cohen WM, Levinthal DA. Absorptive capacity: a new perspective on learning and innovation. *Adm Sci Q* 1990;35:128–52.

12 Todorova G, Durisin B. Absorptive capacity: valuing a reconceptualization. *Acad Manage Rev* 2007;32[3]:774–86.

13 Wainwright DW, Waring TS. (2007). The application and adaptation of a diffusion of innovation framework for information systems research in NHS general medical practice. *Journal of Information Technology* 2007;22:44–58.

14 Lepak DP, Smith KG, Taylor MS. Value creation and value capture: a multilevel perspective. *Acad Manage Rev* 2007;32[1]:180–94.

15 Chesbrough H. *Open Business Models.* Boston: Harvard Business School Press; 2006.

16 Sheehan NT, Stabell CB. Discovering new business models for knowledge intensive organizations. *Strategy and Leadership* 2007;35[2]:22–29.

Appendix 3 **Ethics in knowledge translation**

Burleigh Trevor-Deutsch, Kristiann Allen and Vardit Ravitsky

Ethics Office, Canadian Institutes of Health, Ottawa, ON, Canada

---

KEY LEARNING POINTS

- Utility and justice are two ethical principles that provide the foundation of a bioethical framework for knowledge translation (KT).
- These broad principles should be applied in the context of KT through a number of ethical considerations, such as safety of outcomes, equity of benefits and harms, and ethical stewardship and partnerships.

In this section, we propose tools that integrate ethical dimensions into the broader knowledge translation (KT) discussion, thus extending the discourse from "what can be done" to ethical questions of "what *should* be done?" Ethics is already incorporated into the definition of KT used by the Canadian Institutes of Health Research, namely: "the exchange, synthesis and ethically-sound application of knowledge—within a complex system of interactions among researchers and users—to accelerate the capture of the benefits of research for Canadians through improved health, more effective services and products, and a strengthened health care system." This section outlines principles and considerations relevant to this "ethically sound application of knowledge."

KT involves important ethical challenges such as: What principles and values should guide priority-setting in deciding which innovations to promote or support? When is it safe to translate new knowledge? What types of outcomes should be considered and assessed in making such determinations? What are the responsibilities of different stakeholders in the KT process (e.g., researchers, research funders, knowledge brokers, policy makers, decision makers, and the public)? Which KT processes should be subject to ethics oversight and what mechanisms should be created for such oversight?

Knowledge Translation in Health Care: Moving from Evidence to Practice. Edited by S. Straus, J. Tetroe, and I. Graham. © 2009 Blackwell Publishing, ISBN: 978-1-4051-8106-8.

Ethical analysis and evaluation should be central to KT decision making, and a broadly accepted ethics framework would allow stakeholders to appropriately address such questions in a systematic and comprehensive manner.

Bioethics is a subdiscipline of applied ethics that addresses ethical issues raised by health, health care, and biomedical sciences.[1] It is a young, values-based discipline that attempts to analyse and explain the value-laden and often competing forces that bear on whether and how we develop and use new technologies. Thus far, bioethics has focused primarily on the upstream end of the "knowledge-to-action" continuum, that is, on knowledge *creation*. It has developed comprehensive and mature ethical frameworks for research involving human subjects and has begun to address the ethical and social aspects of setting priorities in research.

In contrast, there is considerable work to be done "downstream," where knowledge *transforms* into *action*. As the rate and power of output emanating from knowledge creation increases exponentially [1], those responsible for translating, adapting, and tailoring new knowledge to specific applications can be overwhelmed by the complexity of the decisions they face. This phenomenon has given rise to the new discipline of KT, which seeks to describe, systematize, and optimize the process, thus, closing the knowledge-to-action gap. As the theoretical framework for KT is developed and established, bioethics should join this intellectual endeavor by contributing an ethical framework for KT. This chapter constitutes a step in this direction.

The evolution of bioethics

In the past, decisions regarding health care, health research, and technology development were largely left to experts and professionals such as physicians, researchers, entrepreneurs, and policy makers. Since its inception in the 1960s, bioethics has brought wider perspectives to the decision-making process, first regarding clinical and research practices and then regarding priority setting and resource allocation (both in health care and in determining research agendas). It fostered the input of allied disciplines [2] (e.g., philosophy, law, and sociology) and played a role in framing and clarifying ethical debates around critical issues such as end-of-life decision and genetic engineering. In so doing, it has fostered informed public input into these debates. Thus, bioethics now moves from providing input into the ethical and social debate around knowledge *creation* (what research should be undertaken, encouraged, or promoted) to the ethical and social debate around KT (which innovations should be pursued and supported).

Moreover, bioethics began in response to notorious scandals arising from violation of research subjects' and patients' rights. It focused, at first, on the "individual" who would have remained vulnerable within the health care and research environments without the protection of standards developed on the basis of bioethical principles. This focus on the individual took up most of the intellectual energy of bioethics for 2 decades. Beginning in the 1980s, there was a shift toward questions related to societal perspectives such as priority setting. The vast body of literature that now exists in this area has set the stage for addressing the ethics of KT. Now is the time to develop a comprehensive and conceptually coherent bioethical framework for KT that will contribute to policy debates around these decisions.

A bioethical framework for knowledge translation

A bioethics framework constitutes one of the primary instruments of ethical analysis. It consists of the most relevant ethical principles and considerations that bear on a decision. Ethical principles are general values that underlie fundamental rules that guide ethical analysis [3]. We propose two overarching principles as the basis of a bioethics framework for KT: utility and justice.

Utility includes maximizing benefits and minimizing harms (known in the classical bioethical context as beneficence and nonmaleficence). Justice is a principle of fair distribution of benefits, risks, and costs. Thus, if KT is concerned with the application of scientific knowledge, then ethically sound KT should ensure that scientific innovations are useful in the broadest possible sense and justly applied. Echoing Gregory Larkin's (2007) [4] "calculus of utility and justice," we agree that "responsible KT would recognize that not all innovation is cost effective and not all science should be translated into practice without serious consideration of the social and economic consequences." Embedded within the principles of utility and justice are subsidiary ethical considerations that constitute the lens through which KT decisions and practices should be viewed and analyzed.

Ethical principles and considerations are often in tension with one another. For example, a proposed innovation may maximize benefits to a select group of patients but at the expense of other patients who are, arguably, in greater need. It is often not possible to maximize all positive or desired outcomes. Thoughtful bioethical analysis gives rise to well-reasoned, *ethically justifiable* solutions based on widely held ethically justifiable moral beliefs that are likely to resonate positively with a society that supports them. It does so by offering solutions that optimize as many ethical considerations as possible, while recognizing that others may be compromised, and explaining why.

Optimizing the outcomes of applying the framework requires a broad view of priority-setting that goes beyond that which may be held by individual researchers, institutions, or organizations. It is an "agenda-setting" perspective that balances maximized social utility considerations against social justice considerations so that the supported innovation can produce the greatest benefits and also allow the fairest distribution of those benefits. Such a framework should also contemplate justifiable exceptions because, although it is primarily utilitarian, there will be circumstances in which KT may violate relevant allied ethical notions, such as human dignity or non-commodification of the human body.

Our framework aligns with the emerging field of E^3LSI (ethical, economic, environmental, legal, and social implications of research).[2] This KT framework therefore owes much to E^3LSI theory but also broadens its current scope. Begun as an adjunct to the Human Genome Project, this growing discipline is now firmly positioned at the forefront of analysis of downstream consequences of research application, particularly, but not exclusively in the biomedical sciences [5].

UTILITY

From the bioethics perspective, the principle of utility suggests that any practice or innovation should attempt to maximize benefits while minimizing risks. The tenets of utility as applied to KT should, therefore, include the following:

- The planned outcomes of KT should be beneficial to individuals and to society.
- Where resource allocation choices are made between competing innovations, potential benefit to individuals and society should be taken into account.
- The choice between competing innovations should be based on achieving the greatest benefit for the greatest number.

Safety of outcomes

Among the key ethical considerations within the principle of utility is the safety of outcomes. Within a bioethics framework for KT, these should include the following:

- When determining which innovations to develop, decision-makers should take into account the broadest spectrum of potential outcomes, including unintended ones.
- Within the process of KT, all involved should adhere to the highest international standards of project planning, risk management, and quality assurance to minimize risks due to the proposed innovations.

KT decision makers and other key stakeholders need to understand the responsibility they bear to help avoid harmful outcomes that could arise from the inappropriate choice of innovation to pursue and of application. The history of science and technology provides examples of well-intentioned but misguided application of research. The thalidomide tragedy is a case in point.

Ethical and responsible KT should incorporate analysis of the downstream effects of innovation to optimize benefits and to minimize potential negative outcomes. A bioethics-based regard for safety of outcomes should, therefore, consider that unintended harms may materialize. Thus, in keeping with the maxim "first, do no harm," those responsible for determining which innovations to implement and how it should be done should consider the broad spectrum of possible outcomes, including social, economic, and environmental impacts, and should monitor these for adverse effects. In addition, once an innovation is selected for development or application, all reasonable efforts should be made to ensure that research products are as safe as possible, that all reasonable precautions have been taken to minimize potential harms, and that mitigation measures are in place in the event of negative outcome.

Confidentiality, privacy, and consent

Confidentiality and privacy need to be protected and consent needs to be maintained. Within a bioethics framework for KT this means that:
- Personal information regarding research subjects should remain confidential.
- The privacy of research subjects should be respected when seeking information or participation beyond that contemplated in the protocol in which the subjects participated.
- Secondary use of nominative information requires fresh consent unless original consent clearly contemplated ongoing permission to use the data in question.

Where data are derived from human subjects, the donors of these data have rights that decision-makers must protect, possibly for many years following data collection [6]. Although this has long been considered by knowledge creators, its downstream relevance to KT has become apparent only recently. Current thinking in KT rightly promotes more open-access reporting and data-sharing strategies to create an environment in which research ideas and partnerships can flourish. However, ethical issues arise. Increased ease of access to data across multiple platforms, coupled with numerous funding and infrastructure opportunities that encourage research collaboration and data-sharing, can severely complicate efforts to protect privacy and confidentiality of research participants [7]. Secondary and subsequent uses of human data and biological material, for instance, may not have been considered in the process of obtaining free and informed consent of research participants in the original protocol.

JUSTICE

Justice, as the term is employed in bioethics, means that there should be fair (not necessarily equal) distribution of resources among potential beneficiaries [8,9]. Therefore, we propose that the principle of justice as applied to KT should ensure that:

• Benefits resulting from innovations should be fairly distributed among individuals and within and among communities.

Equity of benefits and risks

Among the most salient ethical considerations to help in the assessment of justice is a regard for the equitable distribution of benefits and risks. Thus:

• The burden of risks flowing from KT should be carried by those who stand to benefit from it, and—to the extent possible—not by others.

No technology is without risk. Informed technology users understand and accept this. However, risk may extend beyond the user population, especially where environmental, societal, and economic impacts are concerned [10]. It is unethical to inflict significant risk on those who are unlikely to enjoy the benefits of KT. In many cases, it is not possible to control how and where the products of research are used; however, it is possible to take equity (who stands to benefit or be harmed) into account when making strategic decisions regarding innovation.[3]

Consider, for example, antibiotic resistance [11]. There may always be high-risk subpopulations for which precautionary prescription of antibiotics constitutes best practice. Overprescription, however, has a negative spillover effect on the larger population due to the development of pathogen resistance. This was a predictable and, possibly, avoidable KT-based harm. With the benefit of hindsight, we know that judicious KT should have included, from the outset, cautionary instructions for clinicians and health care seekers about the dangers of antibiotic overuse, resistance, and the potential for developing "super bug" strains that affect the whole population. Considering the equity of benefits and risks could have brought this issue to light.

The two remaining ethical considerations in this framework are more operational and relate *both* to utility and to justice.

Stewardship

- Decision makers and practitioners of KT should optimize the efficient use of resources that contribute to the process.

It goes without saying that the intentional misuse of resources is unethical [12]. However, stewardship also stands for the proposition that inefficient use or waste of resources is equally unacceptable, whether human, financial, temporal, or material. Similarly, not "translating" knowledge with the potential to lead to significant benefits also constitutes unethical waste. These assertions are based on an opportunity-cost rationale. Delays caused by inappropriately invested resources can result in real harm to those awaiting innovative treatments. It is important, therefore, that best efforts be made to enable wise decision making regarding the allocation of KT resources. This assertion is most compelling where KT is publicly funded because it involves a fiduciary duty to the public.

Partnerships

- Partnerships for KT purposes should be entered into where conflicts of interest and conflicts of mission are fully declared and adequately managed.

Given the importance of partnerships to KT, the question of whether a partnership is ethically acceptable merits specific consideration within this framework. KT partnerships may be complex, including researchers, institutions, professional organizations, public and private funders, and the non-profit and for-profit sectors. Relationships among these stakeholders can be fraught with conflicts of interest and of mission [13]. For example, a pharmaceutical company's existing financial or intellectual property interests will influence its choice of which innovations to pursue or promote in the context of a new KT partnership. This may be acceptable in a private-sector setting. However, a public-sector partner would have to consider the wider question of what is best for the public and whether the conflict of public and private missions is manageable. In addition, careful consideration should be given to whether a public–private partnership may result in inappropriate endorsement of specific products or companies. KT decision makers should be alert to such potential conflicts, ensuring they remain within manageable parameters.

Summary and future research

This section proposes a bioethical framework for KT based on overarching ethical principles of utility and justice and outlines several key ethical considerations to guide and optimize benefits while minimizing risks. The functionality of this framework lies not only in its enabling formal ethical analysis, but also in its potential to foster a culture of ethics in the KT community.

We have shown how the ethical framework proposed in this chapter departs from the E^3LSI family of analytical tools in its concern for the *overall* KT process. Although E^3LSI is primarily concerned with the implications of research and its outcomes, the framework proposed here adds a systematic analysis of downstream activities, such as the choice of which innovations to pursue (safety and equity), the appropriate use of resources in the process of innovation (stewardship), or the appropriate mechanisms leading to innovation (partnerships). This framework significantly broadens the established E^3LSI discourse and structures it specifically for KT practitioners: research funders, knowledge brokers, policy makers, decision makers, clinicians, health administrators, and others responsible for choosing between the products of research for wider implementation.

Future research and evaluation in this area could determine the framework's utility as an agenda-setting and strategic planning tool for KT. At the same time, potential unintended constraints on upstream freedom of inquiry, posed by misplaced application of the framework, must be monitored and addressed.

Notes

1   Other subdisciplines of applied ethics include, for example, business ethics, sports ethics, and military ethics.

2   Academic communities within this growing field may self-identify with one of many variations in nomenclature: ELSI (ethical, legal, and social implications) in the United States; ELSA (ethical, legal, and social aspects) in Europe; and GE³LS (genomic, ethical, economic, environmental, legal, and social) in Canada.

3   Note that in the context of research ethics, it *is* ethically acceptable to subject research participants to certain levels of risk even though they may not stand to benefit.

References

1 See, for example, Chapter 2 of the present handbook: *Knowledge Creation.*
2 Rothman D. *Strangers at the Bedside: A History of how Law and Bioethics Transformed Medical Decisionmaking.* New York: Basic Books, 1991; Jonsen AR. *The birth of bioethics.* Oxford: Oxford University Press; 1998.

3 Beauchamp TL, Childress JF. *Principles of Biomedical Ethics*. 6th ed. Oxford: Oxford University Press; 2008.

4 Larkin G, Hamann CJ, Monico EP, Dequtis L, Schuur J, Kantor W, et al. Knowledge translation at the macro level: legal and ethical considerations. *Acad Emerg Med* 2007;14[11].

5 Penders B, Horstman K, Vos R. A ferry between cultures: crafting a new profession at the intersection of science and society. *EMBO Reports* 2008;9[8]:709–13.

6 Tri-Council Policy Statement: Ethical Conduct for Research Involving Human Subjects. URL http://pre.ethics.gc.ca/english/policystatement/policystatement.cfm.

7 Knoppers BM, Fortier I, Legault D, Burton P. Population genomics: the public population project in genomics (P^3G): a proof of concept? *Eur J Hum Genet* 2008;16:664–5.

8 Marshall P. Human rights, pluralism and international health research. *Theor Med Bioeth* 2005;26[6].

9 Daniels N. *Just Health Care – Studies in Philosophy and Health Policy*. Cambridge: Cambridge University Press; 1985.

10 Hunt G, Mehta M (eds.). *Nanotechnology: Risk, Ethics and Law*, London: Earthscan Press; 2006.

11 Neu HC. The crisis in antibiotic resistance. *Science* 1992; 257[5073]:1064–73.

12 Auditor General of Canada. *Examining Public Spending: A Guide for Parliamentarians* URL http://www.oag-bvg.gc.ca/internet/English/oag-bvg_e_10218.html.

13 Atkinson-Grosjean J. *Public Science; Private Interests: Cultures and Commerce in Canada's Networks of Centres of Excellence*. University of Toronto Press; 2006.

Index

absorptive capacity, 273–4, 275–7
academic detailing, 124
academic outreach, 254
acceptability, of guidelines'
    recommendations, 76
acceptance, of new knowledge
    applications, 285
accountability relations, 222
ACE-I (angiotensin-converting enzyme
    inhibitors), 94–5
achievable benchmarks, 175
ACT (assertive community treatment),
    218–19
action
    putting knowledge into, 3
    strategies useful in promoting,
        199–200
    theories related to, 196–7, 198–9
action cycle, 6, 7, 59
action gaps, 68. See also gaps
action research. See integrated
    knowledge translation (IKT)
action stage, in transtheoretical model of
    change, 199
action-outcomes, in social cognitive
    theory, 197
activist learner, 207
acute bronchitis, decreasing antibiotic
    use for, 178–9
adaptation, 69
adaptation phase, of ADAPTE, 76, 77–8
adaptation theory, 169–70
ADAPTE collaboration, 75

ADAPTE process
    benefits of, 80
    core principles, 75–6
    guideline adaptation with, 77–9
    phases of, 76–9
    tools supporting, 76, 79
ADAPTE tool, 39
adaptive and responsive capacity, 274,
    275–7
administrative databases, 62–3, 65
adult learning, 209–10
adults, as goal-oriented, 210
adverse events, patient safety
        information preventing, 143
affective domain, of learning, 207
affinity diagram, 64
aftercare planning module, of ADAPTE,
    79
Agency for Healthcare Research and
    Quality (AHRQ), 263
AGREE instrument, 38, 39, 77, 78
AGREE Next Steps initiative, 38
ALLHAT study, 257
analytical thought, 200
androgogy, 209
antihypertensive medications, 257
applicability, of guidelines'
    recommendations, 76
application, of knowledge, 236
Appraisal of Guidelines Research and
    Evaluation (AGREE)
    Collaboration. See AGREE
    instrument

approaches, linking research to action, 270
arthritis self-management education, 141
articles, screening of full-text, 19
assertive community treatment (ACT), 218–19
assessment
    KT (knowledge translation), 271–2
    subjective forms of, 68
assessment module, of ADAPTE, 78
asthma
    monitoring tool, 134
    self-management programs, 141
    symptoms, 254
Atlantic Health Promotion Research Centre KT Library Web site, 50
attitudes
    barriers and facilitators involving, 87–8
    determined by perceptions of consequences, 198
    intention as a function of, 197
    related to KT interventions, 103
    as a sustainability factor, 169
Attitudes Regarding Practice Guidelines tool, 84, 86
attractiveness proof, 283
audit and feedback
    interventions, 126–30
    versus receipt of achievable benchmark data, 175
Australian National Institute of Clinical Studies, 238–9
autocorrelation, 256
awareness-agreement-adoption-adherence model, 115

balance sheet approach, for costs and benefits, 264
barriers
    assessing, 86
    to change, 98–9
    defined, 85
    identifying possible, 86
    to knowledge use, 83, 154
    linking KT interventions to, 99–101
    to physician adherence to clinical practice guidelines, 84–5
    taxonomy of, 87–8
    types of, 85
BARRIERS Scale, 84, 89, 90
Bayesian meta-analysis, 21
behavior
    barriers and facilitators involving, 88
behavior reinforcement, in learning, 208
behavioral control, 197–8
behavioral factors, 104
behaviorist approaches, to learning, 208
beliefs about capabilities and consequences, 103
benchmarking exercises, for organizations, 287
beneficence, 293
benefits
    determining, 263
    equity with risks, 296
    fair distribution of, 293
    maximizing, 293
Berwick, Donald, 228
bias, 20, 22
bias assessment, risk of, 19–20
bioethics, 292–3
Brett's Nursing Practice Questionnaire, 153
Bridging the Know-Do Gap, 271
bronchitis, decreasing antibiotic use for, 178–9
business process re-engineering (BPR), 145, 146
buzz groups, 118
Bzdel Resource Guide, 48

Campbell Collaboration, 16, 47
Canadian Health Services Research Foundation, 50, 125
Canadian Institute for Health Information (CIHI), 220–1

Canadian Institutes of Health Research, 291

Canadian Medical Association, 48

Canadian Neonatal Network, 238

capabilities, knowledge as, 216–18

capacities, associated with KT, 272

case examples, of KT interventions, 174–81

CDSSs (computerized decision support systems), 132, 134–5

Centre for Health & Environment Research KT Database Web site, 50

certification, maintenance of, 120

CHAMP, randomized trial, 254

change
  cognitive psychology theories of, 196–203
  modes of, 145
  programs, variable implementation of, 147
  theories, 185

change management interventions, 145

chart audit utility, 134

chart audits
  measuring clinical care against review criterion, 127
  practical considerations, 128
  questions to consider when beginning, 67
  reviewing and assessing health records, 65

cholecystectomy, by laparoscopic surgery, 219

chronic disease management, impacting CME, 120

chronic heart failure, primary care for, 94–5

CIHR KT Clearinghouse Web site, 52

CINAHL, 48

claims databases. *See* administrative databases

classical theories of change, 185

clinical databases, 65

clinical practice guidelines
  adapting for local use, 73–6
  barriers to physician adherence to, 84–5
  customizing, 74
  defined, 84–5
  developing, 36–7
  impact of, 37–8
  quality of, 38–9
  resources helping in the development of, 37

Clinical Practice Guidelines Framework for Improvement, 83, 84–5
  classification of barriers based on, 85
  conducting barrier assessment studies, 89
  extending, 85–6

clinical scenarios, in CME activities, 118

CME (continuing medical education), 113–14
  courses, online, 119
  current trends in, 120–1
  defining, 114
  process for, 115–16
  purposes of, 114–15

The Cochrane Central Register of Controlled Trials, 18

The Cochrane Collaboration, 16, 47, 250

Cochrane Effective Practice and Organisation of Care Group (EPOC) Web site, 50

Cochrane Review, of audit and feedback, 128, 129

codification, knowledge as, 220–2

cognition and task characteristics continua, 200, 201

cognition modes, 201

cognitive continuum theory, 200–1

cognitive dissonance theory, 101

cognitive domain, 206–7

cognitive factors
  related to KT interventions, 102–3
  role in predicting behaviors, 196

cognitive psychology theories, of change, 196–203
cognitivist approaches, to learning, 208–9
collaborative research. *See* integrated knowledge translation (IKT)
commercialization, 4
communities of practice, 220, 238
online, 119
community of practice strategy, 287
community-based participatory research. *See* integrated knowledge translation (IKT)
comparison arms, for randomized controlled trials, 252–3
competency assessments, of care providers, 67–8
complex adaptive systems theory, 169–70
complex interventions
defined, 160
external validity of, 163
framework for evaluating, 159–63
computerized decision support systems (CDSSs), 132, 134–5
concepts, in conceptual models, 84
conceptual knowledge use, 152, 156
conceptual models
assessing knowledge use, 83, 84–6
defining, 84
of implementing knowledge, 185
confidence interval (CI), in a forest plot, 23
constructivist approaches, to learning, 209
constructs, in psychological theories, 201–2
contemplation stage, in transtheoretical model of change, 199
contestable decision making, 222
contextual features, affecting audit and feedback, 129
contextual variables, affecting delivery of an intervention, 163

continuing education
versus KT, 4
research examining effectiveness of, 211–12
continuing medical education. *See* CME (continuing medical education)
continuous quality improvement, 228
controlled before-after studies, 255, 256
coordinated implementation model, 185, 271
coproduction of knowledge. *See* integrated knowledge translation (IKT)
cost-benefit analysis, 262
cost-effectiveness analysis, 262
cost-effectiveness data, 262–3
costs
determining, 263
fair distribution of, 293
cost-utility analysis, 262
criteria, displaying probabilities within patient aids, 40–1

data
analyzing from studies, 20–1
extracting from studies, 20
feedback mechanisms, for sustainability, 170
methodologies for synthesizing, 29
summarizing and presenting, 133–4
databases
commonly searched for health-related research, 18–19
national, 62
searching large, 48
decentralization, in organizations, 217
decision and selection module, of ADAPTE, 78
decision makers
diffusing knowledge through, 151–2
involving in complex interventions, 162–3

decision making
  enhancing uptake in, 24
  example of contestable, 222
  research evidence informing, 4
  theories related to, 197, 200–1
deep venous thrombosis and pulmonary
  embolism (DVT/PE), 176
Delphi procedure, 61, 97–8
Deming, W. Edwards, 228
depression, implementing guidelines on,
  100–1
descriptive theories. *See* classical theories
  of change
determinants
  of change, 109, 185
  of effectiveness, 99
  of sustainability, 166
development group, for clinical practice
  guidelines, 37
diabetes self-management education,
  141
diagnostic test review, 25
diffusion, 3, 185
  of innovation, 85, 89
  of knowledge, 236
direct costs, 263–4
dissemination, 3. *See also* knowledge
  dissemination
  of review results, 23–4
  strategy, 287
disseminative capacity, 273, 274,
  275–7
distance education techniques, 119
diuretics prescription, rates of, 257
DKTC (dynamic knowledge transfer
  capacity) model, 272–7
domain knowledge, 102
Donabedian framework, considering
  chart audits, 65
dosing regimens, 142
Dreyfus model, 209
DVT/PE (deep venous thrombosis
  and pulmonary embolism),
  176

dynamic knowledge transfer capacity
  (DKTC) model, 272–7

E^3LSI (ethical economic, environmental,
  legal, and social implications of
  research) theory, 294, 298
economic evaluation, 261–5
economic information, in guideline
  development, 262
economic proof, 283
education
  broad meanings of, 113–14
  conceptualizing as an intervention,
    115
  process for, 115–16
  purposes of, 114–15
  related to informatics interventions,
    132–3
  Web-based, 133
educational detailing. *See* educational
  outreach
educational interventions, 113–21. *See
  also* interventions
  active, 95
  aligning to the stage of learning, 115,
    116
  effecting KT, 116–20
  evidence for, 211–12
  passive, 95
educational materials, compared to
  patient decision aids, 39
educational outreach, 124
educational theories, 206–12
Effective Practice and Organization of
  Care (EPOC), 52
electronic brainstorming, 100
electronic medical records systems
  (EMRs), 134
eligibility criteria, 19, 258
EMBASE, searching, 18
end-of-grant KT. *See* dissemination
endogenous knowledge, 217
end-users, evaluating patient decision
  aids, 41

English language, as a barrier, 89
environmental factors, 88
EPC (Evidence-Based Practice Centre)
    program, 16
epidemiological data, 62
epidemiology reviews, 26
EPOC (Effective Practice and
    Organization of Care), 52
equity, in strategic decisions regarding
    innovation, 296
erosion, related to lack of sustainability,
    168
ethical challenges, 291–2
ethical or human subjects protection
    review, 229
ethical principles, 293
ethical proof, 283
ethics, in knowledge translation,
    291–8
evaluation schema, for CME, 120, 121
evaluation strategy, for KT
    interventions, 157
Evaluation Utilization Scale, 153
evaluations, developing, 156
evidence
    identifying, 46
    uptake at the point of care, 74
evidence-based clinical guidelines, 261
evidence-based clinical
    recommendations, 257
Evidence-Based Practice Centre (EPC)
    program, 16
evidence-based professional strategy,
    287
evidence-informed decisions, 264
exchange, 3
exchange efforts, 239
exogenous knowledge, 217
expert organizations, underperformance
    by, 216
experts, associated with knowledge, 216
explanatory phase, of the MRC
    Framework, 161
exploratory methods, 100–1

exploratory phase, of the MRC
    Framework, 161
expressed needs, 61
external communication, 106
external validity
    of complex interventions, 163
    of intervention study designs, 250, 251
extrinsic sources of motivation, for
    learning, 207–8

facilitators
    assessing, 86
    defined, 85
    to knowledge use, 83, 95
    taxonomy of, 87–8
feasibility, of an evaluation, 156
feedback
    delivery of, 128–9
    engagement level with, 129
    factoring into intervention design, 211
    higher-intensity, 129
    as important to learning and skill
        acquisition, 210
felt needs, 61
filters. *See* search filters
final production module, of ADAPTE,
    79
finalization phase, of ADAPTE, 76, 78–9
financial incentives
    providing to physicians, 95
    related to KT interventions, 107–8
financial interventions, 96
financial risk sharing, 107
financial sustainability factors, 169
flexibility, 105
flow diagram, 21, 22
forest plot, 21, 23

gaps
    bridging know-do, 269–72
    identifying, 61, 62
    knowledge-to-action, 5, 60–1
    measuring, 61–8
    reasons for existence of, 68–9

generalizability
  establishing, 258
  of intervention study designs, 250, 251
generalizable knowledge, 157
  versus local, 250
generative capacity, 273, 274, 275–7
GIN (Guidelines International
  Network), 48
Google, 49
Google Scholar, 49
grey literature, 19, 49
group sessions. *See* large group sessions
Guide to Monitoring and Evaluating
  Health Information Products and
  Services, 271
guideline(s)
  adapting, 74, 75
  implementing, 263
  quality, defined by AGREE, 38
guideline development. *See* clinical
  practice guidelines
Guideline Implementability Assessment
  (GLIA) tool, 39
guideline-driven care, uptake, and
  adherence to, 73–4

Hand Hygiene Guideline, 86
health care
  knowledge use in organizations and
    systems, 216–22
  as a societal system, 270–1
health care organizations
  knowledge use in, 216–22
  operating at the middle level, 145
health care provider level outcome
  measures, 155, 156
health literacy interventions, 138–9
health literature, searching for evidence,
  46
health technology assessments, 47
health-evidence.ca site, 47
heart failure treatment, improving, 97
Home Care authority, 241
hospital, identifying gaps, 63

hot water heaters, setting of, 241
HTAi Vortal, 49
human genome epidemiology reviews,
  26
humanist approaches, to learning,
  209–11

ICC (intracluster correlation
  coefficient), 255
IHI (Institute for Healthcare
  Improvement), 228
IKT. *See* integrated knowledge
  translation (IKT)
impact, of knowledge implementation,
  154–8
implementability, of recommendations,
  37
implementation
  indicators measuring for KT
    interventions, 98
  intentions, 198–9
  of knowledge, 236, 285
  process, 145
  strategy, for clinical practice
    guidelines, 38
implementation science, 3, 13
improvement evaporation, 168
incentive systems, 217
incremental ratios, 264
indicators
  becoming trapped by a system of,
    221–2
  measuring KT intervention
    implementation, 98
indirect costs, 263, 264
indirect implementation, of knowledge,
  285
individual studies, knowledge
  translation focusing on, 15–16
individuals, knowledge managers
  targeting, 286
inflation factor, 255
informatics interventions, 131–2
information behavior, 102

initiative decay, 168
innovation
  analysis of downstream effects, 295
  attributes of, 85
Institute for Healthcare Improvement
  (IHI), 228
Institute for Innovation and
  Improvement, 221
Institute of Knowledge Transfer UK Web
  site, 50
Institute of Medicine, 226
institutionalization, 167
instrumental knowledge use, 152, 153,
  156
instruments. *See* tools
integrated knowledge translation (IKT),
  239–41
intention
  to act, 198
  to engage in behavior, 197
interaction, between the presenter and
  participants, 118
interaction in professional teams, 104
interactivity, in CME events, 118
interrupted learning process, 118
internal validity
  establishing, 251–7
  of intervention study designs, 250–1
International Patient Decision Aids
  Standards Collaboration (IPDAS),
  41
Internet, searching for KT material, 49
interpersonal communication networks,
  124
interrupted learning process, 118
interrupted time series, 255–7
intervention review, 25
interventions. *See also specific types of
  interventions*
  defining in the MRC Framework, 161
  facilitating uptake of research, 95
  implementing clinical practice
    guidelines, 37–8
  promoting greater uptake, 147
  in a review process, 18

intracluster correlation coefficient
  (ICC), 255
intrinsic motivation, 207
intuition, 200
IPDAS Collaboration, 41

Joanna Briggs Institute, 16, 47
journals, publication in peer-reviewed,
  23–4
Juran, Joseph, 228
justice, 293, 296–7

Keenan Research Centre Web site, 52
key individuals, 105
KM (knowledge management)
  approach, 280–1
  defined, 280
  framework, 288, 289
  steps for developing strategies, 286
  strategy, 287
  studies, 280–1
know-do gap, bridging, 269–72
knowledge
  adapting, 73–80, 284
  approaches to disseminating, 237–9
  appropriation of value of
    communicated, 284–5
  barriers and facilitators involving, 87
  as capabilities, 216–18, 223
  as codification, 220–2, 223
  communication of developed, 283–4
  dissemination and exchange of, 235
  first-generation, 13
  funnel, 6, 13
  inquiry, 6
  linking to action, 269–71
  networks, 238
  as process, 216, 218–20, 223
  searching for existing, 53
  second-generation, 13
  third-generation, 13
  tools, 6, 7, 41
  transformation processes, 281
  users, 240

knowledge base, 147
knowledge brokers, 125, 217, 237–8
knowledge creation
    component of the
        knowledge-to-action cycle, 36
    funnel, 6, 13
    output emanating from, 292
    phases of, 6–7, 13
knowledge dissemination. *See also*
    dissemination
    defined, 236
    fundamentals of, 236–7
    knowledge manager questions
        regarding, 284
knowledge exchange. *See also* integrated
    knowledge translation (IKT)
    described, 239–40
    focusing on end-of-grant KT, 239
    integrating with mutual learning, 235
    uptake and, 13
knowledge management. *See* KM
    (knowledge management)
knowledge managers
    positioning organizations with respect
        to KT, 286
    sets of questions for, 284
knowledge push and knowledge pull. *See*
    linear approaches
knowledge synthesis, 6–7, 13
    approaches to, 15–16
    finding, 47–8
    qualitative versus quantitative data,
        21
    results of, 21
    types of, 29
knowledge to action. *See* KT (knowledge
    translation)
knowledge transfer, 3. *See also*
    dissemination
    compared to knowledge management,
        280
    defined, 280
    planning guide, 237
    as a value creation process, 281

knowledge use, 4
    approaches to, 272
    assessing, 153–4
    assessing barriers and facilitators to,
        83–91
    defined, 270
    differentiating from outcomes, 155,
        156
    evaluating impact of, 154–8
    frameworks for, 152
    impact of, 156
    key concepts of, 216–22
    measuring, 152, 153–4, 156
    models or classifications of, 152
    monitoring, 151–4
    sustaining, 165–71
knowledge users, 240
Knowledge Utilization Resource Guide,
    47
knowledge value chain, 271
knowledge-based opportunities, 281–2
knowledge-to-action framework, 5–7,
    171
knowledge-to-action gaps, 60
knowledge-to-action interventions,
    261–5
knowledge-to-action process, 271
knowledge-to-practice gaps, 5
KT (knowledge translation). *See also*
    knowledge to action,
        implementation
    activities, 236
    assessment, 271–2
    bioethical framework, 293–4
    defined by Canadian Institutes of
        Health Research, 291
    defining, 3–4
    determinants, 5
    ethical and social debate around,
        292–3
    ethics in, 291–8
    formal definition of, 3–4
    identifying literature on, 46
    importance of, 4–5

KT (knowledge translation) (*cont.*)
  informatics interventions improving, 132
  material, existing collections of, 49, 50–2
  model for, 5–7
  moving developed knowledge to the next stage, 283
  overlap with QI, 226–7
  as push, pull, and exchange, 239
  quality of economic evaluations, 262–3
  research, contrasted with QI initiatives, 229
  searching for articles on, 48
  searching for literature about, 49, 53, 54
  steps for developing strategies, 286
  strategies, 4, 288
  using clinical practice guidelines, 36–9
  using educational interventions to effect, 116–20
  using linkage and exchange activities to effect, 124–5
  using patient decisions aids, 39–42
KT (knowledge translation) interventions
  art of selecting, 97
  case examples, 174–81
  deciding to use single or multicomponent, 101, 109
  linking to barriers, 99–101
  linking to objectives, barriers for change, and theory, 102–8
  linking to theory-based factors, 101, 102–8
  methodologies inviting effectiveness, 249–59
  methods for evaluating, 156–8
  objectives for, 97–8
  research evidence on the effectiveness of, 95–7
  selecting, 94–110
  strategies for, 287

tailored versus nontailored, 109
testing with randomized controlled trials, 252
KT clearinghouse Web site, 48
KT Library, providing information from NCDDR, 51
KT Theories group, 194
KT+ Web site, 51
KU-UC (Knowledge Utilization—Utilisation des Connaissances) Web site, 51

large group sessions
  CME as, 114
  as educational intervention, 116
  formatting, 117
leadership
  related to KT interventions, 105
  as a sustainability factor, 169
learning, stages of, 115
learning domains, 206–7
learning experience, multimethod, 118
learning processes, in communities of practice, 220
learning styles, 207
learning theories, 208–11
leg ulcers, improving best practices, 241
librarians, 19, 48
licensure, maintenance of, 120
lifestyle improvement, identifying options for, 96
Li Ka Shing Knowledge Institute, 83
limitations, study and review-level, 22
linear approaches, 270
linkage and exchange activities, 124–5
literature
  searching for KT, 13
  searching grey, 19, 49
  searching health, 46
  searching unpublished, 49
Literature Database, of the Li Ka Shing Knowledge Institute, 83
literature retrieval, documenting, 21, 22
local applicability, of knowledge, 157

local context, adapting knowledge to, 73–80
local knowledge, versus generalizable, 250
local use, adapting clinical practice guidelines for, 73–6
Lorig model, 140–1
lowest common denominator situation effect, 69

maintenance stage, in transtheoretical model of change, 199
mass media campaigns, 138, 139
measurement, approaches to, 269–77
medical records
  patient-held, 141, 142
  underdocumentation of clinical actions in, 128
Medical Research Council (MRC) Framework, 161–2
Medicare, patients eligible for, 65
Medline, 18, 24, 48
MedlinePLUS, 133
mentorship
  models, 211
  programs, 208
meta-analysis, 16, 47
meta-ethnography reviews, 28, 29
metanarrative reviews, 27, 29
methods, promoting KT practices, 249
middle level, of care, 145
mixed-model approach, for reviews, 29
mobile phone technology, 134
Mode 2 research. *See* integrated knowledge translation (IKT)
models, linking research to action, 270
monitoring systems, for sustainability, 170
motivation
  to learn, 207–8
  related to KT interventions, 103
  theories related to, 196, 197–8
motivators, for behavior change, 207–8
multicomponent interventions, 117

multifaceted KT intervention, 101, 109
multiple-arm trials, 252

narrative synthesis, 20
National Cardiac Surgical, Vascular, and Colorectal Cancer databases, 65
National Coordinating Centre for Methods and Tools Web site, 52
national databases, 62
National Disease and Therapeutic Index, 257
National Health Service (NHS), 73
  Economic Evaluation Database (NHS EED), 263
  Institute for Innovation and Improvement, 166
natural units, 262
needs
  classification of, 61
  determining for CME, 116–17
needs assessments
  determining gaps, 61
  the organization level, 65
  of patients, 40
  using subjective, 117
negative feedback, 199
negative outcomes, 227–8
network meta-analysis, 25
networks
  knowledge use within, 220
  as mechanisms for knowledge dissemination and application, 238
  as a sustainability factor, 169
New York Academy of Medicine, 49
NICE (U.K. National Institute for Health and Clinical Evidence)
  producing U.K. guidelines, 48, 73
  promoting use of codified knowledge, 221
  tagging specifications for guidelines, 134
nonmaleficence, 293
nonrandomized designs, 255
nonrandomized studies, 157–8, 251

normative beliefs, 198
normative needs, 61
normative theories. *See* classical theories
    of change
NorthStar, strategies for completing
    chart audits, 66

objectives
    for KT interventions, 97–8
    setting for CME, 116–17
observational evaluations, 157
on-line CME courses, 119
on-line communities of practice, 119
open-access publication, 180
operant conditioning theory, 199
opinion leadership, 124–5
organic properties, of organizations, 217
organization(s)
    characteristics improving
        management of knowledge, 217
    developing strategies to increase
        knowledge use, 215
    entropic nature of, 69
    implementing knowledge within, 145
    knowledge managers targeting, 286–7
organization domain, of the NHS
    sustainability model, 166
organization level, measuring gaps, 65–7
organizational behavior
    health care themes, 145–6
    as a social science, 148–9
organizational capabilities, influencing
    knowledge use, 217
organizational change programs, 146–7
organizational interventions, 96, 144–9
organizational knowledge, creation and
    synthesis, 147–8
organizational or process level outcome
    measures, 155, 156
organizational perspective, on
    knowledge use, 215
organizational pluralism, 219
organizational resources, 107
organizational size, 107

organizational structures, 105–6
organizational theory, 215–23
outcome(s)
    classifying, 35
    for continuing education/continuing
        professional development, 121
    differences in clinically important, 177
    in Donabedian's framework, 227
    increasing focus on health care, 120
    primary versus secondary, 20
    in a review process, 18
outcome criteria, for chart audits, 127
outcome indicators, 155
outcome probabilities, Patient Decision
    Aid presentation, 40
outsiders, identifying problems, 62

panel of experts, reviewing decision aids,
    41
paper records, compared to electronic,
    66
participants, interaction at CME events,
    118
participatory research. *See* integrated
    knowledge translation (IKT)
partnership building, 284
partnerships, as an ethical consideration,
    297
Pathman model, 115–16
patient(s)
    barriers and facilitators associated
        with, 88
    high-quality resources for, 133
    improving participation of, 41–2
    informing, 95
    promoting involvement of, 137
    reminder systems, 133
    safety interventions, 142–3
    self-management, 134
patient decision aids, 139
    barriers to implementing, 42
    components of, 40
    defining, 39
    developing, 39–41

essential elements, 41
impact of, 41–2
quality of, 42
patient level outcome measures, 155,
    156
patient-centered tele-care, 142
patient-directed interventions, 96
patient-held medical records, 141, 142
patient-mediated interventions, 137–44
patient-oriented strategies, 138
PDSA (plan-do-study-act) cycles, 145,
    228
peer groups, 123
peer influence, exposing the learner to,
    116
peer support groups, 141, 142
people-to-document mechanism, 286,
    287
performance
    accomplishment, 197
    increasing focus on health care, 120
    target levels for chart audits, 128
personal health records, 135
personal visits, to health professionals,
    124
person-to-person mechanism, 286, 287
persuasive knowledge use, 152–3
PharmaNet pharmacy database, 134
physicians
    achievable benchmark data for, 175–6
    adherence to clinical practice
        guidelines, 84–5
    financial incentives to, 95
    forces for educational change, 114–15
    information-seeking behavior, 24
physiological feedback, 197
PICO framework, 17–18, 155
placebo interventions, 252
plan-do-study-act (PDSA) cycles, 145,
    228
planned action theories
    action steps, 192–3
    identified, 186
    list of, 187–91

planned behavior, 197–8
planned change, 185, 186
planning models, for change, 97
policy articulation and integration, 169
political science, views of health care, 145
political sustainability factors, 169
population, in a review process, 18
Population, Intervention, Comparators,
    Outcome, and (Study design)
    (PICO[S]), 17–18, 155
population level, measuring gaps at,
    62–3, 65
portable computers, 134
portfolio-based learning, 119–20
positioning step, for KT and KM
    strategies, 286
practice enablers, at CME events, 117–18
practice gaps, 61, 62, 66. *See also* gaps
practice guidelines. *See* clinical practice
    guidelines
practice level, identifying gaps, 62
practices, converting research
    opportunities into improved, 282–3
pragmatic designs, 258
pragmatic learner, 207
pragmatic phase, of the MRC
    Framework, 161–2
PRECEED model, 115
preceptorship programs, 209
precontemplation stage, in
    transtheoretical model of change,
    199
predisposing elements, in PRECEED
    model, 115
preparation module, of ADAPTE, 77
preparation stage, in transtheoretical
    model of change, 199
preparedness to change, 101
prescriptive theories. *See* planned change
primary studies, 13
priority-setting, 293–4
PRISMA (Preferred Reporting Items for
    Systematic reviews and
    Meta-Analyses), 24

privacy, protecting, 295–6
privacy regulations, for health records, 66–7
problem-based learning approaches, 208–9
process, knowledge as, 218–20
process criteria, for chart audits, 127
process domain, of the NHS sustainability model, 166
process evaluation, 157
process indicators, 155
processes-of-care, 177
production of knowledge. See knowledge creation
products, converting research opportunities into improved, 282–3
professional autonomy, 217
professional development, 107
professional interventions, 95. See also interventions
professional networks, 105
proficiency, stages of, 209
prognostic review, 26
Program in Policy Decision-Making, 52
Program Sustainability Index (PSI), 170
psychological theories
    constructs common to, 201–202
    using to overcome barriers to change, 100–1
public interest detailing. See educational outreach
public-private partnership, 297
PubMED, 48
pull efforts, 239
push efforts, 239

QI. See quality improvement (QI)
qualitative analytical approaches, 21
qualitative data, presenting visually, 21
qualitative evaluation methods, 157
qualitative studies, 162, 259
quality, of retrieved guidelines, 76
quality adjusted life year (QALY), 262

quality improvement (QI)
    assessments of, 228–9
    defining, 226
    frameworks for, 227–8
    initiatives as local in nature, 229
    issues and concerns in, 229–30
    merging with KT research, 229
    principles, 228
    relating to knowledge translation research, 226
    techniques, 63
quality indicators
    as a basis for assessing gaps, 60
    categories of, 155
    components of, 60–1
    defined, 60
    developing, 61
    measuring adherence to, 153
quality of care
    defined, 226
    framework for, 60, 155
    quantifying improvements in, 262–3
quality programs, 146
quantitative case survey, 21
quantitative data, presenting, 21
quantitative evaluation methods, 157–8
questionnaires, 153
QUOROM (Quality Of Reporting Of Meta-analyses) Statement, 24

RAND Health, modifying the Delphi method, 61
randomization, units of, 253, 254
randomized controlled trials (RCTs)
    design choices, 252–7
    synthesizing evidence from, 16
randomized trial designs, 251–2, 253
randomized trials, 157
RDRB (Research and Development Resource Base), 52
realist reviews, 27, 29
receptive capacity, 215
receptive context, 145, 147

record-keeping, identifying and selecting studies, 19
redirections, of physicians, 115
reflection, importance to professional practice, 209
reflective learner, 207
reflective practice, 68
regional administrative databases, 62
reinforcing strategies, in the PRECEED model, 115
relationship brokers, 238
relative risk, in a forest plot, 23
reminder systems, 132, 133
reminder-fatigue, from pop-ups, 177
research evidence, 4, 5
research knowledge, 282, 283
research knowledge-based opportunities, 281–2
research opportunities, 282–3
research synthesis, in the 1960s, 15
Research Transfer Network of Alberta (RTNA) Web site, 51
research use, 3
research utilization, 3, 13
Research Utilization Support and Help (RUSH) Web site, 52
research-use behavior, of professionals, 196
resource scarcity, 261
resource toolkit, Web-based, 75
results
  analyzing from studies, 20–1
  conceptualizing satisfactory, 68
  disseminating, 23–4
  increasing the uptake of, 24, 29
  interpreting, 21–3
  presenting from reviews, 21
review(s). *See also* systematic reviews
  disseminating results of, 23–4
  of draft clinical practice guidelines, 36
  format for presentation of, 24
  increasing the uptake of, 24, 29
  presenting results of, 21

review criteria, for chart audits, 127
review questions, 17–18
review reports, quality of, 24
review team, identifying, 16
risk of bias, assessing, 19–20, 21
risks
  equity with benefits, 296
  fair distribution of, 293
role models
  of appropriate behavior, 211
  to support training, 208
routine applications, 285

Safe Kids Canada, 241
safety
  interventions, 142–3
  of outcomes, 294–5
  proof, 283
sample size, for randomized trials, 253–5
scald burns, reducing among children, 241
scaling up, 167, 168
science of spread, 166
scientific evidence, 218
scope and purpose module, of ADAPTE, 77
screening process, 21, 22
SDM (shared decision making), 87–8
search and screen module, of ADAPTE, 77
search engines, 49
search filters, for KT material, 48
self-care interventions, 140–2
self-directed learner, traits of, 115
self-directed learning, in CME, 119–20
self-efficacy, explaining barriers to change, 101
self-management education, 140, 141
self-monitoring, evaluation of, 141–2
self-regulation theory, 128
sensitivity analyses, assessing bias, 20
service improvement models, 146

setup phase, of ADAPTE, 76, 77
shared decision making (SDM), 87–8
short-term, funding opportunities for
  research, 167
SIGLE (System for Information in Grey
  Literature in Europe), 49
single interventions, 101, 109, 117
situation-outcomes, 197
skill development, self-management
  programs providing, 141
skills, related to KT interventions, 104
slippage, 285
small group learning, in CME, 118–19
social analysis, of technology in health
  care, 219
social cognitive theory, 197
social engagement, 37
social influence theory, 101
social influences, 123
social learning approaches, 211
social network, 105, 273
social processes, supporting constitution
  and circulation of knowledge, 218
social system, 272
social utility, 294
societal agenda, 107
societal costs, 264
societal factors, 107
societal system, 270–1
soft networks, 238
soft periphery, 218
specialization, 106
specification, 105
spread, 167
staff domain, of the NHS sustainability
  model, 166
stages of change, theories related to, 197
stakeholders
  in the choice of research question and
    design, 161
  in clinical practice guideline
    development, 36–7
  developing quality indicators, 61
  in KT intervention development, 110

linking KT interventions to barriers,
  100
relevance of results for, 22
statistical synthesis, employing, 20–1
status quo, factors maintaining, 170
stewardship, as an ethical consideration,
  297
sticky knowledge, 168
strategic knowledge use, 152–3
stroke units, 160, 162
structural criteria, for chart audits, 127
structural indicators, 155
structure, of health services, 227
structured approaches, for planning
  change, 97
structure-process-outcome framework,
  227
studies
  analyzing data from, 20–1
  assessing risk of bias of included,
    19–20
  extracting data from individual,
    20
  locating relevant, 18–19
  selection process for, 19
study designs
  evaluating for KT interventions,
    250–1
  in a review process, 18
styles, of learning, 207
subjective needs assessment strategies,
  117
subjective norms, 197, 198
success factors, for collaborative
  research, 240
summaries of evidence, 47
surgical sites, patient marking of, 143
sustainability
  action plan, 168–9
  defined, 166
  degrees of, 170
  of interventions over time, 163
  of knowledge use, 165–71
  models for, 166–7

monitoring, 170
planning, 167–8
strategies, 166–7
terms related to, 167
terms related to lack of, 168
sustained impact, enhancing, 109
symbolic knowledge use, 152
synthesis. *See* knowledge synthesis and systematic reviews
systematic review methodology, 29–30
systematic review team, 16
systematic reviews. *See also* review(s)
bias and confounding in, 22
conducting, 17
defined, 16
focused versus narrative, 29
general methods applying to, 16
as summaries of evidence, 47
traditional, 25–6
types of, 25–8
system/society outcomes, 156

T2 knowledge translation, 51
target level, of knowledge use, 154
targets, for knowledge use, 153–4
task characteristics, 200
tasks, 68
team cognitions, 104
team processes, 104
technical knowledge, 107
technical proof, 283
technological diffusion, 219
technology transfer, 4, 287
termination stage, in the transtheoretical model of change, 199
terms
KT, 13
KT activities/components, 54
KT-related, 53, 54
for the same concept in KT, 49, 53, 54
theoretical learner, 207
think-pair-share interaction, 118

thromboprophylactic measures, underuse of, 176
time points, in an interrupted time series, 256
tools
for assessing knowledge use, 86, 89
knowledge, 6, 7, 41
patient-friendly, 39
total quality management, 145, 146, 228
tranformative learning, 209
transaction costs, 108
translation mechanisms, 286
transtheoretical model of change, 115, 199–200
trials, of new knowledge applications, 285
TRIP–Turning Research into Practice Web site, 49
trusting relationships, among team members, 240
Trusts, in the NHS, 74
tutorials, outline for searching, 48
two-arm trials, 252, 253

UK Centre for Reviews and Dissemination, 47
UK Medical Research Council Framework for Trials of Complex Interventions, 202
UK National Institute for Health and Clinical Evidence. *See* NICE (U.K. National Institute for Health and Clinical Evidence)
ulcus cruris, lifestyle program for patients with, 96
units, randomizing intact, 253
unpublished literature, searching, 49
US Agency for Healthcare Research and Quality, 48
US National Center for the Dissemination of Disability Research library, 51
utility, 293–5

value
  appropriation by end users, 284
  creation, 281
  creation versus appropriation,
    285
  proof, 283
  slippage, 285
variation, in health care delivery across
    patients, 99
verbal persuasion, 197
vertical social connections, 170

Veterans Administration, codified
    knowledge improving
    performance, 221
vicarious experience, 197
vignettes, in CME activities, 118

Web sites
  promoting KT materials or tools, 50–2
  searching, 19
Web videoconferencing tools, 134
Web-based education, 133